Manual of Ocular Fundus Examination

Manual of Ocular Fundus Examination

Theo Dorion, M.D.

Ophthalmologist in Private Practice, Queens, New York; Assistant Ophthalmologist Surgeon, Wyckoff Heights Medical Center, Brooklyn, New York; Former Attending Surgeon in Ophthalmology, Physicians Hospital, Queens; Former Senior Attending in Ophthalmology, University Clinical Hospital of Ophthalmology, Bucharest

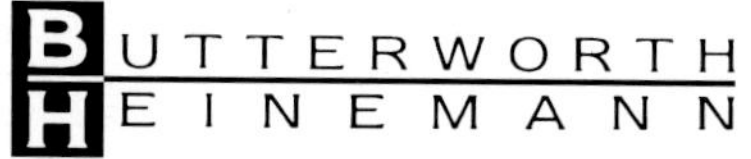

Boston•Oxford•Johannesburg•Melbourne•New Delhi•Singapore

Every effort has been made to ensure that the drug dosage schedules within this text are accurate and conform to standards accepted at time of publication. However, as treatment recommendations vary in the light of continuing research and clinical experience, the reader is advised to verify drug dosage schedules herein with information found on product information sheets. This is especially true in cases of new or infrequently used drugs.

Recognizing the importance of preserving what has been written, Butterworth–Heinemann prints its books on acid-free paper whenever possible.

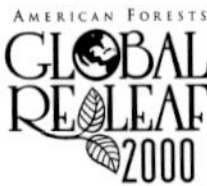

Butterworth–Heinemann supports the efforts of American Forests and the Global ReLeaf program in its campaign for the betterment of trees, forests, and our environment.

Library of Congress Cataloging-in-Publication Data

Dorion, Theo.
Manual of ocular fundus examination / Theo Dorion.
p. cm.
Includes bibliographical references and index.
ISBN 0-7506-9987-6
1. Fundus oculi--Diseases--Handbooks, manuals, etc. 2. Fundus oculi--Examination--Handbooks, manuals, etc. I. Title.
[DNLM: 1. Retinal Diseases--diagnosis handbooks. 2. Choroid Diseases--diagnosis handbooks. 3. Optic Nerve Diseases--diagnosis handbooks. 4. Ophthalmoscopy--methods handbooks. 5. Fundus Oculi handbooks. WW 39 D698m 1998]
RE545.D67 1998
617.7'3--dc21
DNLM/DLC 98-2711
for Library of Congress CIP

British Library Cataloguing-in-Publication Data
A catalogue record for this book is available from the British Library.

The publisher offers special discounts on bulk orders of this book.
For information, please contact:
Manager of Special Sales
Butterworth–Heinemann
225 Wildwood Avenue
Woburn, MA 01801-2041
Tel: 781-904-2500
Fax: 781-904-2620

For information on all Butterworth–Heinemann publications available, contact our World Wide Web home page at: http://www.bh.com/

10 9 8 7 6 5 4 3 2 1

Printed in Hong Kong

To my wife, Venera, for all her support during the writing of this book

To my daughters, Roxana and Florentina

Contents

Preface

The idea to write this book came to me many years ago as I was preparing to take the American Board of Ophthalmology examination. At that time, it was difficult to find a reference book that covered all the clinical, histopathologic, and therapeutic aspects of ocular fundus disorders.

I wrote this book as a practical, comprehensive, yet concise guide—a book where one can quickly and easily find up-to-date information, along with illustrations of fundus conditions and diseases. Toward that end, I reviewed many ophthalmology textbooks, manuals, atlases, and journals published in the United States and around the world during the last 25 years.

This book is designed for a wide audience. In addition to ophthalmologists, optometrists, medical students, and residents, this manual is intended for any health care professional, including general practitioners, internists, emergency room physicians, pediatricians, endocrinologists, and obstetricians, who performs ocular fundus examinations in the office, hospital, or elsewhere.

Chapter 1 describes the method of examination of the ocular fundus by direct ophthalmoscopy and provides clinical and histologic descriptions of the normal fundus. Chapter 2 covers the ocular signs seen most frequently in the ocular fundus—their appearance, significance, clinical interpretation, and histopathology. The remainder of the book covers the more than 200 ocular disorders that can affect the optic nerve, macula, retinal vessels, and peripheral retina, and encompasses a wide variety of etiologies, such as vascular, inflammatory, degenerative, tumoral, parasitic, metabolic, or toxic. These chapters describe systemic diseases with significant ocular components. Each disease or disorder is described comprehensively but concisely—by definition, etiology, pathogenesis, clinical appearance, symptoms, diagnosis and differential diagnosis, histopathology, and treatment.

This book is also intended to be a visual learning tool for the teaching of ocular fundus findings. Typical fundus disorders are illustrated in more than 150 color drawings. The drawings are labeled to provide a quick source of information for establishing a correct diagnosis and an appropriate therapeutic approach.

As there is always a risk of oversimplification in any such concise book, I would gladly accept any suggestions or comments for improving future editions.

Theo Dorion, M.D.

Acknowledgments

I would like to acknowledge my gratitude to all who made this book possible. My special thanks to Arnold S. Statsinger, M.D., former chairman and director of the Department of Pathology at Wyckoff Heights Hospital, Brooklyn, New York, and Addagada C. Rao, M.D., chairman and director of the Department of Surgery at the same hospital, for all their support over the years, which helped me to overcome sometimes difficult periods in my professional life. My sincere appreciation to Stevens M. Podos, M.D., chairman and director of the Department of Ophthalmology at Mount Sinai Medical School, New York, for his encouragement at the beginning of my ophthalmologic career in the United States. Many thanks to my assistants, Mona C. Capusan, Dominique A. Vlad, and Elena I. Georgescu, for their help with manuscript preparation.

Finally, I express my appreciation to the staff of the Medical Division of Butterworth–Heinemann, especially to Karen Oberheim for her ideas on extending the scope of this manual and to Jana Friedman for her helpful editing suggestions.

1

Ocular Fundus Examination

Direct Ophthalmoscopy

Direct ophthalmoscopy is a method of examining the fundus of the eye with the ophthalmoscope, an instrument invented by Hermann von Helmholtz in 1850 in Germany. To perform this examination, the ophthalmologist must be positioned in front of the patient. The ophthalmoscope is maintained at approximately 6 in. (15 cm) from and 25 degrees to the right side of the patient's right eye and at the same distance from and degrees to the left side of the patient's left eye. The examiner looks at each of the patient's eyes in turn, using his or her right eye for viewing the patient's right eye and his or her left eye for viewing the patient's left eye. The examiner should take care to avoid touching the hair, face, or any other part of the patient's body during the examination.

The patient is asked to keep both eyes open. The examining room must be partially or completely darkened. Before the examination, the patient's pupil should be dilated if there are no contraindications. Cyclopentolate 1.0% (Cyclogyl), tropicamide 1.0% (Mydriacyl), or phenylephrine 2.5% (Mydfrin) can be used but will affect the accommodation. The examiner should refrain from dilating the pupil if there is a shallow anterior chamber or if the patient has intraocular lens implants.

The ophthalmologist takes the ophthalmoscope in hand and holds it vertically, close to his or her own eye and approximately 6 in. from the patient's eye. The patient, who should not wear eyeglasses or contact lenses during the examination, is asked to look at the opposite wall, over the examiner's shoulder, and to fixate a distant target, holding the eyes as steady as possible. If both the examiner and the patient have normal visual acuity, the lens on the illuminated hole of the ophthalmoscope is set to 0. If either party has refractive errors, the ophthalmoscope lens must be adjusted accordingly until the fundus details are clearly visible.

The cornea, the anterior chamber, and the lens are viewed at a distance—usually approximately 15 in. from the patient—so any of the media can be explored. Then, the eye is gradually approached until a **red reflex** appears. This phenomenon is a combination of the reflex of the choroidal vasculature and the retinal pigment epithelium (RPE). When light enters the eye, it is reflected back from the fundus along its entry path. If the ophthalmologist is placed approximately in the path of the reflected light, the otherwise black pupil will be filled with a glow, called the *red reflex* or *fundus reflex*. Most ophthalmoscopes project a beam of light of approximately 1 disc diameter (dd). Once the details of the fundus can be seen clearly, the examiner follows a blood vessel to its origin at the optic disc. This is the point from which the examination is begun.

The disc, vessels, and macula are examined in this order. Then the background, retina, choroid, vitreous, and sclera are evaluated. All these structures are brought into focus according to the refractive error of the patient and the examiner. In high myopia, the size of the image will be greatly increased, as opposed to hypermetropia, in which the image will appear much smaller. By direct ophthalmoscopy and assuming a dilated pupil, the fundus can be examined as far anterior to the equator as 1.5 mm from the ora serrata. To examine the entire retina, indirect ophthalmoscopy, which has a wider field and allows for enhanced depth perception, must be used.

The optic disc is examined for clarity of its contour, shape, color, cupping, elevation, and the condition of the vessels on it. The disc may appear smaller in far-sighted and larger in near-sighted patients.

The vessels are evaluated for transparency, the effect of intraocular pressure (e.g., an arteriovenous [AV] compression, called *nicking*), focal narrowing of the arteries, tortuosity and widening of the veins, hemorrhages, and exudates. The central retinal vein usually pulsates spontaneously, but the central retinal artery does not. Therefore, *any arterial pulsation is pathologic*. The ratio between the diameters of the artery and the vein (**A/V ratio**) is assessed; this ratio normally is 2 to 3, the vein being wider. Also examined are the width of the blood column, the vessel walls, the quality of the blood flow within the vessels, and the contour of the vessels.

The macula is examined by moving the projected light approximately 2 dd temporal to the optic disc. The patient is asked to look at the light. The foveal reflex, nerve fibers, and small vessels are noted. By using the green light, called the *red-free filter*, the examiner can see the retinal vessels standing out as black against a green background.

Finally, the background, choroid, vitreous, and sclera are examined to the far periphery. The size of any lesions noted are measured by using the disc diameter as reference. The elevation of a lesion is measured according to the difference between the lens power that clearly focuses the top of the lesion and the power that clearly focuses an adjacent normal fundus area: A change of *3.00 diopters (D)* is equivalent to approximately *1 mm* of elevation.

Appearance of the Normal Ocular Fundus

The normal fundus is depicted in Figure 1-1.

Optic Disc

The disc is the optic nerve head, the site at which the optic nerve enters the eye or the site where the nerve fibers from the entire retina converge to leave the eye (Figure 1-2). It is located at the posterior pole, is composed of nonmyelinated fiber, and has no other retinal structure; hence, it is nonsensory and is called the *blind spot*.

The disc appears as a round or oval area with sharp margins and is vertically oriented, its height generally exceeding its width. It may also be round, elongated, ovoid, or irregular. The normal disc is flat, so the nerve fibers do not rise above the retinal level.

The normal disc is pink or orange, with a pale yellow cup at its center. The temporal half of the disc always is paler than the nasal half, is more transparent, and contains fewer capillaries and thinner papillomacular bundle fibers.

The small, pale, conical central depression is called the *physiologic cup*. It often is enlarged temporally, is the palest part of the optic disc, and contains less prominent capillaries and fewer fibers than the rest of the disc. The size of the cup varies from 30% to 90% of the size of the disc but generally, in the normal eye, is approximately one-third of the disc diameter. The ratio between the diameter of the cup and the diameter of the disc is called the *cup-to-disc ratio*, or **C/D ratio**. Hence, the normal C/D ratio

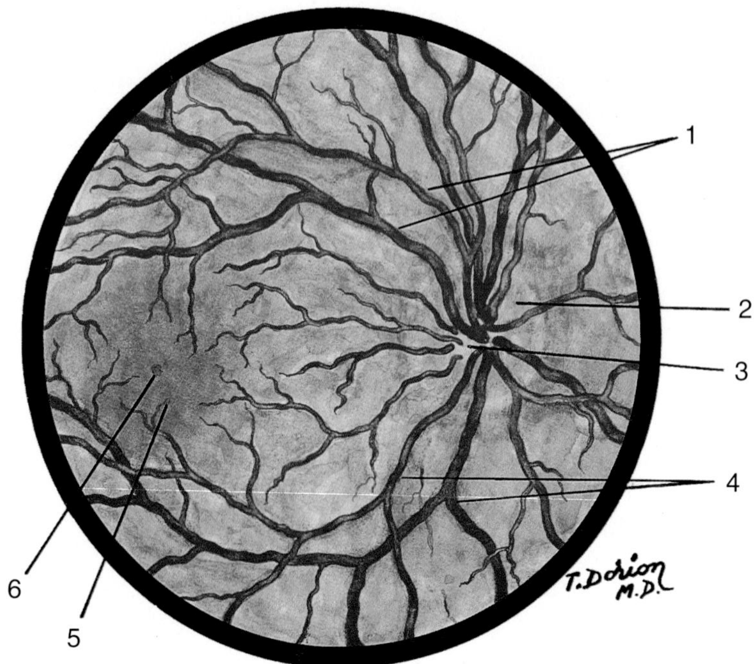

Figure 1-1. *Normal ocular fundus. (1) Superior vascular arcades. (2) Optic disc. (3) Physiologic cup. (4) Inferior vascular arcades. (5) Macula. (6) Foveola.*

may be noted as 0.3–0.9. In any individual, the eyes usually have symmetric cups. Cup asymmetry in excess of 0.5 mm raises the suspicion of glaucoma. The depth of the cup also may vary from shallow to deep enough to expose the lamina cribrosa. The cup is lined with astroglial cells, and its bottom may appear fibrous owing to the fibers of lamina cribrosa or sclera. The area between the margin of the cup and the margin of the disc is called the **neuroretinal rim.** The rim surrounds the cup uniformly and is larger inferiorly but diminishes gradually from the temporal to the superior to the nasal margins, such that it is thinnest nasally.

The disc is smaller in hypermetropia and larger in myopia. Its usual diameter is approximately 1.5 mm. The disc's size serves as a reference for the measurement of any lesions or of the distance between lesions.

The disc margins generally are discretely demarcated, but they may merge gradually into the surrounding retina without any clear-cut edge.

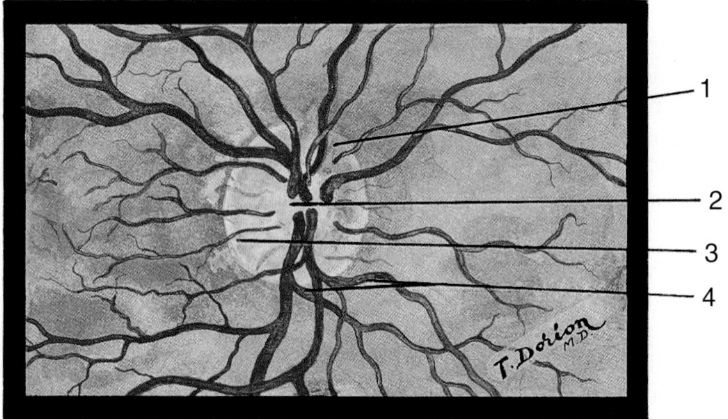

Figure 1-2. *Optic disc. (1) Neuroretinal rim. (2) Physiologic cup. (3) Halo. (4) Central retinal vessels traversing straight across the disc margin.*

Its temporal, upper, and lower margins are more sharply defined, whereas the nasal margin is less distinct. Occasionally, a white border between the choroidal vasculature and the retinal opening, which represents a **scleral ring**, or a sickle-shaped crescent, may be present. The distance between the temporal margin of the disc and the center of the macula is approximately 3.5 mm (or approximately 2 dd).

The disc's appearance varies with patient age, being paler in children, pink with bright reflex in young adults, and pale with a hollow surface, drusen or pigment, and a diminished reflex in the elderly.

Vessels

The primary vessels of the eye are the **central retinal artery** and the **central retinal vein**. Sometimes, as a normal variation of the vasculature, there is also a **cilioretinal artery**. The blood supply of the retina derives from two sources: retinal vessels and choroidal vessels. The two systems do not anastomose.

Retinal Vessels

Retinal vessels are direct vessels (arteries and veins) that run from the central retinal artery, which is the first branch of the internal carotid artery, supplying the inner half of the retina. These vessels do not have autonomic nerve fibers; rather, their constriction and dilation are based solely on autoregulation, which is vascular resistance pressure to blood flow and carbon dioxide tension (P_{CO_2}).

Central retinal vessels, artery and vein, enter and exit the eye within the optic nerve. The greater vessels are located in the retinal nerve fiber layer. The central retinal vessels bifurcate at the disc into *superior* and *inferior branches*, which divide themselves further into *temporal* and *nasal branches*. Each of the resulting four major branches is named for the retinal quadrant it serves: superior temporal, superior nasal, inferior temporal, and inferior nasal. The retinal vessels form two major arcades: the **superior arcade**, composed of the superior temporal artery and vein, and the **inferior arcade**, composed of the inferior temporal artery and vein. At the first bifurcation, the arteries become *arterioles* and the veins *venules*. In this book, we will refer only to arteries and veins. In the disc, the retinal veins exhibit pulsation, called *physiologic venous pulsation*, that is synchronous with the heartbeat and is visible at the disc surface. This pulsation is due to a periodic collapse of the vein wall and may be increased by slight pressure on the globe. Again, normally there is *no* spontaneous central retinal artery pulsation.

The retinal arteries are end arteries: They do not anastomose with any other arteries in the eye. Neither do retinal veins anastomose with any veins of the ciliary body at the ora serrata, where there is a narrow avascular zone. The arteries branch in an acute angle.

Retinal arteries are bright red because they carry oxygenated blood, and their medial coat reflects the light, producing a light reflex that runs parallel to the axis of the artery. The artery has a thicker wall than the veins, which gives a shiny reflex stripe. Retinal veins are duskier and wider than the arteries (A/V ratio: 2:3). The width of a vessel is usually uniform and can be inferred from the size of the blood column. Because the walls of the retinal vessels are normally invisible, we see only the blood column (except on or near the disc, where some sheathing of the vessels may occur, making the vessel walls visible). Normally, the veins taper smoothly in diameter from the disc to the retinal periphery. At or near the disc, however, the normal retinal vessels may have thickened walls and may compress one another.

At the AV crossings, the arteries cross the veins, and their size and lumen remain unchanged; the veins are not concealed or congested distal to the AV crossing. The cilioretinal artery, when it exists, derives from the posterior ciliary artery, the circle of Zinn, or a choroidal artery but *not* from the central retinal artery. In a case of central retinal artery occlusion, the cilioretinal artery is spared, allowing maintenance of central vision and a corresponding visual field.

As mentioned earlier, the retinal vessels are examined for their size, shape, caliber (e.g., narrowing, compression, occlusion, engorgement), contour, course, pulsation, and tortuosity, and for aneurysms, perivascular hemorrhages, and exudates.

Choroidal Vessels

Choroidal vessels are indirect vessels that supply the outer half of the retina and the RPE by diffusion, throughout the choriocapillaris. The arteries appear red, are characterized by a bright streak reflex, are uniformly broad in caliber and rich in hue, and course in sinuous curves, branching at wide angles. They normally are narrower than the veins by a ratio of 2 to 3. In old age, the arteries are narrowed further, follow a straighter course, and branch at an acute angle. The macula has a rich choroidal vasculature but lacks retinal vessels.

The veins follow the course of the arteries. They are wider and darker and are characterized by a light reflex that is duller than that of the arteries.

Capillaries

Capillaries are located in two retinal layers: The ganglion cell layer is superficial, whereas the inner nuclear layer is deep. Retinal capillaries are small (approximately 7 μm in diameter) and have tight endothelial junctions. Choroidal capillaries are larger (approximately 30 μm in diameter) and bear fenestrations close to Bruch's membrane. Immediately behind the lamina cribrosa, some capillaries from the central retinal artery connect with the arteries from the choroidal vasculature. Around the optic disc, within the sclera, some short ciliary arteries form an arterial circle that connects with the central retinal artery; this is called the *circle of Zinn*. Occasionally, as a normal variation of the vasculature, a cilioretinal artery is seen. This cilioretinal artery appears as a large twig from the circle of Zinn that hooks around the edge of the disc to enter the retina.

Macula

The macula is a depression of the retinal posterior pole and measures approximately 6 mm in diameter. It is the most sensitive area of the retina and is the site of fine central vision (normally 20/20). Its center is located

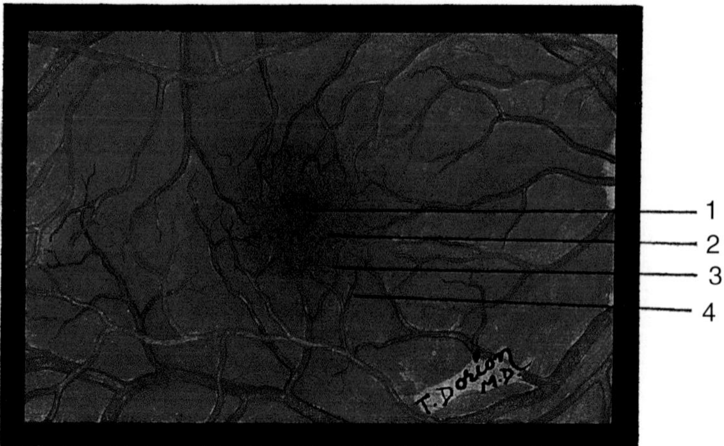

Figure 1-3. *Macula. (1) Foveola. (2) Fovea. (3) Perifovea. (4) Parafovea.*

nearly 2 dd (3 mm) temporal to and approximately 0.7 mm below the disc. The macula is divided arbitrarily into four areas, from the periphery to the center: *parafovea*, *perifovea*, *fovea*, and *foveola* (Figure 1-3).

The **parafovea** is the peripheral area and the largest of the four regions of the macula, measuring slightly more than 0.5 dd. The **perifovea** surrounds the fovea and is approximately 500 μm in diameter. The perifovea may contain a ganglion cell layer that is seven times thicker than normal and that gradually disappears as the foveola is approached. The foveola is an avascular area. A xanthophyll pigment usually is present.

The **fovea** is a red, round area, darker than the rest of the retina, of approximately 1 dd (or 1.5 mm), in which the ratio of cones to rods decreases from the periphery to the center. No retinal vessels course through it, as its nutrition is supplied by diffusion, partly from the surrounding retinal vessels and partly from the choroidal vessels. It is located close to the insertion of the inferior oblique muscle. The fovea appears as an ill-defined, shallow bowl that is red and darker than the surrounding retina, having a concave, sloping floor and forming a slightly oval ring called the *clivus*. The fovea comprises only one retinal layer, the outer plexiform layer of Henle. Under the macula is heavily pigmented RPE and a thickened choriocapillaris. At the clivus of the macula, there is a transition from thick to thin internal limiting membrane and from avascular to vascular retina.

The small, vessel-free central pit in the macula is the **foveola,** which measures approximately 350 µm in diameter. In its center is yet another small depression called the *umbo*. The foveola receives its nutrients from the choriocapillaris. This is the only region of the macula in which no rods are found; the foveola contains only cones. The density of cones in the foveola is greater than elsewhere in the macula—approximately 15,000/mm^2—decreasing to 5,000/mm^2 in the peripheral retina. There is a central foveolar light reflex due to the reflection of the structure's concave surface, which, in old age or in drug-induced retinopathy, may become dull. In young people, a tiny, lustrous central yellow point, named the *macula lutea*, is seen.

Background

The normal background appears orange-red, owing to the pigmentation of the RPE and to the blood in the choriocapillaris and the choroidal vasculature. The background glitters, has a brilliant light reflex, and is uniformly pigmented. The pigmentation varies with age and with the amount of melanin in the RPE, which usually matches the complexion of the patient. Patients with medium or dark skin usually have more choroidal pigment, causing the background to appear darker, especially at the posterior pole; it may also appear streaked, tessellated, or tigroid because of an uneven distribution of melanin and the contrast between the choroidal pigment and blood. Such patients may also have a pigmented rim at the disc margin. In patients with very fair skin, the background is lightly pigmented, the choroidal vessels are markedly prominent, and the four large vortex veins, which are usually invisible in patients with more skin pigment, may be seen.

Retina

The retina is the innermost of the three coats of the eyeball, the other two being the choroid and the sclera. The retina consists of 10 anatomic layers and may be considered to be made up of two parts: the *pigmented retina* or *nonsensory retina*, which is the outer part, formed by the layer of RPE, and the *sensory retina*, also called the *neuroretina* or the *neuroepithelium*, formed by the remaining nine layers. Four types of tissue make up the retina: *neural*, formed by perceptive and integrative cells derived from the central nervous system (CNS); *glial*, formed by supportive cells also derived from the CNS; *vascular*, formed by retinal vessels that link retina to the systemic circulation; and *RPE*.

Ten Retinal Layers

The 10 layers of the retina, from the outer side of the choroid to the inner side of the vitreous, are as follows (Figure 1-4):

1. RPE
2. Photoreceptors, or rod and cone layer
3. External limiting membrane
4. Outer nuclear layer
5. Outer plexiform layer
6. Inner nuclear layer
7. Inner plexiform layer
8. Ganglion cell layer
9. Nerve fiber layer
10. Internal limiting membrane

Retinal Pigment Epithelium

The RPE usually is a single, thin brown layer approximately 16 µm thick that extends from the ora serrata to the edge of the optic disc. It consists of elongated, hexagonal, or cuboid cells, pigmented granules of **melanin,** and laminated bodies called *phagosomes* in the cytoplasm. These RPE cells adhere to Bruch's membrane and to themselves by a cement substance called *Verhoeff's membrane.* From each cell's apex, which faces the rods and cones, exit the pigment processes. RPE plays a role in forming the blood-retina barrier between the choriocapillaris and the sensory retina, in phagocytosis, and in metabolism of vitamin A, and has an atrophic, hyperplastic, or hypertrophic response in some diseases.

Photoreceptors

The photoreceptor layer is composed of two types of cells that are sensitive to light: rods and cones. Cones number nearly 7 million, and rods between 75 and 150 million. As stated earlier, the foveola is the only ocular structure that contains only cones.

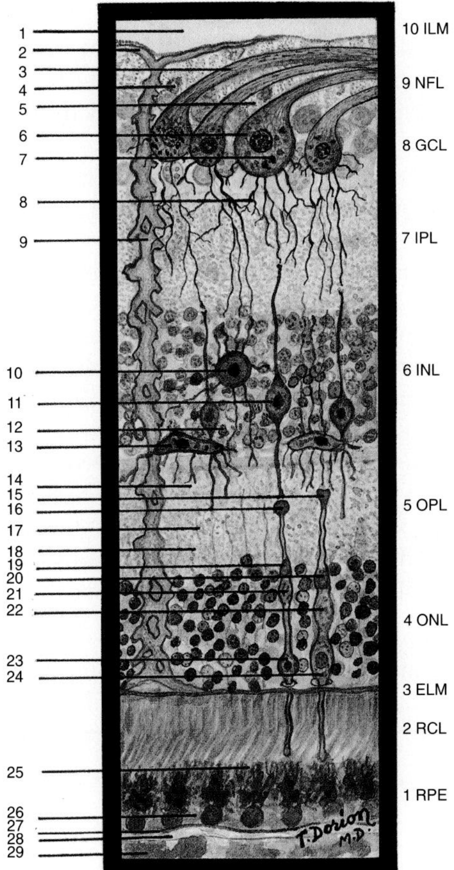

Figure 1-4. *Anatomy of the retina. (1) Vitreous. (2) Footplates of Müller cells. (3) Unmyelinated axons of ganglion cells. (4) Capillary plexus. (5) Microglia. (6) Bodies of ganglion cells. (7) Nissl granules. (8) Synapses between the ganglion cells. (9) Müller cells. (10) Amacrine cell. (11) Bipolar cell. (12) Capillary plexus. (13) Horizontal cell. (14) Inner zone of OPL. (15) Cone's pedicle. (16) Rod's spherule. (17) Middle zone of OPL. (18) Outer zone of OPL, or Henle's fibers layer. (19) Rod's myoid. (20) Cone's myoid. (21) Rod's ellipsoid. (22) Cone's ellipsoid. (23) Rod's cell body. (24) Cone's cell body. (25) Undulating surface. (26) Verhoeff's membrane. (27) Bruch's membrane. (28) Choriocapillaris. (29) Choroid. (RPE, retinal pigment epithelium; RCL, rod and cone layer [photoreceptors]; ELM, external limiting membrane; ONL, outer nuclear layer; OPL, outer plexiform layer; INL, inner nuclear layer; IPL, inner plexiform layer; GCL, ganglion cell layer; NFL, nerve fiber layer; ILM, internal limiting membrane.)*

Rods are longer than cones, are slender, are arranged in parallel, and lie vertical to the retinal layers. They consist of an outer segment, which is 50 μm long and refractile and contains the *visual purple*, and an inner segment, which is thicker and fibrillar and can be divided into two portions: the outer portion (**ellipsoid**), which contains mitochondria, and the inner portion (**myoid**), which contains the Golgi apparatus, ribosomes, and cisternae of the endoplasmic reticulum. The rest of a rod is made up of fibers, the cell body, and a synaptic end called the *rod spherule*, which contains a lamellar structure, the **ribbon**, that provides the spherules with one or two ribbon synapses.

Cones are bigger than rods, have a larger and paler cell body, and are arranged in a single row immediately beneath the external limiting membrane. The cones have no visual purple. Instead, they have pigments that are sensitive to blue, green, and red light. Like rods, cones have an outer segment, which is conical (longer and wider than the rod at its base) and has a blunt, rounded tip and an inner segment, from which a smooth fiber extends to the outer plexiform layer, where it terminates with a thick, triangular club-shaped end called the **cone pedicle**. The pedicle is larger than the rod spherule and contains not one but many ribbon synapses.

External Limiting Membrane

The external limiting membrane it is not a true membrane but a row of dense fibers of rods and cones attached to the Müller cell fibers. It is, in fact, a fine reticulum having small and large orifices that contain rod and cone processes.

Outer Nuclear Layer

The outer nuclear layer is composed of the cell bodies of rods and cones.

Outer Plexiform Layer

The outer plexiform layer (also called the *outer molecular layer*) is composed of the synapses between the rods and cones, bipolar cells, Müller cells, horizontal cells, and amacrine cells. This layer is divided into three zones: (1) the outer zone, or **Henle's fiber layer**, which contains the axons of rods and cones and the Müller cell cytoplasm; (2) the middle zone, which contains the rod spherules and the cone pedicles; and (3) the inner zone, composed of processes of bipolar cells, horizontal cells, and Müller cells. Only the inner zone is truly plexiform.

Inner Nuclear Layer

The inner nuclear layer is composed of four layers of cell bodies, which, from outside to within, are horizontal, bipolar, Müller, and amacrine. The inner nuclear layer houses a capillary plexus.

Inner Plexiform Layer

The inner plexiform layer is composed of synapses between the bipolar cells (which constitute the first-order neurons) and the ganglion cells (which constitute the second-order neurons) and amacrine cells, horizontal cells, and Müller cells. Two types of synapses are found in the inner plexiform layer: (1) ribbon synapses, characterized by a dense lamella surrounded by a halo of vesicles, and (2) conventional synapses, characterized by clusters of vesicles against the presynaptic membrane. The latter do not have a ribbon.

Ganglion Cell Layer

The ganglion cell layer is composed of the bodies of ganglion cells, which are interspersed with neuroglial structures such as Müller cells and with capillaries. The ganglion cells are round or piriform, have multiple dendrites and large nuclei, and contain **Nissl granules** in the cytoplasm. They form a single layer, except in the macular region where they are arranged in many rows. Their long axons form the optic nerve fibers. Ganglion cells are absent from the foveola.

Nerve Fiber Layer

The nerve fiber layer, or **stratum opticum**, is composed of nonmyelinated axons of ganglion cells, as myelinization ends at the lamina cribrosa. The axons run parallel to the retinal surface, are arranged in multiple bundles that form a network that passes through the columns and footplates of Müller cells, and converge toward the optic disc. Microglial tissue is present. In the nerve fiber layer, a capillary plexus also is found.

Internal Limiting Membrane

The internal limiting membrane is the last of the 10 layers of retina. It is a fine, filamentous membrane 1–2 μm thick that is formed by the coalescence of the footplates of Müller cells. This membrane separates the terminal ends of Müller cells from the vitreous and sometimes is difficult to distinguish from the hyaloid membrane, which covers the posterior vitreous surface.

Anatomic Hallmarks of the Retina

The **peripheral retina** is the anterior part of the retina that begins approximately 3 mm posterior to the equator, where the vortex veins pass from the choroid into the sclera, and extends toward the equator to the anterior termination of the retina, at the ora serrata. The distance from the equator to the ora serrata is approximately 3 dd. The **posterior pole** is the retinal area that extends from the optic disc to the equator. The **blood-retina barrier** has two anatomic sites, one at the junction between the endothelial cells of the retinal vessels and the other at the junctions between the RPE cells.

Choroid

The middle coat of the eyeball, lying between the retina and the sclera, is the choroid. Along with the ciliary body and the iris, the choroid makes up the **uvea.** It is of mesodermal origin and is composed largely of blood vessels. The choroid provides the blood supply to the RPE and to the outer half of the sensory retina. It extends from the ora serrata to the optic disc, is 0.1 mm thick anteriorly and 0.25 mm thick at the posterior pole, and is firmly attached to the sclera at the optic nerve and at the points of exit of the vortex veins.

The choroid is composed of five layers. In order from the sclera to the retina, these layers are as follows (Figure 1-5):

1. The **suprachoroid**, or **lamina fusca,** is an avascular layer that connects the sclera to the choroid and is composed of fine, elastic, collagenous lamellar fibers that form a **syncytium.** In this choroidal layer, there are melanocytes, endothelial cells, smooth-muscle fibers, and nerves.

2. **Haller's layer** is located near the sclera and contains large, valveless veins that lead to the vortex veins.

3. **Sattler's layer** contains medium-size veins, arterioles, and collagenous stroma characterized by numerous elastic fibers, melanocytes, and fibroblasts.

4. The **choriocapillaris** is a fine, flat, dense meshwork of interlacing large capillaries measuring approximately 21 µm in diameter and bearing small fenestrations in their walls. The choriocapillaris is lobular and features a feeding artery in its center and a draining vein at its periphery. Its stroma is composed of collagen and elastic fibers. This structure provides the blood supply to the outer retina and protects it from ischemic death.

5. **Bruch's membrane,** also known as **lamina basalis** or **lamina vitrea,** is the innermost part of the choroid. It is nearly 7 µm thick and is generally transparent. Bruch's membrane separates the chorio-

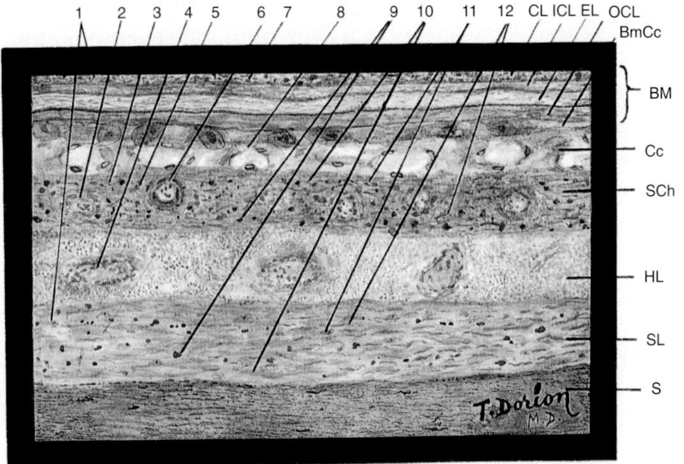

Figure 1-5. *Histologic findings in choroid. (1) Collagen fibers. (2) Medium veins. (3) Collagenous stroma. (4) Large veins with no valves. (5) Fibroblasts. (6) Arterioles. (7) Mucopolysaccharides. (8) Large capillaries with wall fenestrations. (9) Melanocytes. (10) Elastic fibers. (11) Endothelial cells. (12) Smooth-muscle fibers. (CL, cuticular layer; ICL, inner collagenous layer; EL, elastic layer; OCL, outer collagenous layer; BmCc, basement membrane of choriocapillaris; BM, Bruch's membrane; Cc, choriocapillaris; SCh, suprachoroid; HL, Haller's layer; SL, Sattler's layer; S, sclera.)*

capillaris from the RPE and derives from both the choroid and RPE. This membrane consists of five layers; in order from the retina to the choroid, these layers are (a) the cuticular layer, composed of collagen fibers surrounded by **mucopolysaccharides** and located near the RPE; (b) the inner collagenous layer, composed of collagenous tissue; (c) the elastic layer, composed of elastin fibers; (d) the outer collagenous layer, composed of the basement membrane of endothelial cells and located near the choroid; and (e) the basement membrane of choriocapillaris.

The choroid is served by the long posterior ciliary arteries, which nourish the anterior uveal tract, and the short posterior ciliary arteries, which nourish the posterior uveal tract. Its veins are of increasing diameter as they lead to the four vortex veins behind the equator, one in each quadrant. The vortex veins empty into the superior and inferior ophthalmic veins, which drain into the cavernous sinus.

The nerves of the choroid are sympathetic nerves that pass through the ciliary ganglion without synapse and are distributed to the short posterior and long anterior ciliary nerves.

Vitreous

The vitreous is a transparent, semisolid gelatinous mass that occupies two-thirds of the globe. It is uniform, colorless, structureless, inert, and elastic, and is characterized by low optical density. It has no nerves and consists of approximately 99% water.

It may be divided embryologically into three forms. **Primary vitreous** develops in two stages: Primary ectodermal vitreous is associated with the lens capsule formation, whereas primary mesodermal vitreous is associated with the hyaloid vascular system. **Secondary vitreous** probably is derived from Müller cells and composes most of the vitreous body. **Tertiary vitreous** comprises the zonule.

Vitreous is considered to be composed of a solid and a liquid phase. The *solid phase* contains a network of whorls of fine fibrils of collagen type 4, which lacks the usual 640-Å periodicity. The fibrils are arranged randomly in a loose syncytium and do not join or branch but intersperse with the liquid phase. The collagen network has no electrostatic potential. The *liquid phase* contains a viscoelastic colloidal network of **hyaluronic acid**, featuring long, coiled molecules that enclose a large amount of water. They are likened to springy steel wool. The hyaluronic acid network has a high negative potential.

The normal volume of vitreous is in the range of 4–5 ml but can be as high as 6.5 ml. The vitreous transmits light, holds the lens in place, and maintains the sensory retina in apposition to the RPE. It is attached strongly to the retina at the ora serrata, at the edges of the optic disc, and at the macula. It also is adherent at retinal scars, areas of lattice degeneration, or cystic retinal tufts, but it has no firm attachment at the disc surface. Rather, at the disc surface there is a tunnel-shaped space called the *area of Martegiani* that extends toward the vitreous and may become continuous with **Cloquet's canal.**

The vitreous base, or **vitreoretinal symphysis,** is an annular band of adhesion approximately 3–4 mm wide that extends forward from the ora serrata to 2 mm on the **pars plana** and backward 2–4 mm on the retina. This base is the strongest attachment of vitreous to the retina.

No internal limiting membrane is found under the vitreous base. The base is generally considered to consist of an anterior and a posterior portion. The *anterior vitreous base* is the area between the ora serrata and the origin of the anterior hyaloid artery, whereas the *posterior vitreous base* is an area between the ora serrata and the retina in which a posterior vitreous detachment does not produce any damage to the retina. The posterior vitreous base usually cannot be seen.

Vitreous cortex, or **hyaloid**, is the peripheral region of the vitreous that contains large, flat vitreous cells called *hyalocytes*, a few fibrocytes, collagen, and hyaluronic acid suspended in a large amount of water. Anterior hyaloid lines the ora serrata and is hollowed to conform to the posterior convexity of the lens. Sometimes this portion of the vitreous attaches to the posterior capsule of the lens to form an annular zone of adhesion, called *Weigert's ligament*, that is approximately 8–9 mm in diameter. The fibrils of anterior hyaloid are oriented perpendicular to the ora serrata. Posterior hyaloid lines the entire retina. Its fibrils are oriented parallel to the retina.

Sclera

The sclera is the outermost layer of the eye, a dense fibrous structure composed almost entirely of irregular, randomly arranged bundles of collagen (types I, II, and VIII) and elastic tissue. It is a firm, protective coat for the posterior five-sixths of the eye and preserves the shape and rigidity of the eye, keeping vision stable during eye movement. The sclera also prevents scattered light from entering the eye. The sclera is continuous anteriorly with the cornea at the limbus, and posteriorly with the optic nerve at the lamina cribrosa.

The sclera is opaque and has a dull white color because of a lower mucopolysaccharide content than that of the cornea. The sclera also differs from the cornea in that its collagen fibers are variable in size and less regular in their arrangement, it has greater birefringence and a greater water content, and there is an absence of fixed spacing in the stroma. Its capacity to regenerate itself is poor.

The sclera is fully hydrated when containing approximately 65–70% water. If dehydration reduces the water content to less than 40%, it can result in a concentration of proteoglycan, which changes its refractive index to one that is closer to that of collagen, and the sclera becomes translucent. An increase to more than 80% water content may cause the sclera to appear bluish.

The sclera is approximately 1.2 mm thick at the posterior pole surrounding the optic nerve, decreases gradually in thickness to 0.6 mm at the equator, and is approximately 0.8 mm thick at the limbus. The sclera is thinnest immediately beneath the insertions of the recti muscles, where it is only 0.3 mm thick.

The sclera has two large openings: the *anterior scleral foramen* and the *posterior scleral foramen*. The anterior scleral foramen is located at the corneal junction. Its inner surface has a scleral spur to which the ciliary muscle is attached. Slightly anterior to this spur is the **canal of Schlemm**. The posterior scleral foramen is located 3 mm medial to the posterior pole, permitting the passage of the optic nerve. It is cone-shaped, 1.5–2.5 mm in diameter on the inner surface and 3.0–3.5 mm on the outer surface of the sclera. The posterior scleral foramen is bridged by the most posterior portion of the sclera, a silver-colored modified structure called the *lamina cribrosa*. The lamina cribrosa is formed of collagen fibers and nerve axons and is lined with microglia. Many small orifices around the lamina cribrosa transmit short and long posterior nerves and vessels. There are four openings located 4 mm posterior to the equator and between the recti muscles, one for each vortex vein. The vortex veins drain the choroidal veins. There are also a number of small openings for nerves.

The sclera is divided into three layers: the episclera, the scleral stroma, and the lamina fusca.

The episclera (or **Tenon's capsule**) is the outermost layer of the sclera, which acts as a synovial membrane for smooth eye movement. It is a fibroelastic structure composed of moderately dense connective tissue, which is loosely connected to the stromal sclera by fine strands of collagen. It has two layers: the inner, deeper visceral layer, which is tightly adhered to the scleral stroma and contains a network of vessels, and the outer, *superficial* or *parietal* layer, which fuses with the conjuctiva and the muscle sheath near the limbus. The two layers are connected by loose, delicate connective tissue lamellae.

The episclera is richly vascularized by small vessels, in a deep and superficial plexus of anterior ciliary arteries. These vessels anastomose at the limbus with the conjunctival vessels. The deep episcleral vessels cannot be blanched by epinephrine 1% solution or phenylephrine 10% solution eye drops, whereas the conjunctival vessels can be. The episclera, permeable to water, protein, and glucose, provides part of the sclera's nutrition; the rest of the sclera's nutrition is provided by the choroid.

The scleral stroma is an avascular, dense, fibrous tissue composed of closely packed interlacing bundles of collagenous fibers from 10 µm to

15 μm in diameter and 100 μm to 150 μm in length, which are oriented parallel to the limbus, and elastic fibers, which cross randomly over each other. There are fibroblasts, more numerous in the superficial layers, which connect to one another by protoplasmic processes to form a *syncytium*. The fibers of the sclera tend to run in concentric circles near the cornea and the entrance of the optic nerve, whereas in other places, such as at the insertion of the extraocular muscles, they become more meridional, forming complicated loops running with backward convexity parallel to the surface.

The lamina fusca is the innermost portion of the sclera, adjacent to the choroid. It blends with the suprachoroidal and supraciliary lamellae of the uveal tract. It is composed of small bundles of collagen fibers, fibroblasts, elastic tissue, and a large number of dendritic melanocytes, which give it its brownish color.

The sclera is supplied by blood vessels derived from the long posterior and anterior ciliary vessels, which are present almost entirely in the episclera, and from the choroidal vasculature. Scleral sensory innervation derives anteriorly from the long ciliary nerves, which may form loops (called *Axenfeld loops*) at the nasal and temporal limbus, and posteriorly from the short ciliary nerves which enter the sclera close to the optic nerve. Vasomotor ciliary nerve fibers that accompany the blood vessels are also present.

Vascular Changes

The retinal vessel wall is lined by endothelial cells, which resemble muscle cells and fibroblasts except that they have fewer nuclei. The cells are disposed irregularly, are circular, oblique, or longitudinal, are nonfenestrated, and are tightly joined, so that the vessels may provide a blood-retina barrier similar to the blood-brain barrier. Capillaries have a single layer of continuous epithelial cell lining surrounded by an interrupted layer of **pericytes**, covered at their external membrane by a basement membrane. Vascular changes can take the form of changes in the light reflex; changes in shape, size, caliber, or course of the vessels; and changes that occur at the AV crossing points (Figure 1-6).

Changes in the light reflex include **widening of the light reflex**, which appears as a broader and softer light reflex, with less distinct borders, instead of a bright central line. Widening may be due to irregularities in the caliber of the artery. The **copper-wire reflex** might occupy most of the width of the artery and appears as a burnished, metallic copper

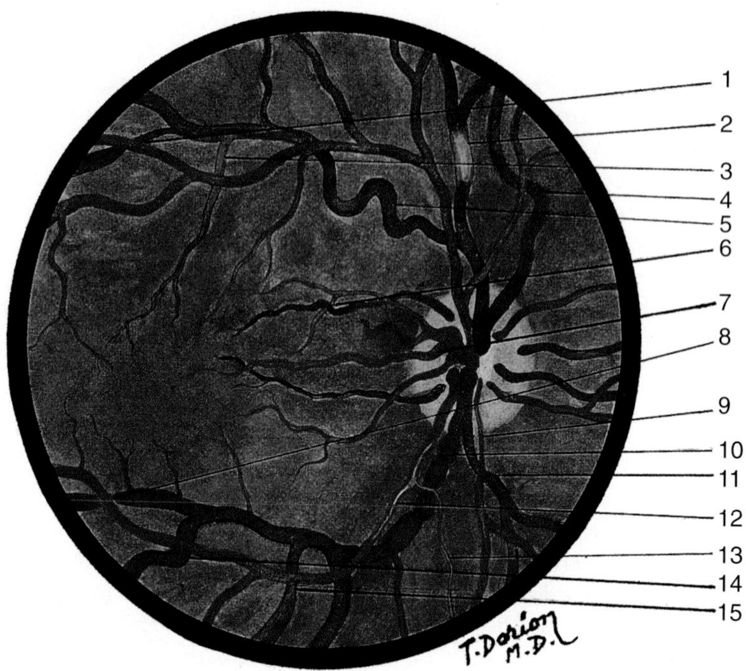

Figure 1-6. *Vessels and vascular changes. (1) Stenosis. (2) Sheathing. (3) Depression. (4) Salus' sign. (5) Tortuosity. (6) Humping. (7) Anomalous arterial branch. (8) Nicking. (9) Copper-wire reflex. (10) Sausage-shaped vein. (11) Gunn's sign. (12) Silver-wire reflex. (13) Arterial attenuation. (14) Deviation. (15) Banking.*

wire. The **silver-wire reflex** has the appearance of a whitish tube containing a red fluid. This reflex may be attributable to a replacement fibrosis, which obscures the blood column to the artery.

A host of changes in shape, size, caliber, and course of vessels can occur. **Narrowing** is a localized irregular constriction of the arterial caliber. In **arterial attenuation**, an artery appears as a thin, red, threadlike artery beyond its second bifurcation and usually disappears from view at the equator. **Anomalous branching** occurs occasionally at the central retinal artery. **Tortuosity** is a condition of increased length and diameter of retinal vessels, which make an arcuate course. A special form is the *prepapillary vascular loop*, which sometimes projects into the vitreous. **Sheathing** is a fibrous coat around a vessel's wall. It may be partial, appearing as a ribbon of red blood within the lines of one or both sides of the wall, or total, appearing as a white, fibrous cord with no visible red blood column. *Parallel sheathing* is lateral sheathing. A **sausage-shaped vein** is a marked, interrupted, dilatation of a vein caused by irregularities in the vein's wall.

At the AV crossings, the artery and the vein usually have a common adventitial sheath, the artery crosses over the vein, and the venous lumen is narrowed. Changes in this area can be classified as early (a simple deflection of a vein), moderate (a partially cut vein), or marked (a completely cut vein that leaves a space on either side of the artery). **Loss of transparency** is the earliest change, in which the vein can no longer be seen beneath the artery. **Nicking** is a localized constriction of vessels, with a tapering concealment of the vein that is narrowed, though its lumen remains normal. The venous blood column appears to terminate abruptly on either side of the AV crossing. **Banking** is a dilatation and swelling of a vein peripheral to the AV crossing, due to impeded circulation. The vein takes on the appearance of an hourglass, with constriction on both sides of the crossing, or of an aneurysmal swelling. **Depression** is a slight variation in color of a vein for some distance on either side of the artery but without any evidence of compression or circulatory impediment. The vein may be deflected deep into the retina. **Gunn's sign** is a compression of the vein in which the vessel is depressed, narrowed, and deviated downward and laterally. **Humping** is an abrupt elevation of the vein over the artery, usually due to a thickening of the arterial wall. **Stenosis** is compression of the vein that produces an obstruction of the distal segment, which then becomes dilated and swollen. **Deviation of the vein** is a displacement of the vein: The vessel turns abruptly in its course just as it reaches the artery, making an S-shaped bend and, just beyond the artery, resumes its normal course. **Salus' sign** is an arcuate deviation of the vein at a right angle; the vessel gradually becomes smaller and thinner until a segment of the vein is concealed.

Suggested Reading

Becker RA. Hypertension and Arteriosclerosis. In W Tasman, EA Jaeger, MM Parks, et al. (eds), Duane's Clinical Ophthalmology, vol 3. Philadelphia: Lippincott–Raven, 1996;13:1–22.

Bloom W, Faucett DW. A Textbook of Histology (10th ed). Philadelphia: Saunders, 1975;937–959.

Glaser JS. Anatomy of the Visual Sensory System. In W Tasman, EA Jaeger, MM Parks, et al. (eds), Duane's Clinical Ophthalmology, vol 2. Philadelphia: Lippincott–Raven, 1996;43:1–56.

Jonas JB, Papastathopoulos K. Ophthalmoscopic measurement of the optic disc. Ophthalmology 1995;102:1102–1106.

Kozart DM. Anatomic Correlates of the Retina. In W Tasman, EA Jaeger, MM Parks, et al. (eds), Duane's Clinical Ophthalmology, vol 3. Philadelphia: Lippincott–Raven, 1996;1:1–18.

Leishman R. The Cardiovascular System. In A Sorsby (ed), Modern Ophthalmology, vol 2 (2nd ed). Philadelphia: Lippincott, 1972;447–508.

Macleod D. Vitreous and Vitreoretinal Disorders. In DJ Spalton, RA Hitchings, PA Hunter (eds), Atlas of Clinical Ophthalmology (2nd ed). London: Wolfe, 1994;12.11.

Montgomery DMI. Measurement of optic disc and neuroretinal rim areas in normal and glaucomatous eyes. Ophthalmology 1991;98:50–59.

Quigley HA, Katz J, Gilbert D, Sommer A. An evaluation of optic disc and nerve fiber layer examinations in monitoring progression of early glaucoma damage. Ophthalmology 1992;99:19–28.

Reeh MJ, Reeh M, Wobig JL, Wirshafter JD. The Globe. Ophthalmic Anatomy. San Francisco: American Academy of Ophthalmology, 1981;130–154.

Reinecke RD, Farrel TA. Fundamentals of Ophthalmology (2nd ed). San Francisco: American Academy of Ophthalmology, 1987;92–114.

Spalton DJ. The Optic Disc. In DJ Spalton, RA Hitchings, PA Hunter (eds), Atlas of Clinical Ophthalmology (2nd ed). London: Wolfe, 1994;17.23.

Spalton DJ, Marshall J. The Normal Retina. In DJ Spalton, RA Hitchings, PA Hunter (eds), Atlas of Clinical Ophthalmology (2nd ed). London: Wolfe, 1994;13.2.

Warwick R. Anatomy: Section I. Orbit, Globe, and Its Central Connections. In A Sorsby (ed), Modern Ophthalmology, vol 1 (2nd ed). Philadelphia: Lippincott, 1972;37–170.

2

Ocular Signs

Arterial Attenuation

Arterial attenuation is a constriction of an artery, *focal* or *generalized*, and occurs more commonly in young patients with hypertension who do not develop fibrosis. It is caused by a vascular spasm. The attenuation appears as a narrowed artery (diminished arterial diameter), sometimes like a thin, red thread, starting beyond the second bifurcation. It may disappear when the arterial blood pressure returns to normal.

Asteroid Hyalosis

Asteroid hyalosis (also known as *Benson's disease* and *hyalitis*) is a benign, usually unilateral, vitreous degeneration of unknown etiology, in which multiple particles of calcium soaps, phospholipid, and sulfur are present in the vitreous (Figure 2-1). Asteroid hyalosis is not associated with any systemic disease. It appears as myriad highly refractile, birefringent crystals, or silvery or golden dots that are spherical, stellate, or discoid (like snowballs) and are suspended in a normal vitreous. They swirl during eye movement but always return to their original position.

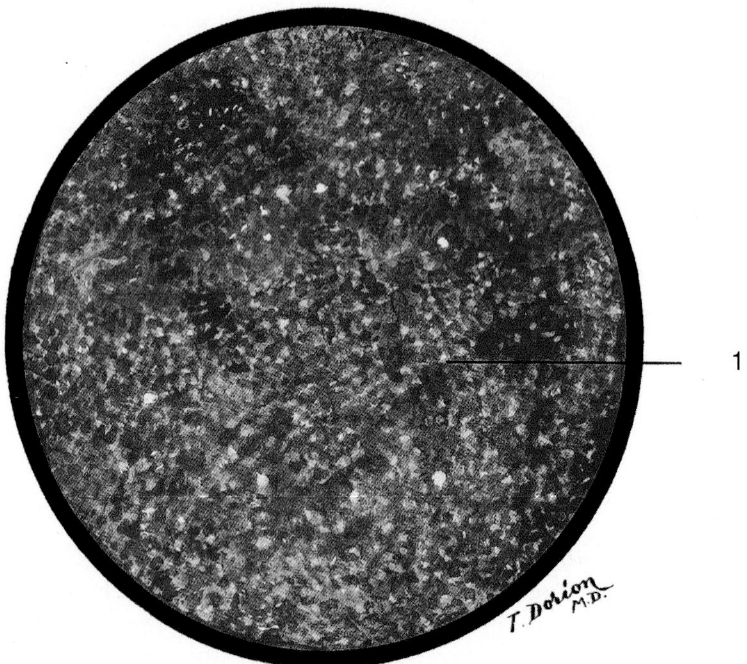

Figure 2-1. *Asteroid hyalosis. (1) Calcium soaps, phospholipid, or sulfur suspended in a normal vitreous.*

Beaten Bronze Atrophy

Beaten bronze atrophy is a macular atrophy that usually occurs in Stargardt's disease (fundus flavimaculatus) or in cone-rod dystrophy. It is due to a slowly progressive macular degeneration, which may cause atrophy of the retinal pigment epithelium (RPE), with complete disappearance of the pigment cells, photoreceptors, or choriocapillaris. It also can be associated with areas of pigment proliferation and calcium deposition.

Beaten bronze atrophy appears as oval or elliptic patchy areas of depigmentation in the macula, with brownish foveal spots that are sharply delineated, surrounded by a garland of small, irregular white-yellow flecks, some of which are confluent. Calcium deposits that vary in size, are linear or fishlike, and often aggregate in clusters also are seen; these give the appearance of a beaten metal. The foveal reflex is

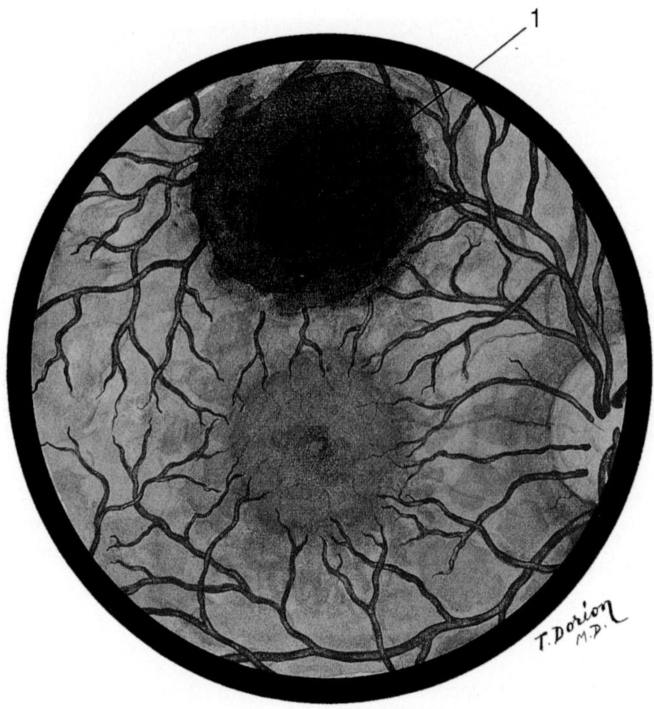

Figure 2-2. *Black sunburst. (1) Ovoid circumscribed lesion, composed of hyperplasia and hypertrophy of retinal pigment epithelium, and hemosiderin.*

pronounced, altered from normal, tapetal-like, and polychromatic. Choroidal vessels are visible.

Black Sunburst

Black sunburst is a heavily pigmented lesion of the midperipheral retina (Figure 2-2) and occurs usually in nonproliferative sickle cell retinopathy. It probably is caused by an occlusion of an artery and a recent infarction, which may produce preretinal, intraretinal, or subretinal hemorrhage that later may dissect into the subretinal space, simulating a pigment migration.

Black sunburst appears as a black, ovoid, circumscribed lesion (or lesions) of approximately 0.5–1.0 dd in size, with irregular spiculate or

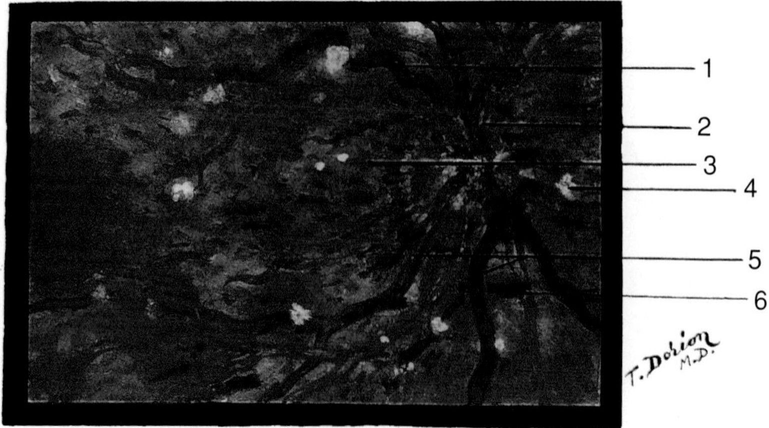

Figure 2-3. *Blood-and-thunder. (1) Tortuous veins. (2) Congested optic disc. (3) Superficial flame-shaped hemorrhages. (4) Cotton-wool spots. (5) Dilated retinal vessels, arteries, and veins. (6) Preretinal hemorrhage.*

stellate borders and a perivascular deposition of melanin pigment and yellowish granules.

Areas of RPE atrophy, RPE hyperplasia, pigment migration, and hemosiderin develop after intraretinal and subretinal hemorrhages.

Blood-and-Thunder

Blood-and-thunder is an extensive hemorrhage of the posterior pole (Figure 2-3). It occurs in occlusion of the central retinal artery or in venous occlusion. Multiple gross, massive hemorrhages of different types and sizes are seen around the optic disc. There are preretinal, superficial, flame-shaped or striate hemorrhages or deep intraretinal hemorrhages, which may occupy a large portion of the posterior retina.

The retinal vessels are markedly dilated, the veins tortuous and irregular. The optic disc is congested and edematous, usually with blurred, indistinct margins and a flat, blood-filled physiologic cup. Scattered cotton-wool spots (soft exudates with fluffy margins), caused by infarction in the retinal nerve fiber layer, are present throughout the posterior pole.

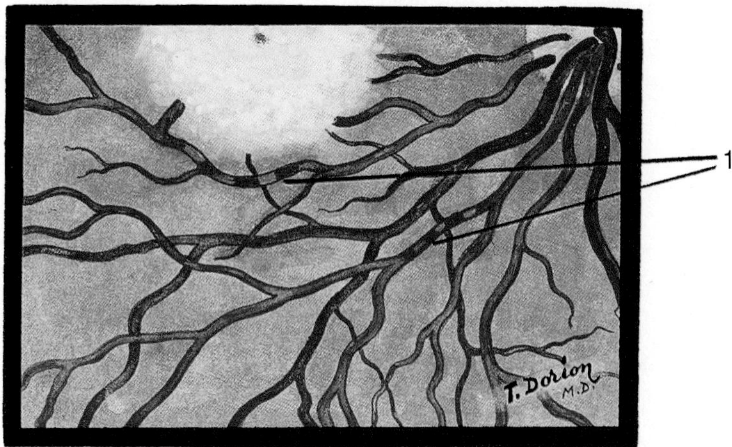

Figure 2-4. *Boxcarring vessels. (1) Segmentation of arterial blood flow, in a central retinal artery occlusion.*

Boxcarring Vessels

Boxcarring vessels are a segmentation of the blood flow in the retinal arteries (Figure 2-4) that generally occur in central retinal artery occlusion but may affect the veins also. Several portions of the artery demonstrate a sluggish circulation, as evidenced by a to-and-fro movement of the blood, and are interspersed with other segments of the artery that are empty.

Bull's-Eye Macula

Bull's-eye macula is a degenerative macular lesion that resembles a target or a bull's-eye (Figure 2-5). It occurs usually in chloroquine retinopathy, cone-rod dystrophy, Spielmayer-Vogt-Batten-Mayou disease, Laurence-Moon-Bardet-Biedl syndrome and, rarely, in Leber's congenital amaurosis. Bull's-eye macula is caused by an atrophic macular degeneration of the RPE beneath the foveola as well as in the perifoveolar region.

Bull's-eye macula appears as a fine granular pigment accumulation in the center of the macula, which in time becomes a hyperpigmented spot surrounded by an annular patchy depigmented area that usually

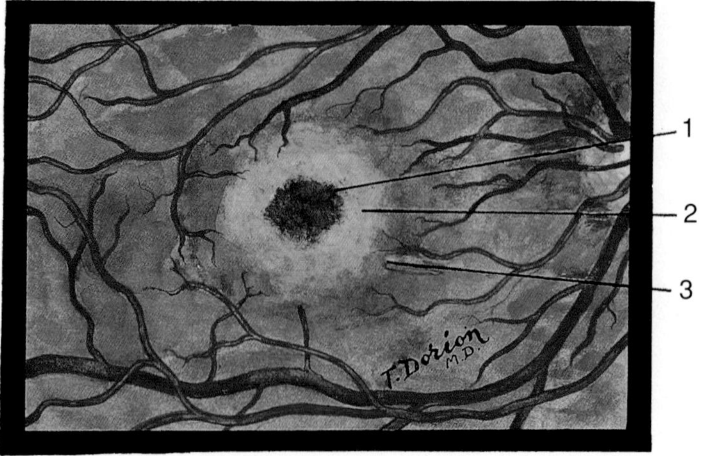

Figure 2-5. *Bull's-eye macula. (1) Pigment accumulation in macula. (2) Depigmented retinal pigment epithelium atrophy. (3) Hyperpigmented perifoveal area.*

is horizontal and is more prominent inferiorly. This depigmented zone is surrounded in turn by a perifoveal hyperpigmented area, which gives the lesion its characteristic appearance.

Candle Wax Drippings

Candle wax drippings are granulomatous exudates, which occur generally in sarcoidosis. They are due to an accumulation of inflammatory cells (sheathing) around the retinal vessels. Candle wax drippings appear as multiple, small, discrete, round or oval, white-yellow exudates located along the branches of the veins, usually in the form of strings of pearls at the posterior pole.

Cattle Trucking

Cattle trucking is a sign of retinal circulation stagnation (Figure 2-6), which occurs usually in central retinal artery occlusion. A clumping of the blood column is seen in the arteries, which are markedly narrowed and irregular in caliber, with sludgy and segmented blood flow.

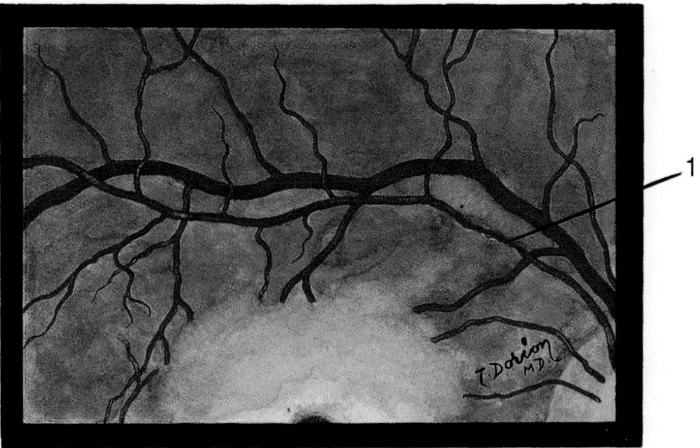

Figure 2-6. *Cattle trucking. (1) Clumping and narrowing of artery.*

Cherry-Red Spot

Cherry-red spot is a macular retinal infarction that occurs in central retinal artery occlusion. It also describes an accumulation of anomalous products in some metabolic storage diseases, such as Tay-Sachs, Sandhoff's, Niemann-Pick, or Farber's disease (Figure 2-7). The lesion is due to infarction of the ganglion cell layer and the nerve fiber layer, usually in the perifoveolar and parafoveolar regions, which produces a retinal edema. *This does not occur in the foveola*, from which the nerve fiber and ganglion cell layers are absent (Figure 2-8). In the metabolic storage diseases just mentioned, there is a deposition of some material in the ganglion cell layer in the perifoveolar and parafoveolar regions.

Cherry-red spot appears at the foveola as a small, round, red, orange, or red-brown spot, usually less than one-third disc diameter in size, with irregular margins. Its location at the foveola determines the degree of visibility of the normal choroid. It is surrounded by a milky white, edematous and opaque retina that involves the perifoveolar and parafoveolar regions.

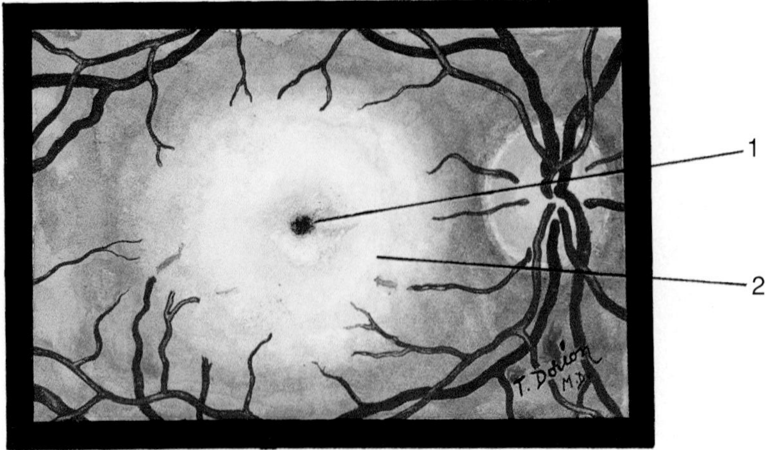

Figure 2-7. *Cherry-red spot. (1) Visible red choroid in foveola. (2) Opaque, cloudy, edematous retina.*

Comet Tail

Comet tail is a depigmented area in the midperipheral retina (Figure 2-9) that occurs commonly in glioma, familial adenomatous polyposis, or Turcot's syndrome. It is due to a disturbance at the level of the RPE. It appears as a small, yellow-white, triangular, curvilinear patch, usually comet tail–shaped, of approximately 0.5–1.0 dd in size, located adjacent to an oval area of chronic RPE hypertrophy in the midperiphery of the fundus.

Copper-Wire Reflex

The copper-wire reflex is an alteration of vessel wall transparency that occurs often in elderly patients with hypertension and moderate arteriosclerosis. It is generally due to a blending of the yellow fat products and the red blood column in the arteries, which may produce a thickening of the vessel wall. It appears as an abnormal wider and brighter light reflex of the arteries, a burnished, metallic, copperlike streak (Figure 2-10) that may occupy most of the width of the vessel. The blood

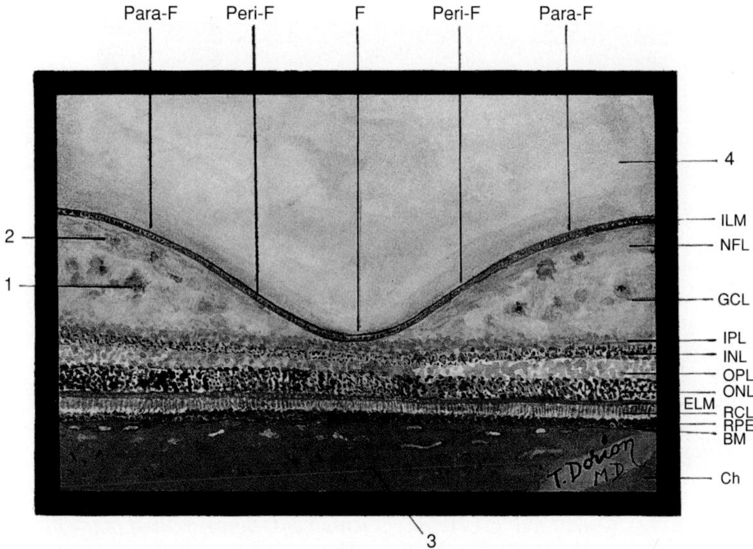

Figure 2-8. *Cherry-red spot: histopathology. (1) Edema and infarctions in nerve fiber layer. (2) Edema and infarctions in ganglion cell layer. (3) Choroid, visible as a red spot at foveola. (4) Vitreous. (F, foveola, a nerve fiber layer and ganglion cell layer–free zone; Peri-F, perifoveolar area; Para-F, parafoveolar area; ILM, internal limiting membrane; NFL, nerve fiber layer; GCL, ganglion cell layer; IPL, inner plexiform layer; INL, inner nuclear layer; OPL, outer plexiform layer; ONL, outer nuclear layer; ELM, external limiting membrane; RCL, rod and cone layer [photoreceptors]; RPE, retinal pigment epithelium; BM, Bruch's membrane; Ch, choroid.)*

column is present but is intermingled with the intravascular lipids and is better seen by looking perpendicularly through the surface of the wall.

Cotton-Wool Spots

Cotton-wool spots (also known as *soft exudates* or *cytoid bodies*) are retinal microinfarcts that usually occur in diabetes, hypertension, retinal vein occlusion, papilledema, collagen diseases, anemia, leukemia, and hyperviscosity syndromes. They are due to spasms of precapillary arterioles or to a fibrinoid necrosis, which may cause an endothelial abnormality. That, in turn, may produce an occlusion of an arteriole,

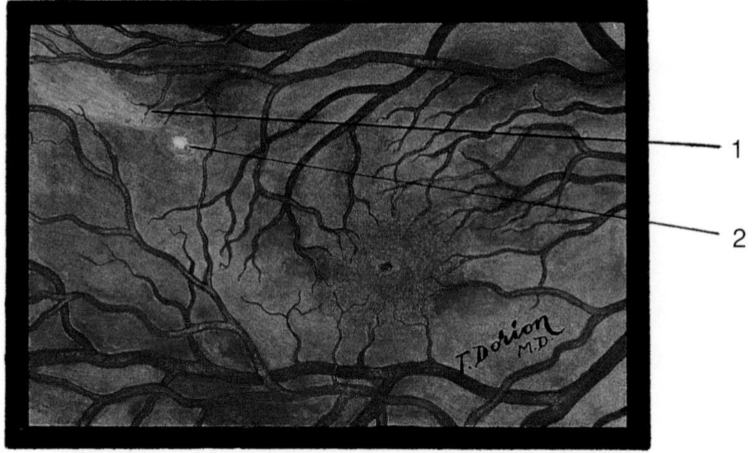

Figure 2-9. *Comet tail. (1) Hypopigmented curvilinear retinal pigment epithelium atrophy. (2) Oval chronic retinal pigment epithelium hypertrophy.*

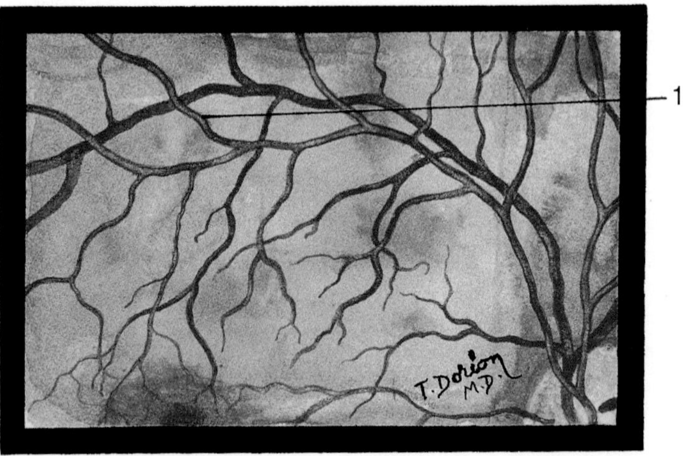

Figure 2-10. *Copper-wire reflex. (1) Metallic, burnished, abnormal light reflex of artery.*

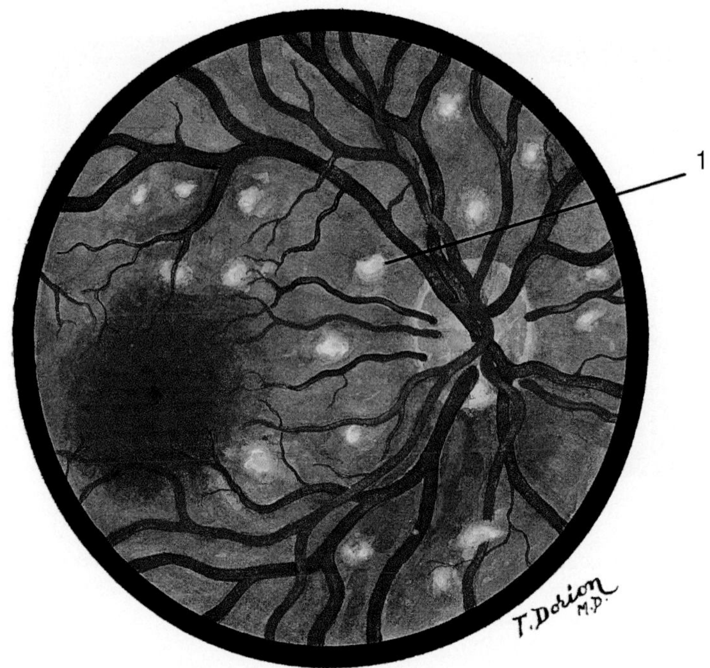

Figure 2-11. *Cotton-wool spots. (1) Microinfarcts of ganglion cell axons in retinal nerve fiber layer.*

followed by a secondary ischemia that interrupts the axonic flow, resulting in an infarction of the ganglion cell axons located in the retinal nerve fiber layer (Figure 2-11), with focal accumulation of axoplasmic debris.

Cotton-wool spots appear as multiple, pale, gray-white, slightly elevated spots, with blurred, feathery, indistinct, irregular soft margins. They usually are located at the posterior pole around the optic disc. Because of their appearance as a swollen end-bulb, they have been likened to a cell nucleus—hence the name *cytoid bodies* (Figure 2-12).

Crescent

A crescent is a congenital or acquired, progressive or stationary, depigmented lesion at the margin of the optic disc that occurs more com-

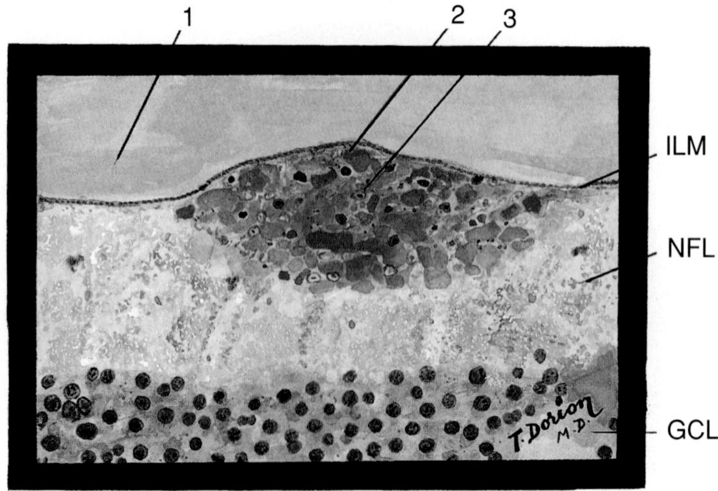

Figure 2-12. *Cotton-wool spots: histopathology. (1) Vitreous. (2) Microinfarcts of nerve fiber layer. (3) Ruptured enlarged ganglion cell axons, called* cytoid bodies. *(ILM, internal limiting membrane; NFL, nerve fiber layer; GCL, ganglion cell layer.)*

monly in high myopia. It may be due to failure of development of the RPE at the margin of the disc, which results in RPE atrophy and choroidal atrophy that is not covered completely by the choriocapillaris and the RPE; or to a misalignment of several layers of the retina, choroid, and sclera; or to an oblique insertion of the optic disc.

A crescent appears as a semilunar, white-yellow patch located at the margin of the disc, usually inferiorly and temporally, peripapillary or sometimes circumpapillary (Figure 2-13). It measures approximately one-third disc diameter but may be up to several disc diameters in width. The optic nerve head may appear oval, with its long axis parallel to the crescent. Occasionally, a second choroidal crescent, outside the original crescent, may be present as a result of disturbed pigmentation. Sometimes, when the temporal crescent is large, there may be a light reflex on the opposite side, which occurs mostly in young patients as a result of a pilling up of the nasal retina, called the *Weiss-Otto reflex*. Retinal vessels may be stretched temporally. Choroidal vessels may be prominent.

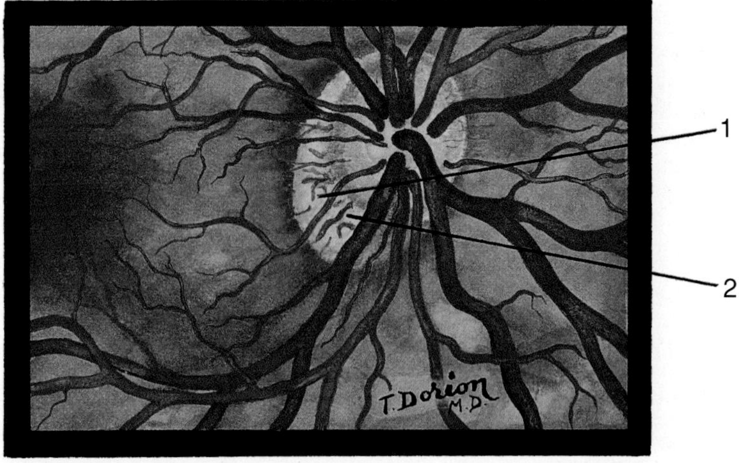

Figure 2-13. *Crescent. (1) Semilunar, white-yellow patch located at the margin of the disc, usually inferiorly and temporally. (2) Temporally stretched retinal vessels.*

Dalen-Fuchs Nodules

Dalen-Fuchs nodules are inflammatory choroidal exudates that occur in several stages in sympathetic ophthalmia and sarcoidosis. They appear as multiple small, yellow-white nodules (Figure 2-14) that are focal or confluent, round or oval, have fluffy margins, and are widespread, distributed at the posterior pole and localized beneath the RPE or above Bruch's membrane. A large area of hypopigmented RPE atrophy often is found among them.

The nodules are caused by the inflammatory process of the diseases in which they occur. The inflammatory process produces an accumulation of giant cells, clusters of epithelioid cells with or without pigment, and lymphocytes, causing a discontinuation and atrophy of RPE, degeneration and misalignment of photoreceptors, and often an obliteration of the choriocapillaris beneath the nodules.

Drusen

Drusen (also called *hyaline bodies* or *colloid bodies*) are congenital or acquired multiple amorphous deposits of cholesterol, calcium, sialic

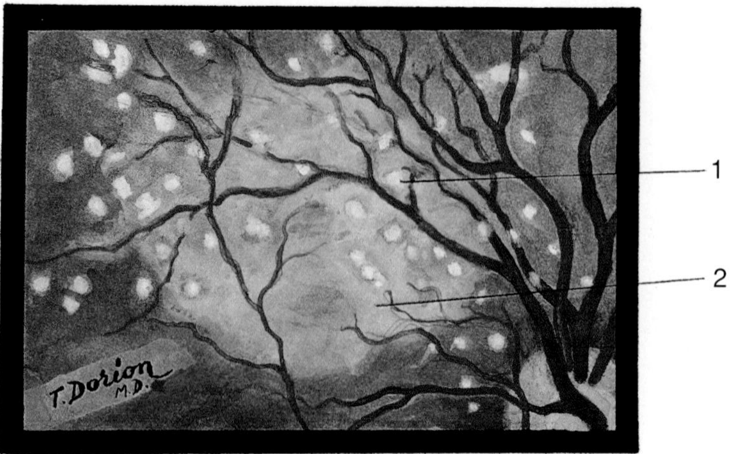

Figure 2-14. *Dalen-Fuchs nodules. (1) Inflammatory choroidal exudates. (2) Depigmented area of retinal pigment epithelium atrophy.*

acid, or cerebrosides, located extracellularly between Bruch's membrane and the RPE in the macula, peripheral retina, or optic disc (Figure 2-15). Drusen of the disc are not related to other drusen of the macula or of the peripheral retina.

The drusen appear as small, usually bilateral, symmetric, discrete, fine, round, granular, yellow circumscribed lesions, almost equal in size. They are clustered in the fundus.

Congenital drusen often are autosomal dominant, due to a familial abnormality, such as an excess of immature neuroglia in the RPE, which may undergo degeneration. *Acquired drusen*, or *secondary drusen*, may be due to changes in the RPE in which the cells cast off part of their cytoplasm by a process called *apoptosis*. They may also be due to an alteration of the axoplasmic transport.

There are various types of drusen: hard, soft, calcified, or basal laminar membranous. *Hard drusen* are small, well-defined, glistening lesions with fine pigment clumps and secondary atrophic patches. They may become confluent to form plaques. *Soft drusen* are larger than hard drusen, pale, yellow, homogenous, and dome shaped, often with overlying pigment. They have indistinct margins and vary in size. *Calcific drusen* or *regressing drusen* are white and harder than any other type of drusen, and they occasionally display pigment stippling. *Basal lamina membranous drusen* are a late form, which may not be identi-

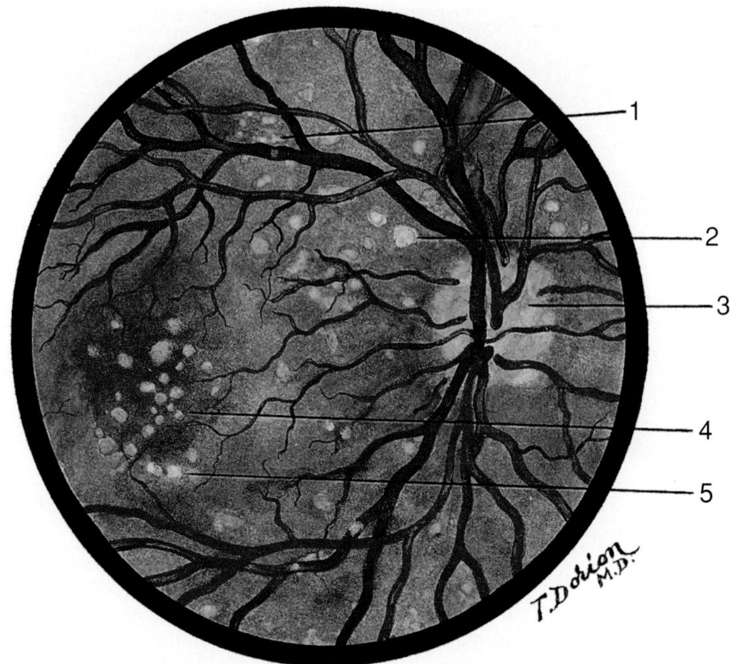

Figure 2-15. *Drusen. (1) Hard drusen. (2) Soft drusen. (3) Disc drusen. (4) Macular drusen. (5) Calcific drusen.*

fiable clinically, composed of hyalinized Bruch's membrane and fibrillar segment long-spacing collagen.

Disc drusen are usually either *ordinary*—laminated calcareous concretions—or *giant*—astrocytic hamartoma located anterior to the lamina cribrosa. They appear as round, crystalline, small, yellow-white formations in the optic nerve head, sometimes without any nodular disc elevation because they are located beneath the nerve fibers. The physiologic cup usually is absent.

Elschnig's Spots

Elschnig's spots are infarcts of choriocapillaris that usually occur in hypertension. They are due to ischemia of the RPE produced by a choroidal artery occlusion. The spots appear as small, yellow-gray, round areas of hyperplasia and hypertrophy of the RPE, have a pig-

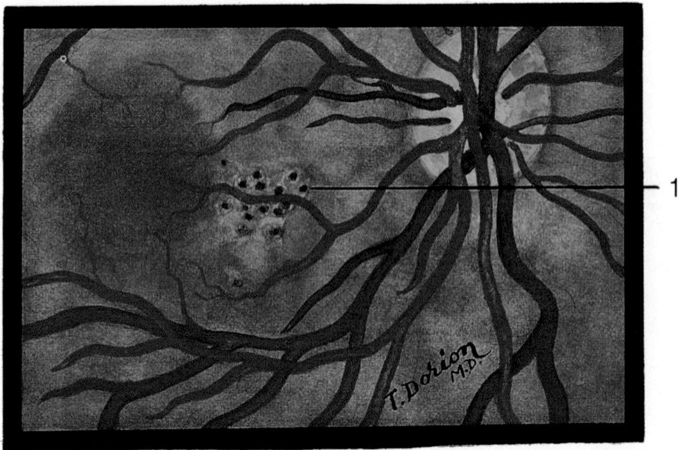

Figure 2-16. *Elschnig's spots. (1) Infarcts of choriocapillaris, with pigmented center and yellow or red halo.*

mented center surrounded by a yellow or red halo, measure approximately one-sixth to one-third disc diameter, and are located at the posterior pole, frequently near the optic disc (Figure 2-16).

Fish Tail

Fish tail is a degenerative lesion of the retina that usually occurs in Stargardt's disease (fundus flavimaculatus). It is caused by an alteration of the retina in which lipofuscin pigment accumulates in the RPE cells, which may become markedly engorged. No other retinal layer is involved.

Fish tail appears as multiple fine, yellow-white angular spots of varying sizes and shapes, either as individual fishlike dots and flecks or as confluent clusters, scattered in the macula or in the postequatorial retina. The condition arises in sequential waves: As the old spots fade, new ones are developing.

Fuchs' Spot

Fuchs' spot is a macular lesion that occurs commonly in high myopia. It is caused by a recurrent choroidal hemorrhage that leads to hyper-

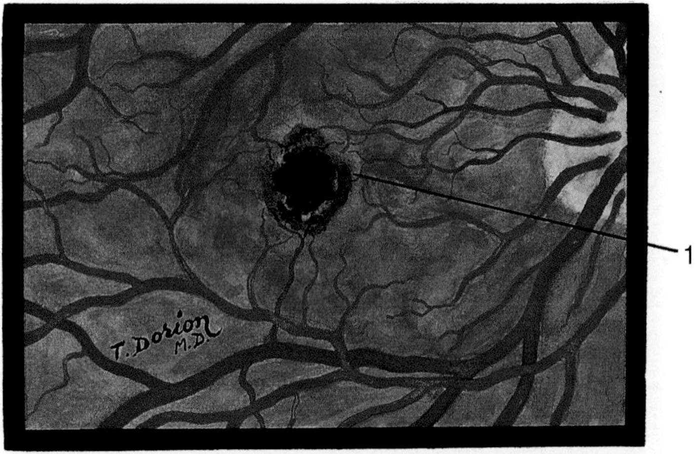

Figure 2-17. *Fuchs' spot. (1) Hemosiderin deposit in macula.*

plasia of the RPE, a proliferation of subretinal and sub-RPE scar tissue, and a chorioretinal degeneration, with depositation of hemosiderin in the macula.

Fuchs' spot appears as a black, round or elliptic macular lesion (Figure 2-17), may be bilateral, measures approximately one-third disc diameter (but varies in size and can be larger), is slightly elevated and sharply circumscribed, and has irregular margins. Occasionally, it may be covered by fibrosis, giving it a gray, green, yellow, or red appearance. In time, the spot becomes less distinct and is surrounded by a thin halo of chorioretinal atrophy. It may occur in an area overlying a previous choroidal neovascular membrane.

Ghost Vessel

A ghost vessel is a retinal vessel that has no blood in the lumen (Figure 2-18). It usually occurs in syphilis, after the inflammation has subsided. It appears as a white cord of varying length, with a permanently closed lumen. It is different from a *periphlebitis*, which conceals the blood column but does not occlude it.

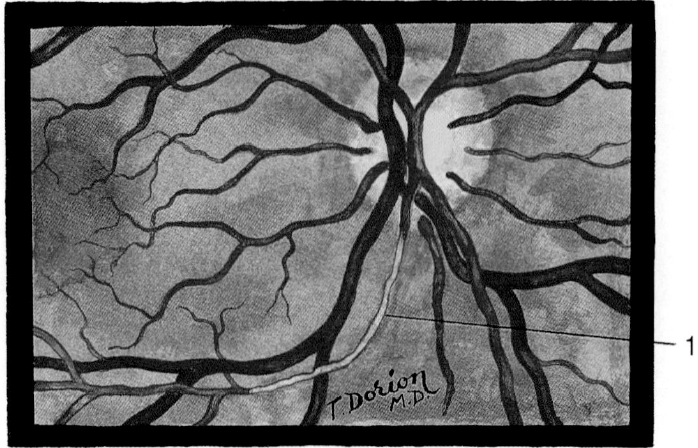

Figure 2-18. *Ghost vessel. (1) Retinal vessel without blood.*

Glaucomatous Cup

A glaucomatous cup is a depression of the optic disc that occurs in glaucoma (Figure 2-19) and that differs from the physiologic cup in size, shape, color, and appearance of the neuroretinal rim and retinal vessels.

Size

The cup may be entirely enlarged, but a large cup alone is not diagnostic of glaucoma. Usually, the disc appears to be vertically elongated, with a cup-to-disc (C/D) ratio greater than 0.6 or with an asymmetry of cupping greater than 0.2 between the eyes. In advanced glaucoma, the cup may be markedly enlarged, so that the C/D ratio may be almost 1.0.

Shape

The cup may be round, oval, or eccentric. It often may expand outward, and the disc may recede backward in a movement of the disc surface called *saucerization*. The cup may slope away such that the nasal slope is steeper than the temporal slope. Occasionally, the deepening of

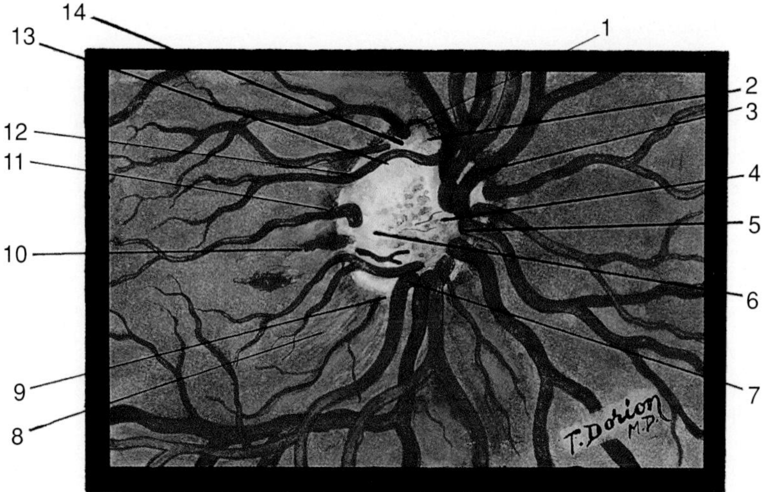

Figure 2-19. *Glaucomatous cup. (1) Notching. (2) Undermining of cup's edge. (3) Nasal shift of major vessels. (4) Fenestrations of lamina cribrosa evident. (5) Disappearance of large central retinal vessels under neuroretinal rim. (6) Optic nerve atrophy. (7) Bending of major vessels. (8) Nerve fiber defect. (9) Thinning of inferior temporal rim. (10) Flame-shaped splinter hemorrhage. (11) Bending of small vessels. (12) Saucerization. (13) Cup larger than area of pallor. (14) Vertical extension of pallor and cupping.*

the cup causes the lamina cribrosa to bow posteriorly and makes its gray fenestrations evident; this is called the *laminar dot sign.*

Sometimes, the cup expands downward vertically to the inferior pole in an inverted teardrop shape. There may also be a pit or a focal loss of the lamina cribrosa, located centrally in an excavated disc. An acquired optic nerve pit at the 5-o'clock or 6:30-o'clock area, usually at the outer edge of the disc, may be considered diagnostic of glaucoma.

Color

The cup is paler in its vertical diameter and may be pinkish or whiter than normal for a long time until, in advanced glaucoma, a portion of the cup (the temporal and nasal sides) becomes much paler and dusky with a gray-white pallor.

Neuroretinal Rim

The neuroretinal rim is the portion of the optic disc located between the margin of the cup and the margin of the disc. The rim usually is paler than the adjacent retina and is localized in a quadrant, the nerve fibers being visible. In glaucoma, the neuroretinal rim becomes progressively thinner, starting at the temporal and inferior side. It is not uniform as it surrounds the cup and may be partially or completely absent. As the cup extends to the rim, notching—a pitlike focal enlargement of the cup or an erosion of the disc in the upper temporal area or at the inferior pole—may develop. Notching may give the disc a slightly oval shape. There may be slitlike generalized or localized *striations* of the rim owing to the nerve fiber loss.

Retinal Vessels

Retinal vessels usually are displaced to the nasal half of the disc and lie on the floor of the cup, the temporal side being more vascularized. They bend sharply as they pass the edge of the disc and may disappear under the rim. In advanced glaucoma, there may be a hooking of the vessels under the scleral rim, with diffuse loss of nerve fibers, called *bean-pot cupping*. Flame-shaped superficial splinter hemorrhages may occur at the disc margin, most of them located between the artery and the vein at the inferotemporal quadrant. Some hemorrhages are transient, but others may recur. As the glaucoma progresses, a loss of normal fiber striations, called *nerve fiber defect,* may occur in a late stage.

Histopathology

In glaucoma (Figure 2-20), the ganglion cells suffer axonal damage as they pass through the lamina cribrosa. Astroglia and microvessels are lost. Neovascularization, dilatation of the vessels, or optic nerve atrophy may be present. In a late, advanced glaucoma, the lamina cribrosa is displaced backward, bowed away from the eye, and stretched. The neuroretinal rim also is displaced toward the lamina cribrosa.

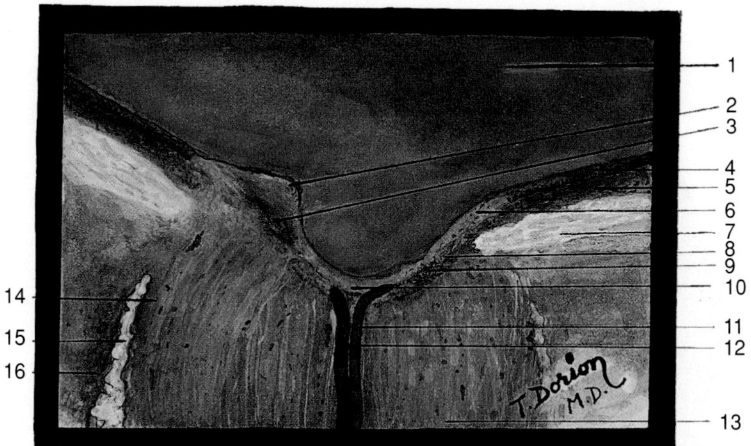

Figure 2-20. *Glaucomatous cup: histopathology. (1) Vitreous. (2) Neuroretinal rim displaced toward lamina cribrosa. (3) Dilatation of vessels. (4) Retina. (5) Choroid. (6) Retinal portion of optic nerve. (7) Sclera. (8) Lamina cribrosa displaced posteriorly and stretched. (9) Neovascularization. (10) Optic nerve atrophy with loss of astroglia and microglia. (11) Central retinal artery. (12) Central retinal vein. (13) Optic nerve. (14) Dura mater. (15) Subarachnoid space. (16) Pia mater.*

Grouped Pigmentation

Grouped pigmentation (also known as *bear's tracks, cat's pawprints,* and *melanosis of the retina*) is a benign, unilateral, stationary, nonfamilial, pigmented degeneration of the retina (Figure 2-21) that is of no clinical significance. It is due to hypertrophy of the RPE cells, which are densely pigmented with spherical granules of melanin that migrate in a region usually occupied by the photoreceptors, which have degenerated or are absent.

Grouped pigmentation appears as several grouped, sharply delineated, flat, round or oval, gray-black pigmented patches, approximately 0.1–3.0 mm in diameter, surrounded by a thin hypopigmented ring. The groups are scattered throughout the posterior pole or may be limited to a sector that is larger at the periphery and strongly resembles bear's tracks.

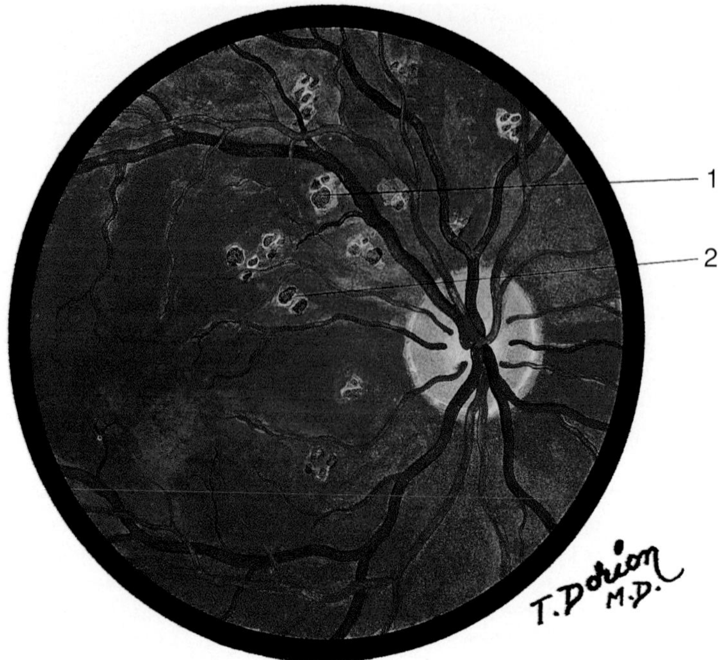

Figure 2-21. *Grouped pigmentation. (1) Retinal pigment epithelium hypertrophy. (2) Hypopigmented ring.*

Gunn's Sign

Gunn's sign is a deviation of a vein at the arteriovenous (AV) crossing (Figure 2-22), which occurs frequently in hypertension. It appears as a vein that is displaced downward and laterally, is depressed or nicked, and is narrowed by the artery, with banking and concealment of the venous blood segment distally to the AV crossing.

Hard Exudates

Hard exudates (also known as *waxy exudates*) are deep intraretinal deposits (Figure 2-23) that usually occur in hypertension, arteriosclerosis, diabetes, anemia, Coats' disease, retinal vein occlusion, angiomatosis retinae, macroaneurysms, radiation retinopathy, and optic neuropathy.

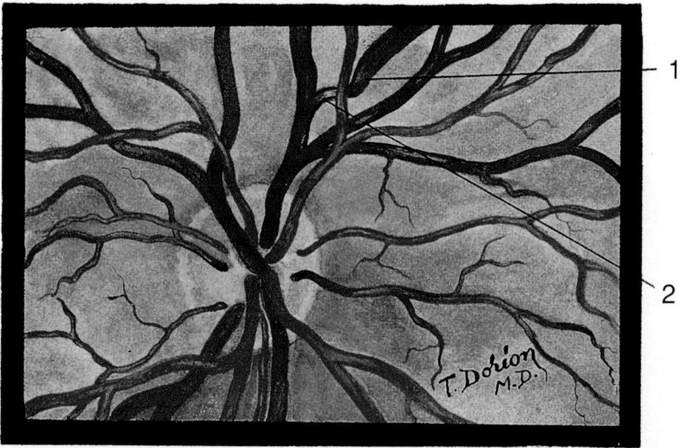

Figure 2-22. *Gunn's sign. (1) Deviated, depressed, and narrowed vein at arteriovenous crossing. (2) Concealment of venous segment, distally to arteriovenous crossing.*

They are due to accumulation of free fat or lipid-laden macrophages and foamy histiocytes (*glitter cells*) and lipoproteins in the outer plexiform layer and inner nuclear layer.

They appear as small, discrete, bright, white-yellow or slightly waxy, refractile, glistening, circumscribed, sharply delineated individual dots. Alternatively, they may appear as clusters, as confluent patches, or as a partial or complete ring surrounding macroaneurysms or zones of retinal edema. They usually are located at the posterior pole, near or around the macula, or are scattered throughout the fundus, varying in number from a few to 50 or more.

Macular hard exudates generally are of two types: Either they are arranged as a complete or partial circle of yellow-orange, globular, garlandlike patches called *circinate macular retinopathy* that surround the macula, or they are distributed as the spokes of a wheel, termed a *macular star*. They may progress to form larger plaques. The discrete hard exudates may resolve in 4–6 months, but the confluent exudates may not clear for years. Their lateral spread in the retina probably is limited by the Müller cells.

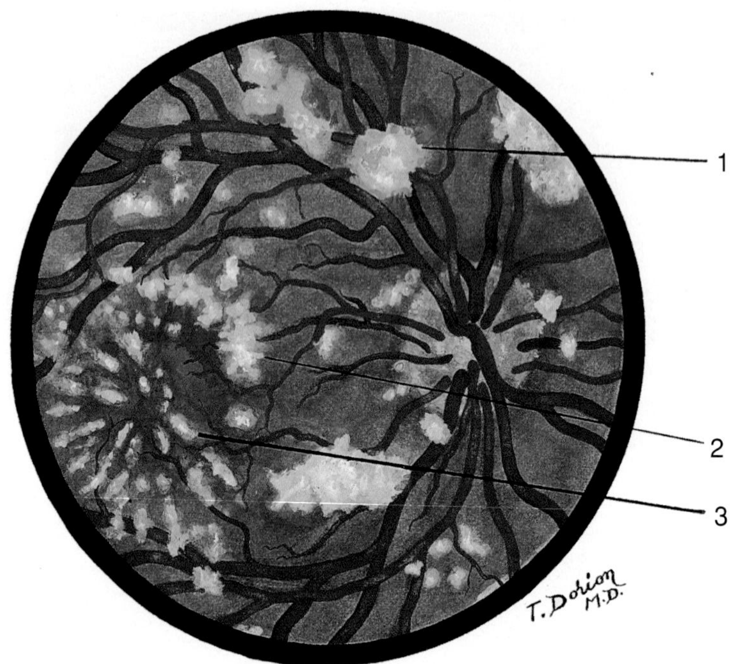

Figure 2-23. *Hard exudates. (1) Deep intraretinal deposits of lipoproteins. (2) Circinate maculopathy. (3) Macular star.*

High Water Marks

High water marks are deposits of proteinaceus material at the level of the RPE located around the optic disc. They often occur after a papilledema resolves. They appear as concentric, circumpapillary, yellowish undulating rings of intraretinal deposits, arranged in two or three rows, which represent the limits of a previous papilledema. Sometimes, they are horizontal.

Hollenhorst Plaque

Hollenhorst plaque is an arterial embolus that arises far from the eye, from an atheromatous plaque of a carotid artery stenosis. It appears as a single or as multiple refractile yellow spots (Figure 2-24) or as a plaque

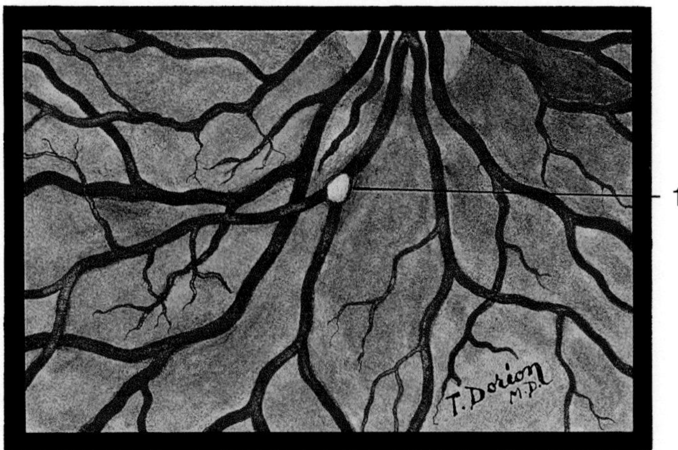

Figure 2-24. *Hollenhorst plaque. (1) Cholesterol or fibrin embolus at artery bifurcation.*

of cholesterol or fibrin, with irregular, sharp margins, located almost always at the bifurcation of retinal arteries and occluding the vessel's lumen. The Hollenhorst plaque may be larger than the vessel itself.

Intraretinal Microvascular Abnormalities

Intraretinal microvascular abnormalities (IRMAs) are irregularities in the caliber of the small vessels and vascular communications. They occur usually in diabetes and are due to an early shunt and collateral vessel formation in nonproliferative diabetic retinopathy.

IRMAs are seen as tortuous, dilated segments of intraretinal microvessels, located more commonly at the periphery of the disc. They measure approximately 31 μm in diameter, which is approximately one-fourth of the width of a vein at the disc margin, though occasionally they are larger.

Lacquer Cracks

Lacquer cracks are discontinuities, breaks, tears, or clefts in Bruch's membrane (Figure 2-25) through which connective tissue, hemorrhage,

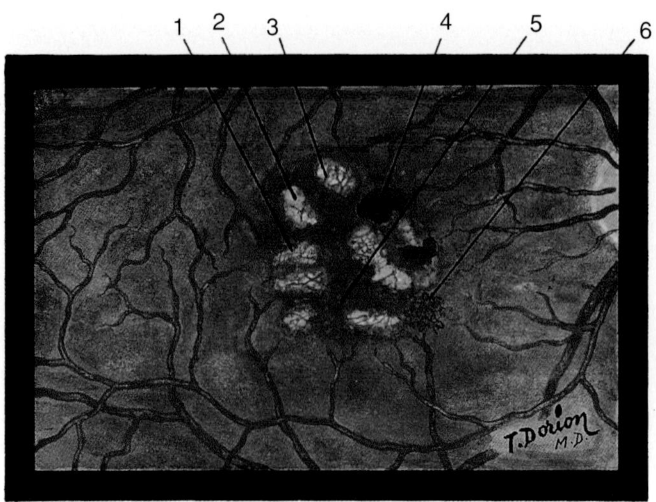

Figure 2-25. *Lacquer cracks. (1) Macular depigmented streaks, representing discontinuities in Bruch's membrane. (2) Retinal pigment epithelium atrophy. (3) Visible choroidal vessels. (4) Subretinal hemorrhage. (5) Connective tissue, which may pass through these breaks. (6) Choroidal neovascularization.*

and choroidal neovascularization may pass and grow beneath the RPE. They occur more frequently in high myopia but also are seen in Marfan's, Ehlers-Danlos, or Stickler's syndrome. Lacquer cracks are due to a stretching of the retina and an atrophy of the RPE.

The cracks appear as multiple linear or stellate, white-yellow subretinal streaks of irregular caliber and variable size, usually branching horizontally but possibly oriented vertically or as crisscrossing lines. They lie deep in the retina at the posterior pole, mostly at the macula. Normal large choroidal vessels may cross over. In the macular area, there may be secondary RPE proliferation, hemorrhage, and subretinal neovascularization, which give rise to a dark disciform degenerative lesion called *Fuchs' spot.*

Leopard Spots

Leopard spots describe a unilateral or bilateral retinal pigmentation, usually rapidly progressive, that occurs in choroidal metastases, in the cerebrohepatorenal syndrome of Zellweger, or after a chronic choroidal

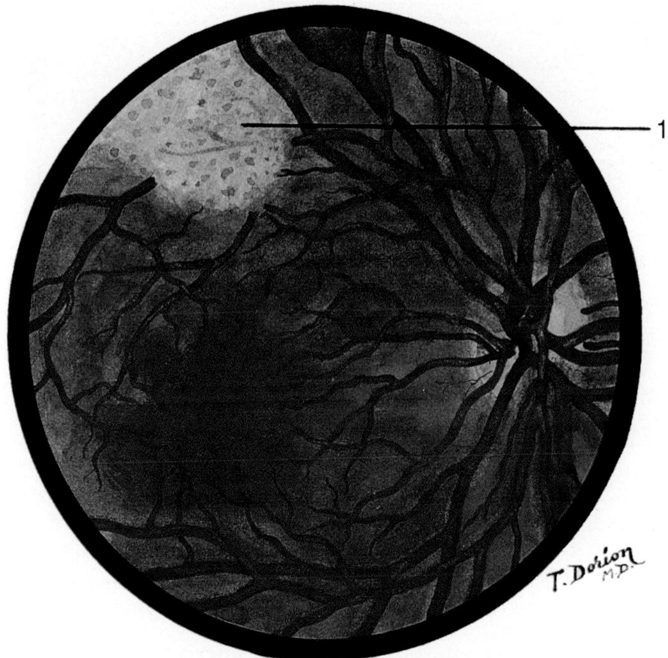

Figure 2-26. *Leopard spots. (1) Peripheral retinal area with elevated amelanotic lesions and pigmented clumps of retinal pigment epithelium.*

effusion. The condition appears as a diffuse, spotty area of pigmentation, with multiple small, slightly elevated amelanotic lesions and scattered pigmented clumps of RPE cells located throughout the peripheral retina, which gives rise to a specific pattern of pigmentation likened to leopard's spots (Figure 2-26).

Macroaneurysms

Macroaneurysms usually are unilateral, congenital or acquired, focal dilatations of the vessels, mostly of the arteries (Figure 2-27), which occur more commonly in women older than 60 years who have ocular or systemic diseases such as hypertension, arteriosclerosis, previous branch retinal vein occlusion, Coats' disease, Eales' disease, or angiomatosis retinae, or even after laser photocoagulation. They prob-

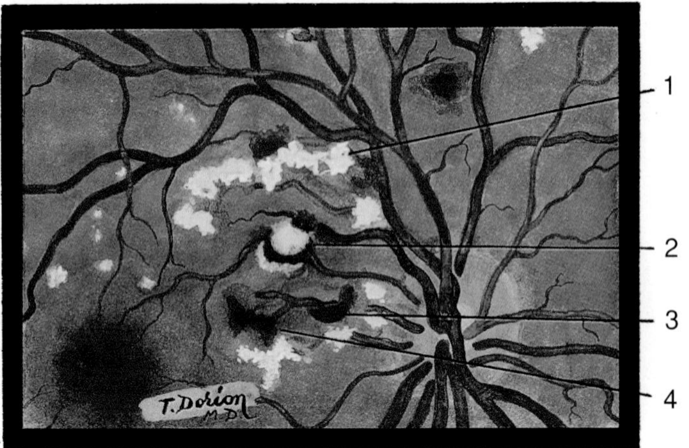

Figure 2-27. *Macroaneurysms. (1) Hard exudates. (2) Dilatation of artery. (3) Preretinal hemorrhage. (4) Subretinal hemorrhage.*

ably are caused by an embolization of the sclerosed vessels that have damaged walls, altered permeability, decreased elasticity, increased intraluminal pressure, and dilatation.

Macroaneurysms appear as multiple, round, spherical or fusiform dilatations of the arteries or larger arterioles of 100–300 μm, up to several times their normal diameter. Occasionally, they pulsate. They may rupture, causing hemorrhage and surrounding retinal edema. Also, there may be hard exudates (in the form of lipid deposits arranged diffusely or circinate in the macula) or macular cysts. Sometimes, macroaneurysms cause a central serous choroidopathy. Occasionally, the hemorrhages occur at two or more levels—preretinal, subretinal, or vitreal—and are called *hourglass hemorrhages*; these may resolve spontaneously.

A symptom of macroaneurysms is decreased visual acuity to counting fingers or worse. Fluorescein angiography may reveal hyperfluorescent saccular dilatation of the artery, capillary nonperfusion, and leakage of the dye. Branch retinal vein occlusion and choroidal neovascularization should be included in the differential diagnosis.

Histopathologically, there is loss of the muscular coat of the artery (Figure 2-28). The artery is spherically dilated, and its wall is thinned and fibrotic. The elastic lamina has a large defect that is filled with a

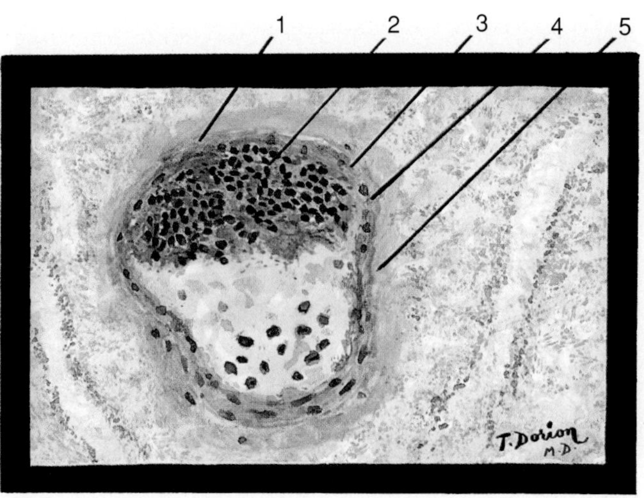

Figure 2-28. *Macroaneurysms: histopathology. (1) Spherical dilatation of artery. (2) Fibrosanguineous exudate. (3) Large defect in elastic lamina. (4) Loss of muscular coat of artery. (5) Thinned vessel wall.*

fibrosanguineous exudate. Preretinal, retinal, and vitreous hemorrhages may be present.

Usually, treatment is not necessary. Laser photocoagulation, adjacent to the macroaneurysm or even directly on it, may be effective; light-gray burns using 200- to 500-μm spots of argon green light are used.

Macrovessel

Macrovessel is a rare, usually unilateral, congenital anomaly of the retinal vessels that may be a part of AV anastomoses (group I of Archer's classification). It is not associated with any midbrain AV malformations. It appears as a large, aberrant retinal vessel, generally a vein (Figure 2-29), particularly located in the macula and crossing normally the horizontal raphe and the macula. Fluorescein angiography may reveal early filling and delayed emptying of the aberrant vessel, as well as a dilated capillary bed surrounding the macrovessel. The rest of the retinal arteries and capillary are intact and are of normal size.

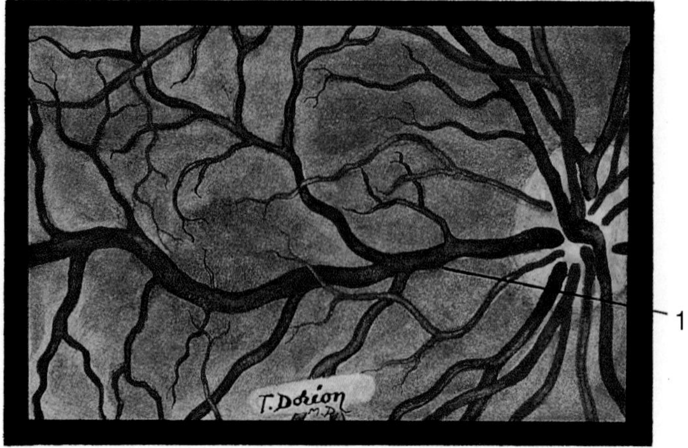

Figure 2-29. *Macrovessel. (1) Large, aberrant retinal vein, crossing horizontal raphe and macula in a normal regular pattern.*

Macular Star

Macular star is an accumulation in the macula of intraretinal hard exudates that describe a starlike pattern (Figure 2-30). This condition often occurs in diabetes, hypertension, retinal edema, angiomatosis retinae, Leber's idiopathic stellate neuropathy, or a resolving chronic papilledema. It is caused by leakage of a plasma lipid and serum residues from arterioles or capillaries in the macular area, more frequently in the presence of a swollen optic disc.

Macular star appears as deep hard exudates arranged in the macula as the spokes of a wheel radiating from a central hub. They are yellow-white or silver-gray in hypertension and waxy in diabetes. Their density varies depending on the fat content. They usually are located beneath the vessels, especially at the nasal side.

Histopathologically, collections are seen of shiny exudates containing lipid-laden macrophages (Figure 2-31), edema residues, histiocytes, and microglia, accumulated in the obliquely oriented outer plexiform layer of Henle. Usually, they are located around diseased vessels, but sometimes they are present also in the inner nuclear layer.

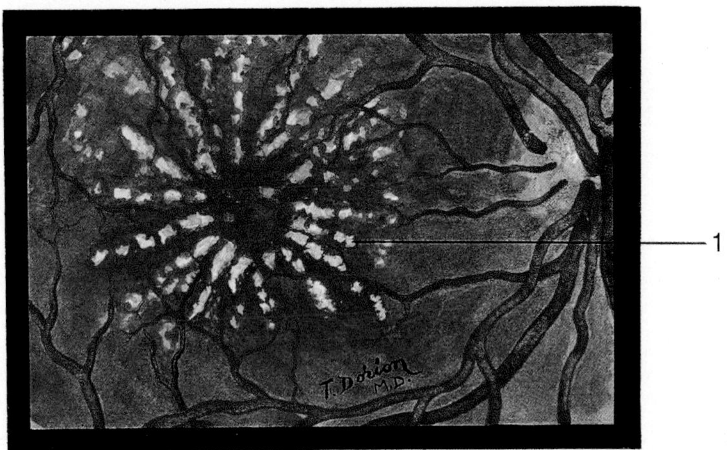

Figure 2-30. *Macular star. (1) Hard exudates in outer plexiform layer of Henle.*

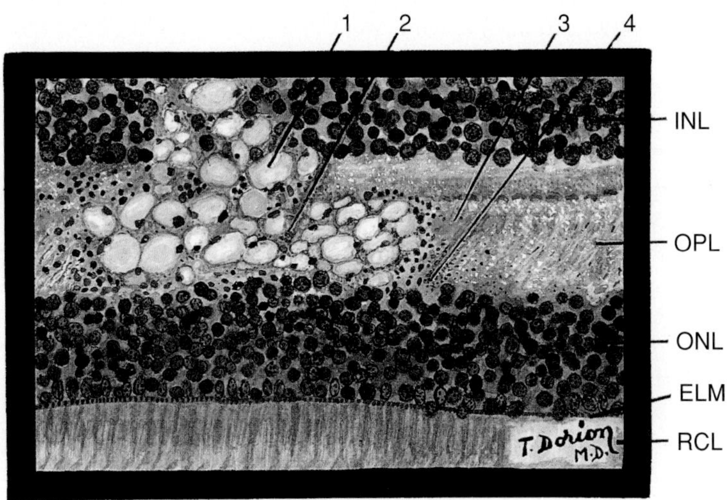

Figure 2-31. *Macular star: histopathology. (1) Fat-filled macrophages. (2) Histiocytes. (3) Edema residues. (4) Microglia. (INL, inner nuclear layer; OPL, outer plexiform layer, or Henle's layer, with obliquely oriented fibers; ONL, outer nuclear layer; ELM, external limiting membrane; RCL, rod and cone layer [photoreceptors].)*

Microaneurysms

Microaneurysms are fine outpouchings of the capillary walls, particularly at the venous side, which may occur in diabetes, Coats' disease, hyperviscosity syndromes, and periphlebitis. They probably are due to hypoxia of the tissue in an abortive neovascularization or to regressed changes (or both) in a previously proliferative vessel or to static engorgement of a weakened degenerative capillary wall.

Microaneurysms appear as multiple tiny, round or ovoid red spots, having sharp margins and measuring 20–200 μm in diameter. They commonly arise from viable *cellular capillaries* and cluster around nonviable *acellular capillaries*, scattered throughout the posterior fundus, far from the retinal vessels and unrelated to them. They have a patent lumen packed with stagnant erythrocytes, which may become occluded with fibrin or basement membrane material. They are thin-walled with loss of pericytes; the ratio between endothelial cells and pericytes may be 2 to 1 or greater (whereas the normal pericyte-to–endothelial cell ratio is 1 to 1). The microaneurysms may hyalinize in time, may bleed, or may convert to minute white dots.

Moth-Eaten Lesions

Moth-eaten lesions are nonprogressive, autosomal recessive, degenerative lesions of the peripheral retina (Figure 2-32) that occur usually in fundus albipunctatus and Groenblad-Strandberg syndrome. They are caused by a degeneration of Bruch's membrane, which becomes thickened in some areas of its cuticular layer.

The lesions appear as multiple small, discrete, punctate, dull, depigmented yellow-white dots, with a slightly irregular mottling, some of them fused and located deep in the retina at the periphery. They spare the macula, the peripapillary area, and the posterior pole. Occasionally, they are radially oriented relative to the macula.

Optic Pit

The optic pit is an anomaly or an incomplete coloboma of the optic disc (Figure 2-33). It is usually congenital, though it may be acquired (as in low-tension glaucoma). Generally, the pit is unilateral and stationary. It may be associated with serous macular detachment, RPE detach-

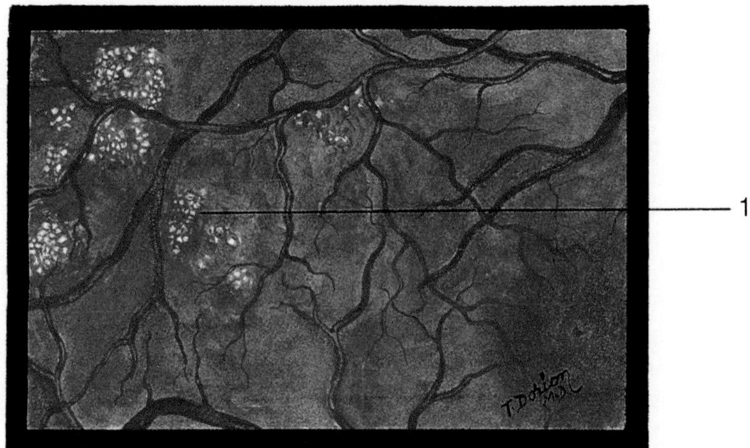

Figure 2-32. *Moth-eaten lesion. (1) Thickening of cuticular layer of Bruch's membrane.*

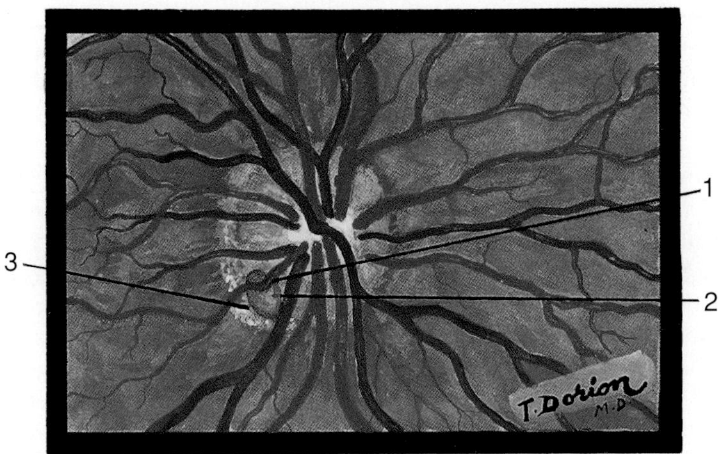

Figure 2-33. *Optic pit. (1) Vessels dive into pit, then course normally. (2) Outpouching of neural tissue. (3) Peripapillary choroidal atrophy.*

ary. It may be associated with serous macular detachment, RPE detachment, macular holes, or retinal cysts.

When congenital, an optic pit may be caused by an embryonic defect of the lamina cribrosa or by an anomalous development of the primordial optic nerve papilla and a consequent failure of peripapillary folds to resolve completely. When acquired, a pit may be due to splitting of the retina from the disc margin toward the macula.

A *congenital optic pit* appears as a small depression that is round, oval, or triangular; gray; darker than the surrounding disc surface; and sharply delineated, or as a craterlike hole within the optic disc. In either case, it is approximately 0.1–0.8 dd in size and is located mostly in the lower temporal quadrant near or over the disc edge, or centrally. It may be shallow or deep—more often of 5 D depth but occasionally as deep as 25 D (8 mm). The disc may be moderately enlarged, may have some surface irregularities, and might exhibit peripapillary choroidal atrophy adjacent to the pit. Retinal vessels dive into the pit and then emerge to continue their normal course. There may be a central serous detachment, hemorrhage, microcysts, pigmentary disturbances, or a full-thickness macular hole that can enlarge over time.

An *acquired optic pit* appears as a focal or polar notching of the disc, which represents a loss of the neuroretinal rim tissue. At that site, lamina cribrosa appears more excavated and sharply delineated, with loss of the laminar architecture. The pit may be extremely pale in contrast to other areas of the disc and may extend to the outer edge of the disc, leaving little or no rim adjacent to the pit. Retinal detachment and optic disc coloboma are not seen.

An optic pit usually is asymptomatic. However, decreased visual acuity and blurred vision can occur, as can metamorphopsia and micropsia.

Evaluation of the visual field may demonstrate a nerve fiber bundle defect or an altitudinal defect. Fluorescein angiography may reveal leakage from the pit, and there may be masking of the background fluorescence at the site of an existing serous macular detachment. Age-related macular degeneration, RPE detachment, and central serous macular detachment should be considered in the differential diagnosis.

Histopathologically, an outpouching of the neural tissue is seen surrounded by a capsule of connective tissue (Figure 2-34). A decreased number of ganglion cells populate the retina toward the side of the pit. The lamina cribrosa may be discontinuous, and the pit may pass posteriorly through such breaks to protrude into the subarachnoid space. Occasionally, a communication between the pit and the orbit or the vitreous occurs.

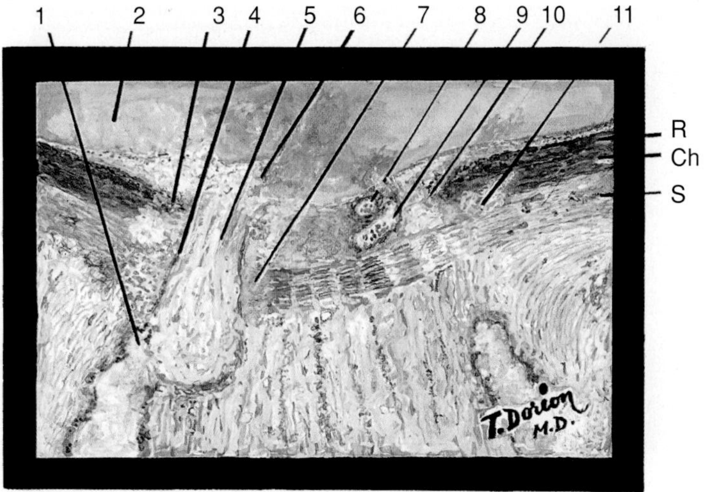

Figure 2-34. *Optic pit: histopathology. (1) Pit protruding into subarachnoid space. (2) Vitreous. (3) Decreased number of ganglion cells toward side of pit. (4) Capsule of connective tissue. (5) Outpouching of neural tissue. (6) Communication between pit and vitreous. (7) Discontinuation of lamina cribrosa with loss of laminar architecture. (8) Central retinal artery. (9) Central retinal vein. (10) Ganglion cells are normal in number on other side of disc, toward macula. (11) Peripapillary choroidal atrophy. (R, retina; Ch, choroid; S, sclera.)*

Treatment is not helpful and usually is not necessary, though laser photocoagulation and **vitrectomy** both have been used.

Peau d'Orange

Peau d'orange is a mottled pigmentation of the retina (Figure 2-35) that usually occurs in Groenblad-Strandberg syndrome and resembles the cutaneous changes of this pseudoxanthoma elasticum disease. It occurs also in malignant melanoma and in Paget's disease. It is caused by a blending of the degenerative yellow alteration of the RPE and Bruch's membrane and the normal orange pigmentation of the fundus.

Peau d'orange appears as multiple irregularly shaped, yellow dots, most of them of similar size, located focally or diffusely at the posterior pole. Sometimes, the dots have a stippling appearance, which might lead one to believe that this condition is a precursor of angioid streaks.

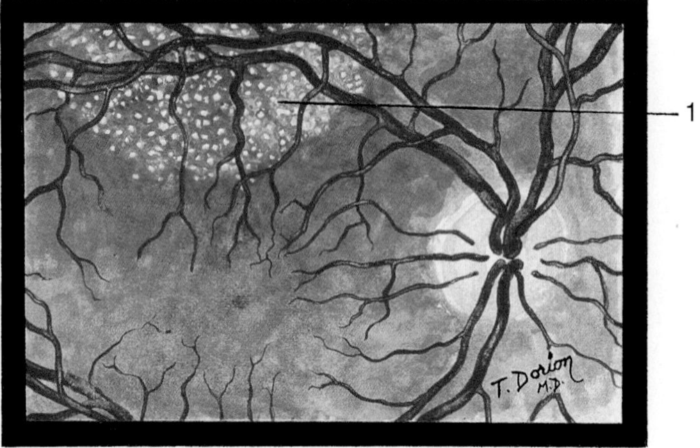

Figure 2-35. *Peau d'orange. (1) Degenerative alterations of retinal pigment epithelium and Bruch's membrane.*

Prepapillary Vascular Loop

A prepapillary vascular loop is a unilateral congenital vascular anomaly of a retinal vessel, a deviation from the vessel's normal course, at the disc (Figure 2-36). The loop is a small vessel (artery or vein), usually having a white sheath of glial tissue, that arises from the optic disc, deviates abruptly, curves, and makes a reverse loop pointing backward toward the disc at a 180-degree angle in a figure-of-eight or in a corkscrew spiral in front of the optic disc surface. It then projects into the vitreous for approximately 1.5–5.0 mm and returns to the disc to continue its normal course. The vessel may arise from a central retinal vessel, from a branch retinal vessel, or from a cilioretinal artery. If a vein, it may pulsate. The optic disc is normal, the superficial capillary plexus of the disc is not dilated, and the nerve fibers are not swollen and do not cover the vessels.

Preretinal Hemorrhage

Preretinal hemorrhage (also called *subhyaloid hemorrhage*) is a hemorrhage located anterior to the retina and posterior to the vitreous (Figure 2-37). It occurs frequently after a subarachnoid hemorrhage or head trauma, in sickle-cell disease, hypertension, blood dyscrasias, and

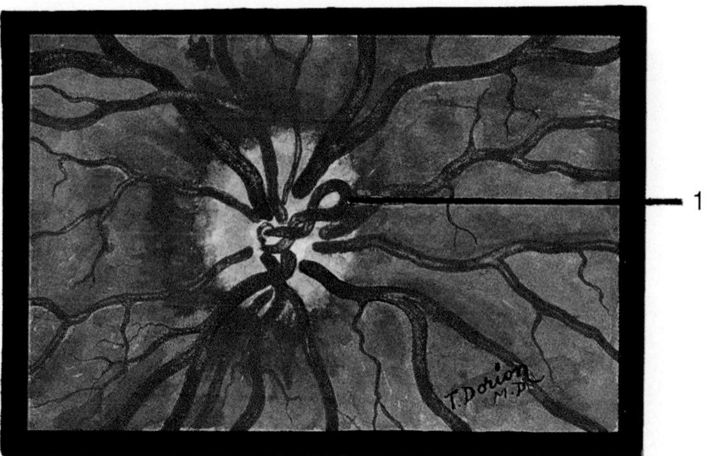

Figure 2-36. *Prepapillary vascular loop. (1) Deviation of a retinal vessel in corkscrew spiral in front of disc surface.*

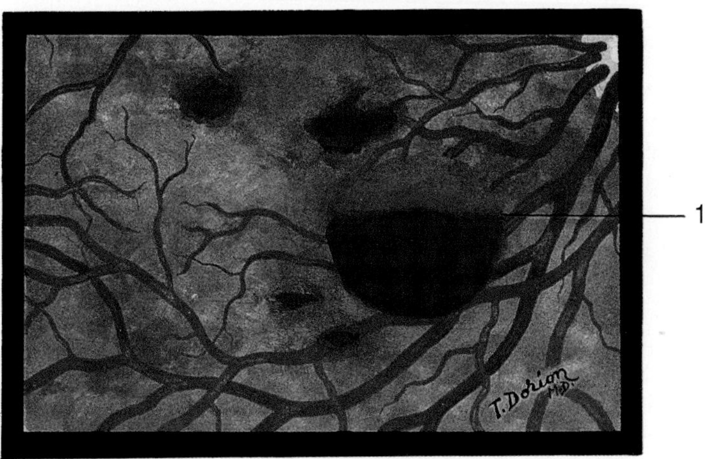

Figure 2-37. *Preretinal hemorrhage. (1) Hemorrhage with a flat horizontal fluid level, resembling a boat profile, located anterior to retina but posterior to vitreous face.*

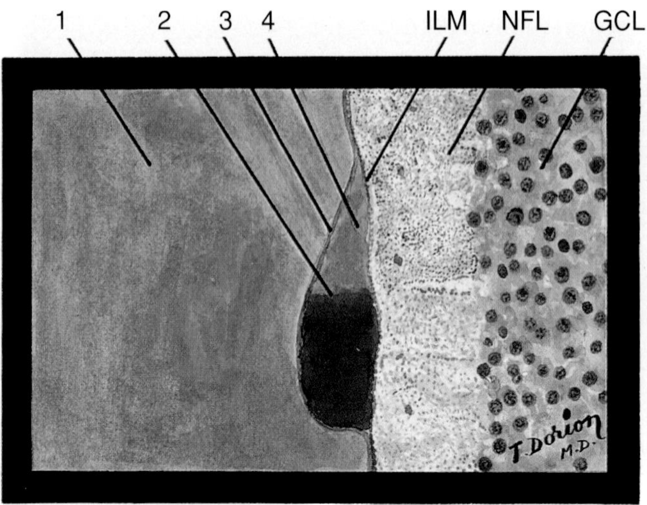

Figure 2-38. *Preretinal hemorrhage: histopathology. (1) Vitreous. (2) Hemorrhage in subhyaloid space, between retina and vitreous, with horizontal fluid level. (3) Vitreous posterior face, called hyaloid membrane. (4) Subhyaloid space. (ILM, internal limiting membrane; NFL, nerve fiber layer; GCL, ganglion cell layer.)*

renal diseases, or in pregnancy after forceps delivery. It may be caused by a sudden increase in intracranial pressure, after bleeding into the subhyaloid space, by damage to the superficial retinal vessels (e.g., direct trauma), by retinal tears, by an abnormality of the vessel's wall, by a disparity between high blood pressure within the vessel and a low ocular pressure surrounding it, by blood cell disorders, or by a rupture of neovascular fronds.

The hemorrhage is large and displays a horizontal fluid level, a flat top, and a rounded bottom because of the effect of gravity, thereby resembling the profile of a boat. A preretinal hemorrhage that is localized adjacent to the optic disc may be diagnostic of a subarachnoid hemorrhage. It usually resolves entirely, but a yellow residue might persist for several months.

Histopathologically, a pocket of blood accumulates into the subhyaloid space, between the retinal internal limiting membrane and the posterior vitreous face (Figure 2-38).

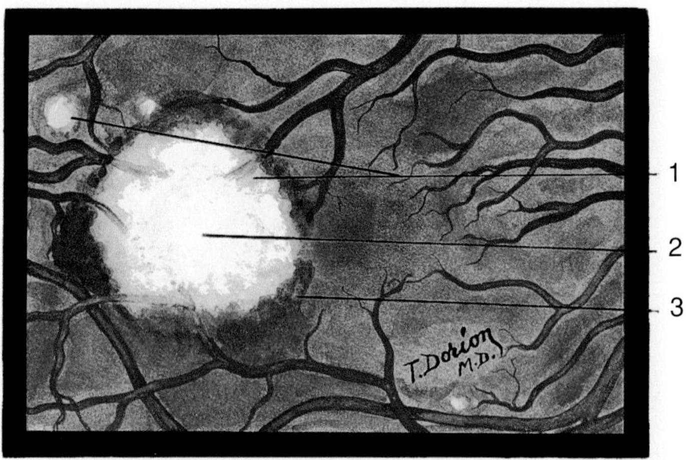

Figure 2-39. *Punched-out lesion. (1) Chorioretinal scar. (2) Bare sclera. (3) Proliferation of retinal pigment epithelium, hypertrophy, and hyperplasia.*

Punched-Out Lesion

A punched-out lesion usually is a scar from a healed chorioretinal lesion (Figure 2-39) and occurs often in toxoplasmosis, histoplasmosis, coccidioidomycosis, some bacterial infections, and choroidal vascular insufficiency. It is due to excessive necrosis of the retina and choroid.

The lesion is round or oval, irregular, yellow white, variably sized, and sometimes similar to paving-stone degeneration lesions, having sharp, well-defined margins and a central area of bare sclera surrounded by clumps of pigment. More frequently, the lesion is located at the posterior pole, but it also is seen in the midperiphery or posterior to the equator.

Histopathologically, RPE is absent from the lesion's center (Figure 2-40). However, at the lesion's periphery there is RPE proliferation, hyperplasia, and hypertrophy. Scars of the choroid and adjacent outer retinal layers also are present. A discontinuity of Bruch's membrane may be seen. There is no choroid neovascularization.

Roth's Spot

Roth's spot (also known as *Litten's sign* and *white-centered hemorrhage*) is a focal retinal hemorrhage having a pale center (Figure 2-41).

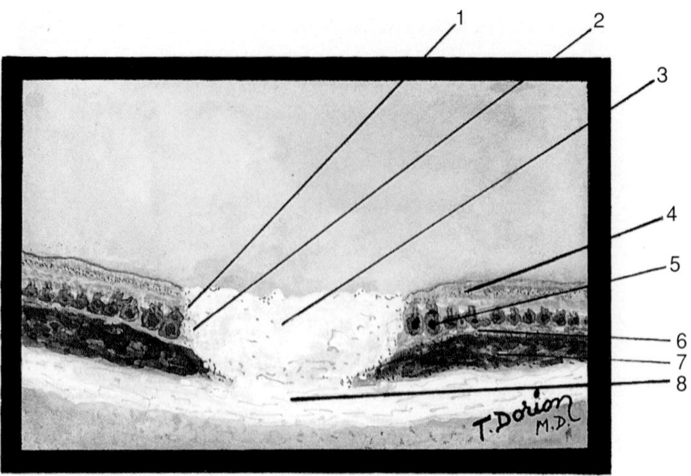

Figure 2-40. *Punched-out lesion: histopathology. (1) Chorioretinal scar. (2) Retinal pigment epithelium absent. (3) Excessive necrosis of retina and choroid. (4) Retina. (5) Hypertrophy and hyperplasia of retinal pigment epithelium. (6) Bruch's membrane discontinued. (7) Choroid. (8) Sclera, bare and visible.*

It occurs in subacute bacterial endocarditis, leukemia, idiopathic thrombocytopenic purpura, pernicious anemia, blood dyscrasias, systemic lupus erythematosus, other collagen diseases, multiple myeloma, diabetes, sickle cell anemia, candidiasis, and other fungal endophthalmitides. It may be produced by a capillary rupture, a retinal infarction in the nerve fiber layer, or an extravasation of a white material such as a microabscess, a plug of fibrin, platelets, leukemic cells, or fungi. Roth's spot appears as single or multiple round or oval white foci surrounded by a ring of superficial hemorrhage scattered throughout the fundus.

Salmon Patches

Salmon patches are preretinal and intraretinal hemorrhages that occur in sickle cell retinopathy, angioid streaks, and Grönblad-Strandberg syndrome. They appear as small, intraretinal or preretinal, round or ovoid spots (Figure 2-42) of approximately 0.25–1.00 dd that initially are red and then turn pink, orange, and white. The spots are scattered

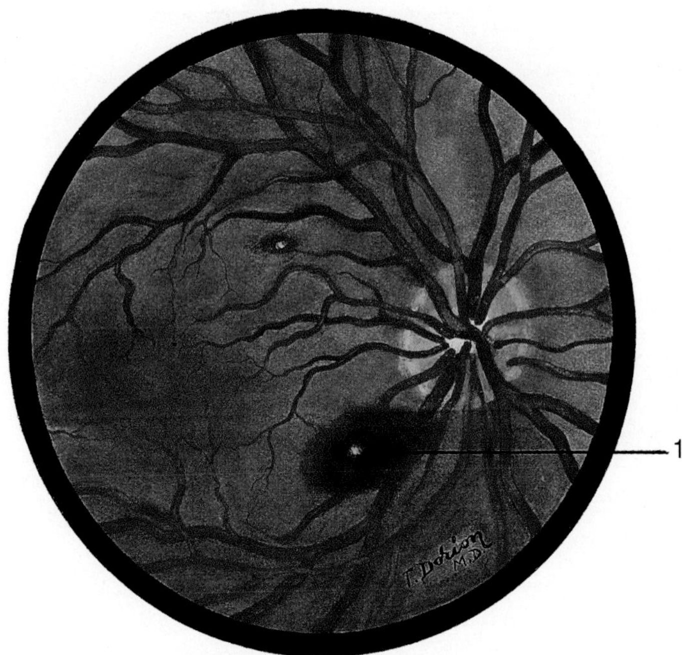

Figure 2-41. *Roth's spot. (1) White-centered hemorrhage with a microabscess, plug of fibrin or platelets, leukemic cells, or fungi in middle of lesion.*

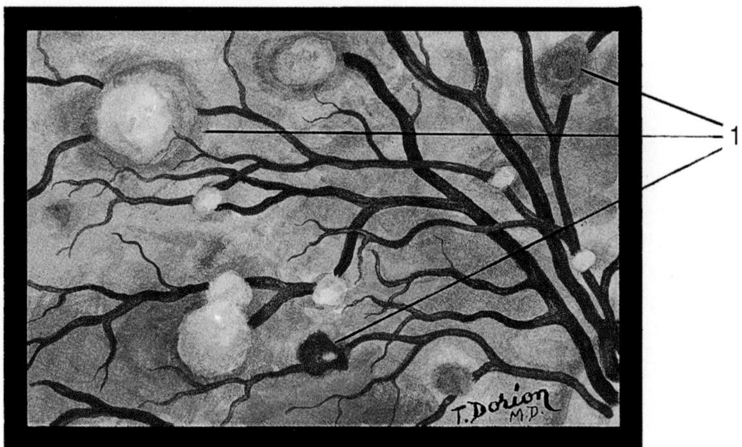

Figure 2-42. *Salmon patches. (1) Preretinal and intraretinal hemorrhages.*

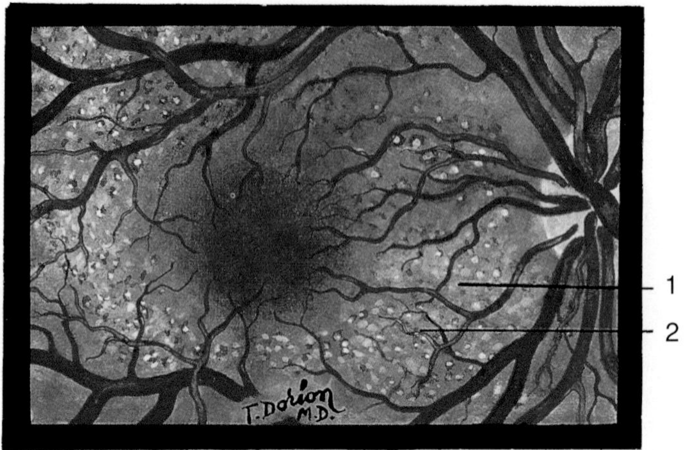

Figure 2-43. *Salt-and-pepper lesion. (1) Atrophy of retinal pigment epithelium. (2) Hypertrophy of retinal pigment epithelium.*

throughout the fundus but usually spare the visual axis. Often, they resolve over days or weeks, leaving focal areas of atrophic split retina, a schisis, or a pigmented retinal scar.

Histopathologically, salmon patches are hemorrhages seen in the subhyaloid space, between the internal limiting membrane and the posterior face of the vitreous, in the nerve fiber layer of the retina, or between the RPE and the sensory retina.

Salt-and-Pepper Lesion

A salt-and-pepper lesion is a slowly progressive hyperpigmentation and hypopigmentation of the posterior pole (Figure 2-43) that occurs in rubella, congenital syphilis, varicella, influenza, cytomegalovirus retinopathy, progressive ophthalmoplegia, retinal aplasia, cystinosis, and choroideremia or secondary to a burned-out retinitis. It is caused by mixed foci of atrophy and hypertrophy of the RPE, usually in alternating areas.

Salt-and-pepper lesions appear as small focal, yellowish, bright clumps of white punctate lesions or exudates surrounded by a minute, brown-pigmented ring, often bone spicule–like, simulating retinitis pig-

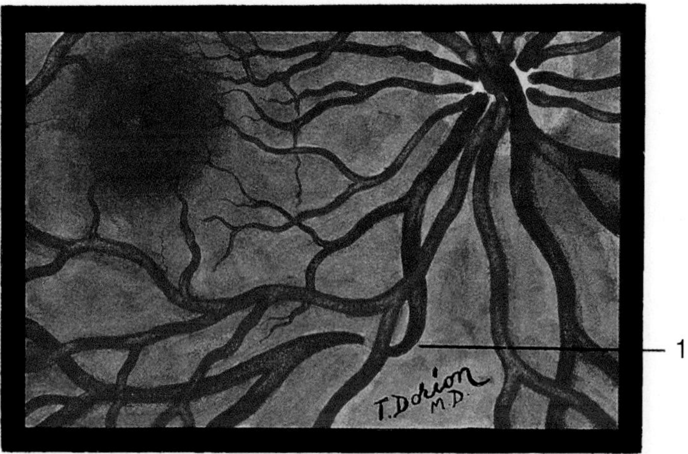

Figure 2-44. *Salus' sign. (1) Deviated vein at right angle, with a segment concealed, at arteriovenous crossing.*

mentosa. The lesions or exudates are scattered diffusely and irregularly throughout the fundus. They may heal spontaneously and do not recur.

Salus' Sign

Salus' sign is a deviation of a vein at the AV crossing (Figure 2-44) and occurs often in hypertension. A vein is deviated at a right angle at the AV crossing, where it gradually becomes smaller and thinner such that a segment of the vein is concealed.

Sea Fan

A sea fan is a retinal arterial neovascularization resembling the marine invertebrate *Gorgonia flabellum* (Figure 2-45) and occurs most often in proliferative sickle cell retinopathy and in proliferative diabetic retinopathy. It may be caused by a capillary infarction in the periphery of the retina, which may cause a chronic retinal ischemia, which in turn may produce an occlusion of the retinal arteries, followed by

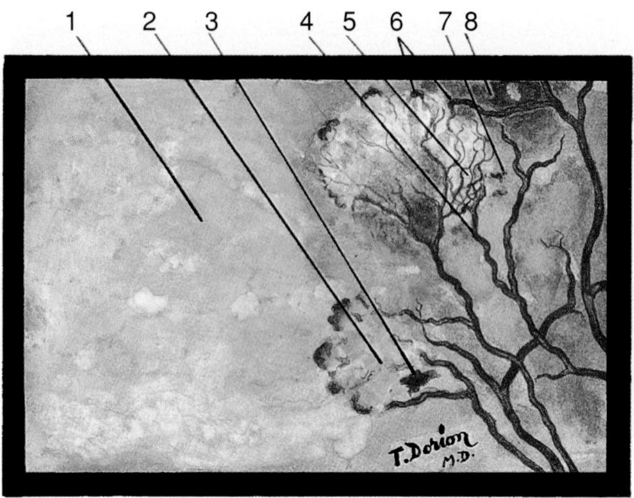

Figure 2-45. *Sea fan. (1) Nonperfused retina. (2) Patches of fibrotic tissue. (3) Intraretinal hemorrhage. (4) Tortuous arteries. (5) Retinal arterial neovascularization. (6) Arteriovenous anastomoses. (7) Preretinal hemorrhage. (8) Perfused retina.*

AV anastomoses and, later, by an arterial proliferation at the junction of perfused and nonperfused retina.

This anomaly appears as white patches of gliotic tissue at the peripheral retina or near the disc that form a prominent neovascular fan, which is pulled forward by detached vitreous gel. It usually is located superotemporally at the equator but may grow circumferentially in other quadrants. It may protrude from the retina toward the center of the eye. The arteries appear more tortuous than do the veins. Preretinal and intraretinal hemorrhages and fibrosis may be present. There may be a spontaneous thrombosis and complete regression of sea fans, or they may progress further to develop new vessels and fibrous tissue.

Fluorescein angiography may reveal hyperfluorescence of the arterial neovascularization and capillary nonperfusion.

Histopathologically, new vessels are seen arising from pre-existing AV anastomoses, located between choriocapillaris and RPE or between RPE and sensory retina.

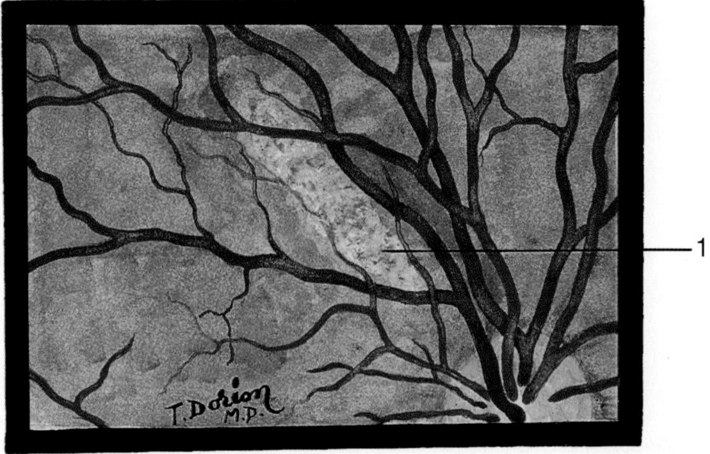

Figure 2-46. *Siegrist's streaks. (1) Chorioretinal atrophy and infarctions, along choroidal vessels.*

Siegrist's Streaks

Siegrist's streaks are pigmentary disturbances and chorioretinal atrophy (Figure 2-46) usually occurring in severe malignant hypertension. They are the result of choroidal infarctions.

Small, pale areas of fine pigment, in flecks, clusters, or yellow-white streaks, are arranged linearly as chains. They measure approximately 1 dd in size and are located along the choroidal vessels, more often at the equator.

Silver-Wire Reflex

The silver-wire reflex is an increased arterial light reflex (Figure 2-47), occurring often in late, marked arteriosclerosis and severe hypertension. It is caused by progression of the fibrous process, which may occupy all the arterial wall's layers and which may obscure the blood column. This reflex also might be caused by an arterial occlusion. It appears as a whitish tube, or a chalky-white artery, having a marked silver light reflex and containing a red fluid.

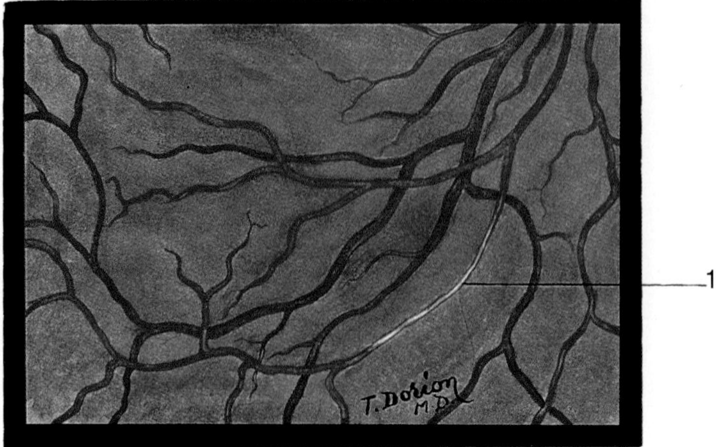

Figure 2-47. *Silver-wire reflex. (1) Increased light reflex of an arteriosclerotic artery.*

Smoldering Retinitis

Smoldering retinitis is a localized, mobile, inflammatory process of the retina (Figure 2-48). It involves the layers of the sensory retina but not the RPE and occurs in cytomegalovirus retinopathy. It is an outcome of an incomplete response to medical treatment of cytomegalovirus.

It appears as an opaque, white, granular line, of variable shape and size, located at the posterior pole along the border of a previously healed cytomegalovirus retinitis. It advances over time, moving in a sequential, creeping pattern to at least 1,000 μm from its original location and increasing in opacity.

Snowballs

Snowballs (also called *snowbank*) are microabscesses in the vitreous (Figure 2-49), seen usually in sarcoidosis, pars planitis, and candidiasis. They are caused by the inflammatory processes or fungal infections associated with these diseases.

Snowballs are seen as spherical, coarse clumps of gray-white, opaque cellular aggregates, composed of fibrovascular tissue and scattered mononuclear inflammatory cells, located deep in the lower vitreous.

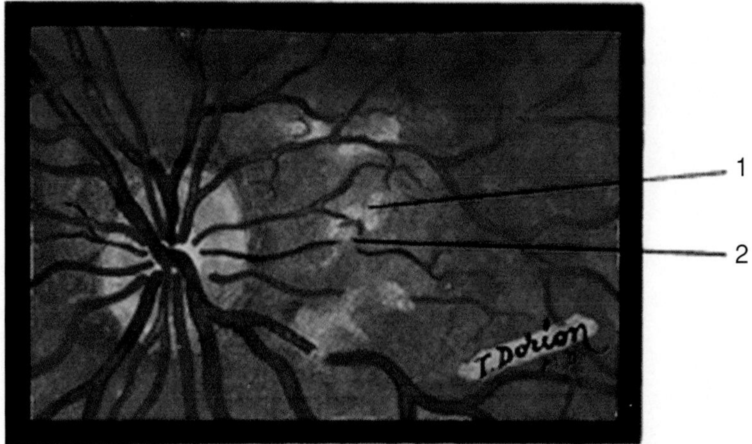

Figure 2-48. *Smoldering retinitis. (1) Moving inflammatory process of sensory retina. (2) Healed cytomegalovirus retinitis lesion.*

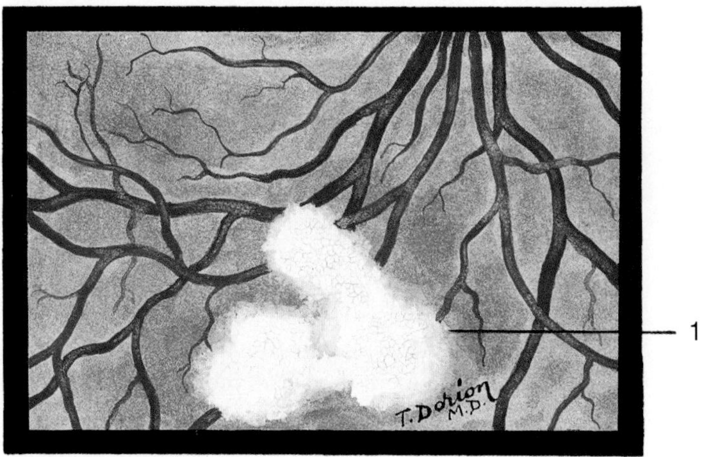

Figure 2-49. *Snowballs. (1) Vitreal microabscesses.*

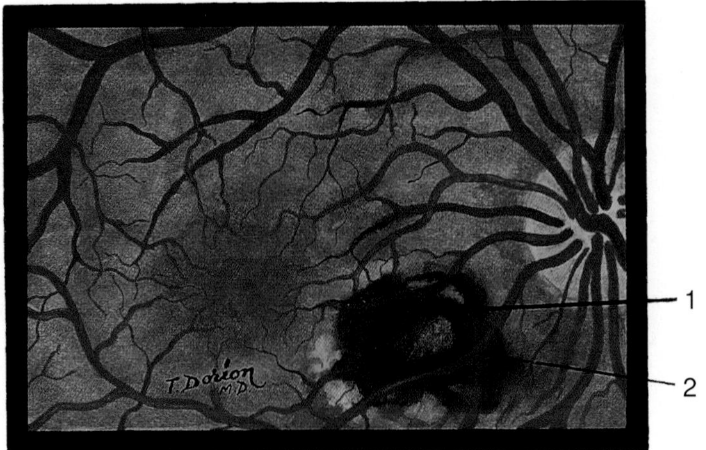

Figure 2-50. *Subretinal hemorrhage. (1) Blood accumulated between retina and choroid. (2) Retinal vessels coursing normally over it.*

Their size and shape vary. Frequently, they appear in chains, like a string of pearls, and cast a shadow on the retina. Alternatively, they may form massive infiltrates or fluffy exudates or appear as a membrane over the peripheral retina, ora serrata, and pars plana.

Subretinal Hemorrhage

Subretinal hemorrhage is a hemorrhage located between the retina and the choroid (Figure 2-50). It occurs most commonly in toxoplasmosis, myopia, age-related macular degeneration, and bleeding disorders, postoperatively, after traumatic choroidal rupture, secondary to subretinal neovascular membrane, or after an excessive Valsalva's maneuver. Subretinal hemorrhage may be an extension of a choroidal hemorrhage or due to a choroidal subretinal neovascular membrane or the passage of abnormal vessels from the choroid into the retina.

The hemorrhage appears as a large, extremely dark gray or purple-red, dusky, often blotchy, ameboid, elevated area with well-defined margins but *no fluid level.* It may vary in size and shape and may be located anywhere in the fundus, including the optic disc and the macula. Retinal vessels course normally over the subretinal hemorrhage.

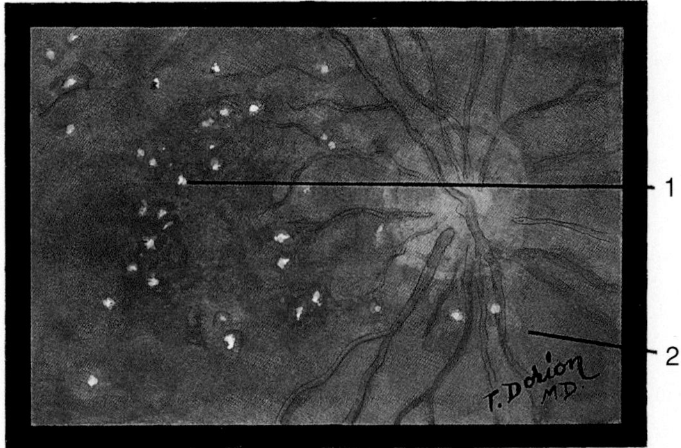

Figure 2-51. *Synchisis scintillans. (1) Cholesterol crystals. (2) Liquefied vitreous.*

It may mimic a choroidal melanoma. After a few weeks, it becomes depigmented to a whitish hue.

Sunset Glow

Sunset glow is a bilateral depigmentation of the fundus that occurs in the third stage, the convalescent stage, of Vogt-Koyanagi-Harada syndrome. It is caused by marked pigment loss from the RPE during the healing process of the disease. There is pigmentary dispersion—a mixture of small, dark yellow pigment deposits interspersed with white depigmented spots of varying sizes—located at the peripheral retina, at the equator, in the peripapillary region, or sometimes in the macula, which gives rise to a setting-sun picture.

Synchysis Scintillans

Synchysis scintillans (also known as *cholesterolosis bulbi*) is an accumulation of cholesterol crystals in the vitreous (Figure 2-51) that occurs after trauma, surgery, or vitreous hemorrhage, more commonly in men

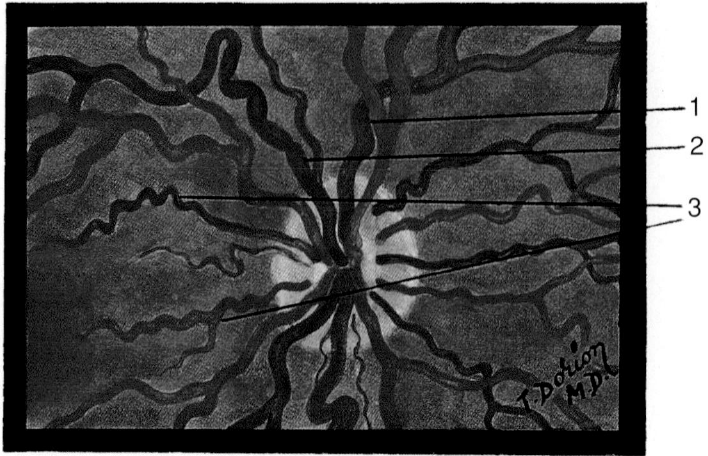

Figure 2-52. *Tortuosity. (1) Dilated, twisted, deviated vessels. (2) Sausage-like vein constrictions. (3) Corkscrewlike arteries and veins.*

before 40 years of age. The appearance is of multiple, flat, glistening, polychromatic, yellow-white or golden, highly refractile cholesterol crystals floating freely in a liquefied vitreous. The crystals move with eye movement and usually settle in the lower vitreous when the eyes are motionless. These particles consist of degenerative material and are not attached to the vitreous fibrils. Occasionally, free hemoglobin spherules may be seen in the vitreous.

Tortuosity

Tortuosity is a change in the course of retinal vessels (Figure 2-52) and may be congenital or acquired. Increased venous pressure or a marked decrease in intraocular pressure can incite tortuosity, as can an increase in the serum protein level (as in blood dyscrasia), hyperviscosity syndromes, and multiple myeloma; an increase in the number of red cells (as in polycythemia vera); or a fibrous replacement in the arterial walls. Tortuous arteries and veins will be seen to be deviated, twisted, irregularly contoured, corkscrewlike, engorged, and increased in length and diameter. Blood column flow is sludgy. Veins appear focally narrowed or occluded at the AV crossings, resemble a string of sausages, and display a diffuse, increased red or purplish hue.

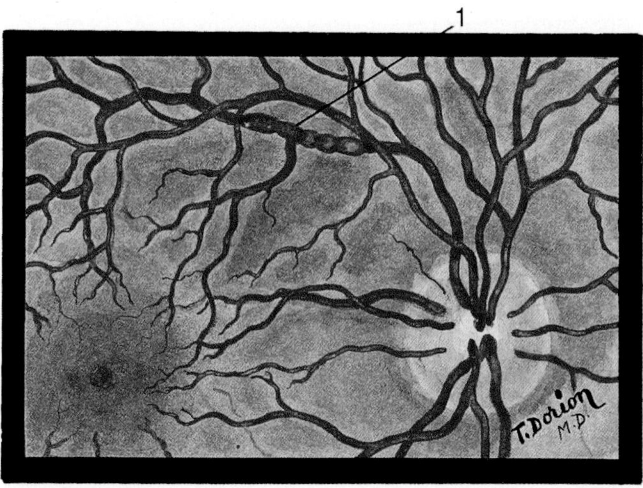

Figure 2-53. *Venous beading. (1) Segmental dilatations of a vein, resembling a string of beads.*

Congenital tortuosity is an autosomal dominant disease, called *hereditary retinal artery tortuosity,* in which there is extreme tortuosity of the retinal arteries although the veins remain normal. Generally, in congenital tortuosity, no other vascular changes are seen.

Acquired tortuosity occurs frequently in heart diseases such as coarctation of the aorta, in which there is a diffuse corkscrew tortuosity of the arteries that may increase with age. Hypertension also is commonly associated with acquired tortuosity, although the tortuosity commonly is limited to the macula. In acquired tortuosity, other alterations usually occur in the vessel walls and, because the arteries and veins share a common adventitial sheath at the AV crossing, changes may occur at this site as well.

Venous Beading

Venous beading is a localized dilatation of veins (Figure 2-53) and can be congenital (a bilateral autosomal dominant vascular abnormality) or acquired (which may occur in nonproliferative diabetic retinopathy, Alport's syndrome, occlusive carotid artery disease, hypertension, hyperviscosity syndromes, angiomatosis retinae, or papilledema). Venous beading may be caused by increased venous pressure or markedly decreased intraocular pressure, which can produce dilatations of portions of the vein, which in turn may cause a sluggish retinal venous circulation.

In venous beading, there is a segmental, irregular increase of venous caliber that resembles a string of beads and that pulsates normally with pressure on the globe.

White with Pressure

White with pressure is a change in fundus color, from its normal orange-red to yellow-white or translucent gray-white, during a scleral depression or indentation. It occurs more frequently in persons older than 70 years, especially in myopes, in retinoschisis, posterior vitreal detachment, vitreous liquefaction, choroidal detachment, and retinal tears. A mild vitreal traction from vitreoretinal adhesions can be the inciting event.

White with pressure appears in varying shapes and lengths and forms a small, isolated area to a circumferential band having smooth or scalloped margins. The anomaly sometimes is migratory and usually is located in the superior and temporal quadrants (often in the presence of staphyloma) or at the posterior edge of a lattice degeneration. Its posterior margin is very sharp, whereas the anterior margin fades into the peripheral retina. Occasionally, there may be an island of normal retina within its borders, which may be mistaken for a retinal break. The retina may lose its transparency so that the choroidal vasculature may no longer be visible.

White without Pressure

White without pressure is a benign bilateral area of whitening of the peripheral retina that may frequently be present in the general population and in the elderly in the absence of any scleral depression or indentation. It also is known to occur in sickle cell retinopathy, posterior vitreous detachment, vitreous liquefaction, and lattice degeneration. The lesion has no clinical significance.

Vitreous-retina interaction may be the cause. Such an interaction might produce disorganization of the RPE with pigment proliferation and migration, accumulation of fluid between the RPE and sensory retina, disruption or absence of the internal limiting membrane, vitreous strands, and cortical vitreous condensation.

White without pressure appears as pale bands located in the superior and temporal peripheral retina. It may be *focal*, surrounding an island of normal retina, or *circumferential*, on the entire perimeter of the retina. Its borders may be smooth or scalloped, the posterior margin being sharper and better delineated as a demarcation line. Immediately posterior to that area, there may be a darker red retina, which may extend from the ora serrata to 3 dd posteriorly or to the equator or, rarely, to the temporal vascular arcades. Areas of retinal degeneration may be present.

Suggested Reading

Ackerman AL. Retinal Problems in Systemic Diseases. In W Tasman, EA Jaeger, MM Parks, et al. (eds), Duane's Clinical Ophthalmology, vol 5. Philadelphia: Lippincott–Raven, 1996;42:1–5.

Benson WE, Tasman W, Duane TD. Diabetes Mellitus and the Eye. In W Tasman, EA Jaeger, MM Parks, et al. (eds), Duane's Clinical Ophthalmology, vol 3. Philadelphia: Lippincott–Raven, 1996;30:19–22.

Bernardino VB, Naidoff MA. Retinal Inflammatory Diseases. In W Tasman, EA Jaeger, MM Parks, et al. (eds), Duane's Clinical Ophthalmology, vol 3. Philadelphia: Lippincott–Raven, 1996;10:1–10.

Birge HL. Mycotic Infections. In A Sorsby (ed), Modern Ophthalmology, vol 2 (2nd ed). Philadelphia: Lippincott, 1972;231–250.

Bolling JC, Buettner H. Acquired retinal arteriovenous communications in occlusive diseases of the carotid artery. Ophthalmology 1990;97:1148–1152.

Borruat FX, Bogousslavsky J, Uffer S, et al. Orbital infarction syndrome. Ophthalmology 1993;100:562–568.

Brodsky BC, Ford RE, Bradford JD. Subretinal neovascular membrane in an infant with a retinochoroidal coloboma. Arch Ophthalmol 1991;109:1650–1651.

Brown GC. Congenital Fundus Abnormalities. In W Tasman, EA Jaeger, MM Parks, et al. (eds), Duane's Clinical Ophthalmology, vol 3. Philadelphia: Lippincott–Raven, 1996;8:3–18.

Caird FI, Blach RK. Diabetes Mellitus. In A Sorsby (ed), Modern Ophthalmology, vol 2 (2nd ed). Philadelphia: Lippincott, 1972;289–300.

Callanan DG, Lewis ML, Byrne SF, Gass JDM. Choroidal neovascularization associated with choroidal nevi. Arch Ophthalmol 1993;111:789–794.

Cernea P, Munteanu G. Papilledema. In Opticopatia. Bucharest: Editura Medicala, 1983;145–147.

Chan CC, Palestine AG, Nussenblatt RB. Sympathetic Ophthalmia and Vogt-Koyanagi-Harada Syndrome. In W Tasman, EA Jaeger, MM Parks, et al. (eds), Duane's Clinical Ophthalmology, vol 4. Philadelphia: Lippincott–Raven, 1996;51:1–9.

Charles H. Retinal Vasculitis. In W Tasman, EA Jaeger, MM Parks, et al. (eds), Duane's Clinical Ophthalmology, vol 4. Philadelphia: Lippincott–Raven, 1996;47:1–12.

Damato BE, Spalton DJ. The Uveal Tract. In DJ Spalton, RA Hitchings, PA Hunter (eds), Atlas of Clinical Ophthalmology (2nd ed). London: Wolfe, 1994;9.7.

Diaz-Lopiz M, Menezo JL. Congenital hypertrophy of the retinal pigment epithelium in familial adenomatous polyposis. Arch Ophthalmol 1988; 106:412.

Duker JS. Cytomegalovirus Retinitis. In W Tasman, EA Jaeger, MM Parks, et al. (eds), Duane's Clinical Ophthalmology, vol 3. Philadelphia: Lippincott–Raven, 1996;28A:1–7.

Duker JS, Brown GC. Vascular Anomalies of the Fundus. In W Tasman, EA Jaeger, MM Parks, et al. (eds), Duane's Clinical Ophthalmology, vol 3. Philadelphia: Lippincott–Raven, 1996;22:1–10.

Early Treatment Diabetic Retinopathy Study. Grading diabetic retinopathy from stereoscopic fundus photographs [ETDRS rep. no. 10]. Ophthalmology 1991;98(suppl 9):786–806.

Eshaghpour E, Anisman PC, Goldberg RE, Margargal LE. Ocular Manifestations in Congenital Heart Diseases. In W Tasman, EA Jaeger, MM Parks, et al. (eds), Duane's Clinical Ophthalmology, vol 5. Philadelphia: Lippincott–Raven, 1996;22A:1–12.

Finkelstein D, Clarkson JG, Branch Vein Occlusion Study Group. Branch and central retinal vein occlusion. Focal Points 1987;12:2–12.

Folberg R, Bernardino VB. Pathologic Correlates in Ophthalmology. In W Tasman, EA Jaeger, MM Parks, et al. (eds), Duane's Clinical Ophthalmology, vol 3. Philadelphia: Lippincott–Raven, 1996;7:1–25.

Gass JDM. Some Problems in the Diagnosis of Macular Diseases. In MD Davis, et al. (eds), Symposium on Retinal Diseases. Transactions of the New Orleans Academy of Ophthalmology. St. Louis: Mosby, 1977;261–274.

Glaser JS. Topical Diagnosis: Prechiasmal Visual Pathways. In W Tasman, EA Jaeger, MM Parks, et al. (eds), Duane's Clinical Ophthalmology, vol 2. Philadelphia: Lippincott–Raven, 1996;5:49–59.

Gross FJ, Friedman AH. Systemic Infectious and Inflammatory Diseases. In W Tasman, EA Jaeger, MM Parks, et al. (eds), Duane's Clinical Ophthalmology, vol 5. Philadelphia: Lippincott–Raven, 1996;33:2–12.

Hunter PA. Allergic Eye Diseases, Episcleritis and Scleritis. In DJ Spalton, RA Hitchings, PA Hunter (eds), Atlas of Clinical Ophthalmology (2nd ed). London: Wolfe, 1994;5.26.

Jaeger EA. Retinopathy in the Connective Tissue Diseases. In W Tasman, EA Jaeger, MM Parks, et al. (eds), Duane's Clinical Ophthalmology, vol 3. Philadelphia: Lippincott–Raven, 1996;21:1–6.

Jampol HD. Normal (low) tension glaucoma. Focal Points 1991;9(12):3–10.

Javet JC, Spaeth GL, Katz J, et al. Acquired pits of optic nerve. Ophthalmology 1990;87:1038–1044.

Jonas JB, Fernandez MC, Naumann GOH. Glaucomatous parapapillary atrophy. Arch Ophthalmol 1992;110:214–222.

Keefe KS, Freeman WR, Peterson TJ, et al. Atypical healing of cytomegalovirus retinitis. Ophthalmology 1992;99:1377–1384.

Khawly JA, Pollock SC. Litten's sign (Roth's spots) in bacterial endocarditis. Arch Ophthalmol 1994;112:691–695.

Kornzweig AL. Senescence of the Eye. In A Sorsby (ed), Modern Ophthalmology, vol 2 (2nd ed). Philadelphia: Lippincott, 1972;703–720.

Lam S, Tessler HH. Intermediate Uveitis. In W Tasman, EA Jaeger, MM Parks, et al. (eds), Duane's Clinical Ophthalmology, vol 4. Philadelphia: Lippincott–Raven, 1996;40:1–4.

Lam S, Tessler HH, Lam BL, Wilensky JT. High incidence of sympathetic ophthalmia after contact and noncontact neodymium:YAG cyclotherapy. Ophthalmology 1992;99:1818–1822.

Lopez PF, Maumenee IH, De la Cruz Z, Green R. Autosomal dominant fundus flavimaculatus. Ophthalmology 1990;97:789–809.

MacCumber MW, Floer RW, Langham ME. Ischemic hypertensive choroidopathy. Arch Ophthalmol 1993;111:704–705.

Moyer P. New system recognizes four types of drusen. Ophthalmol Times 1994;9:52.

Munden PM, Sobol WM, Weingeist TA. Ocular findings in Turcot's syndrome (glioma-polyposis). Ophthalmology 1991;98:111–114.

Rubsamen PE, Gass JDM. Vogt-Koyanagi-Harada syndrome. Arch Ophthalmol 1991;109:682–687.

Sanborn GE, Magargal LE. Arterial Obstructive Disease of the Eye. In W Tasman, EA Jaeger, MM Parks, et al. (eds), Duane's Clinical Ophthalmology, vol 3. Philadelphia: Lippincott–Raven, 1996;14:17–22.

Schatz H, Chang LF, Ober RR, McDonald RN. Central vein occlusion associated with retinal arteriovenous malformation. Ophthalmology 1993;100:24–29.

Schneiderman TE, Kalina RE. Subretinal hemorrhage precedes development of angioid streaks. Arch Ophthalmol 1994;112:1622–1623.

Schlaegel TF Jr. Complications of Uveitis and Their Management. In W Tasman, EA Jaeger, MM Parks, et al. (eds), Duane's Clinical Ophthalmology, vol 4. Philadelphia: Lippincott–Raven, 1996;60:1–6.

Sebag J. Vitreous Pathobiology. In W Tasman, EA Jaeger, MM Parks, et al. (eds), Duane's Clinical Ophthalmology, vol 3. Philadelphia: Lippincott–Raven, 1996;42:8.

Sivalingam A, Bolling J, Goldberg RE, et al. Ocular Abnormalities in Acquired Heart Diseases. In W Tasman, EA Jaeger, MM Parks, et al. (eds), Duane's Clinical Ophthalmology, vol 5. Philadelphia: Lippincott–Raven, 1996;22:1–8.

Spalton DJ. Intraocular Inflammation. In DJ Spalton, RA Hitchings, PA Hunter (eds), Atlas of Clinical Ophthalmology (2nd ed). London: Wolfe, 1994;10.2.

Spalton DJ, Schilling JS. The Retina: Vascular Diseases I. In DJ Spalton, RA Hitchings, PA Hunter (eds), Atlas of Clinical Ophthalmology (2nd ed). London: Wolfe, 1994;14.2.

Spalton DJ, Schilling JS. The Retina: Macular Diseases and Retinal Dystrophies. In DJ Spalton, RA Hitchings, PA Hunter (eds), Atlas of Clinical Ophthalmology (2nd ed). London: Wolfe, 1994;16.17.

Spalton DJ, Schilling JS, Schulenburg WC. The Retina: Vascular Diseases II. In DJ Spalton, RA Hitchings, PA Hunter (eds), Atlas of Clinical Ophthalmology (2nd ed). London: Wolfe, 1994;15.2.

Trevor-Roper PD. Blood Dyscrasias and the Reticuloendothelial System. In A Sorsby (ed), Modern Ophthalmology, vol 2 (2nd ed). Philadelphia: Lippincott, 1972;509–522.

Vander JF, Duker JS, Jaeger EA. Miscellaneous Diseases of the Eye. In W Tasman, EA Jaeger, MM Parks, et al. (eds), Duane's Clinical Ophthalmology, vol 3. Philadelphia: Lippincott–Raven, 1996;36:2–10.

Vander JF, Tasman W. Photocoagulation of the Posterior Segment Disorders. In W Tasman, EA Jaeger, MM Parks, et al. (eds), Duane's Clinical Ophthalmology, vol 6. Philadelphia: Lippincott–Raven, 1996;76:1–14.

Weinberg WR. Sarcoidosis. In W Tasman, EA Jaeger, MM Parks, et al. (eds), Duane's Clinical Ophthalmology, vol 4. Philadelphia: Lippincott–Raven, 1996;44:1–2.

Williams GA. Ocular Manifestations of Hematologic Diseases. In W Tasman, EA Jaeger, MM Parks, et al. (eds), Duane's Clinical Ophthalmology, vol 5. Philadelphia: Lippincott–Raven, 1996;23:1–10.

Zhang K, Bither PP, Donoso P, Seideman JG. A dominant Stargardt's macular dystrophy locus maps to chromosome 13q34. Arch Ophthalmol 1994; 112:759–764.

3

Optic Nerve Disease

Papilledema

Papilledema, or choked disc, is an edematous swelling of the optic nerve head that may be acute or chronic. It can occur in the presence of a cranial tumor, which increases the intracranial pressure, called *plerocephalic papilledema*. It also is seen in malignant hypertension and in central retinal vein thrombosis.

Papilledema may be due to an active inflammation after a local irritation. Alternatively, it may be due to a passive transudation through the retinal veins, which may increase the pressure in the central retinal vein, slowing the venous drainage and producing a blockage of the axonal transport at the lamina cribrosa. This slowing and blocking is followed by an accumulation of fluid in the optic nerve, with axonal swelling and separation of the neurofibrils.

Papilledema is seen as a hyperemic optic disc with vascular congestion in the acute stage. The disc is elevated, has a blurred margin starting at the nasal side, and the physiologic cup is obliterated (Figure 3-1). Retinal vessels on the disc surface are displaced forward and are partially buried. The superficial capillary plexus is dilated. Veins are markedly dilated, engorged, and tortuous and, almost always, spontaneous venous pulsation is lost. There may be flame-shaped, striate hemorrhages or subretinal hemorrhages, mostly peripapillary at the nasal side, which may break into the vitreous. Whitish soft exudates, **cotton-wool spots,** are located on the disc surface, in the peripapillary region, or in the central retina. Grayish white striae of **hard exudate**

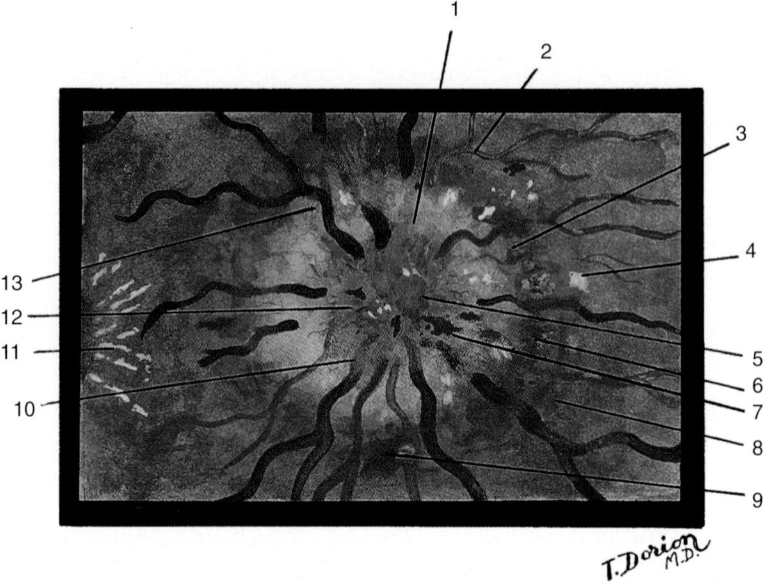

Figure 3-1. *Papilledema. (1) Elevated, hyperemic disc. (2) Arterial attenuation. (3) Blurred margins. (4) Cotton-wool spots. (5) Obliterated physiologic cup. (6) Peripapillary hemorrhages. (7) Flame-shaped hemorrhages. (8) Patton's lines. (9) Subretinal hemorrhages. (10) Partially buried vessels. (11) Macular star. (12) Dilated capillary plexus. (13) Tortuous veins.*

residues, which result from a leakage of plasma lipid from the swollen disc, might be seen in an arrangement that radiates from the macula to form a so-called *macular star*. Sometimes, there are retinal folds, called *Patton's lines*, or choroidal folds, at the edges of the disc. Rarely, peripapillary retinal detachment occurs. In time, the disc may become pale and atrophic.

Symptoms

Visual acuity is usually normal, although sometimes there is a transient vision loss or diplopia. The pupillary light reflex is normal. An enlarged blind spot can characterize the visual field.

Diagnosis

Direct or indirect ophthalmoscopy with a Hruby lens, fundus contact, or 60-D lens is used to make the diagnosis. Computed tomographic (CT) scanning also contributes, as does early magnetic resonance imaging (MRI). *Lumbar puncture is contraindicated in acute papilledema* because of possible brain herniation into the tentorial fissure of foramen magnum, which may press on the medulla and cause sudden death.

Differential Diagnosis

A host of conditions should be considered in the differential diagnosis: optic neuritis; tumor of the disc, orbit, or brain; pseudopapilledema (in hypermetropia); myelinated nerve fibers; drusen of the disc; pseudotumor cerebri; Graves' disease; anterior ischemic optic neuropathy (AION); uveitis; central retinal vein occlusion; postoperative increased intraocular pressure (IOP); Leber's hereditary optic neuropathy; acute glaucoma; ocular trauma; disc anomaly; sinusitis; cardiopulmonary insufficiency; emphysema; cystic fibrosis; congenital heart diseases; sarcoidosis; giant-cell arteritis; and nutritional diseases.

Histopathology

Among the histopathologic findings in papilledema is an increased tissue mass in the optic nerve head, which causes the physiologic cup to disappear (Figure 3-2). Photoreceptors are displaced. The peripapillary space may be filled with a proliferation of a tissue, called the **intermediate tissue of Kuhnt**. In chronic papilledema, nerve fiber degeneration occurs, with local swelling and separation of the neurofibrils, which later may disappear to be replaced by spindle-shaped **cytoid bodies**. The neuroglia may proliferate as may the connective tissue around the vessels. Thickening of the lamina cribrosa is usually present. At a later stage, the optic nerve may become atrophic.

Treatment

Treatment addresses the underlying cause.

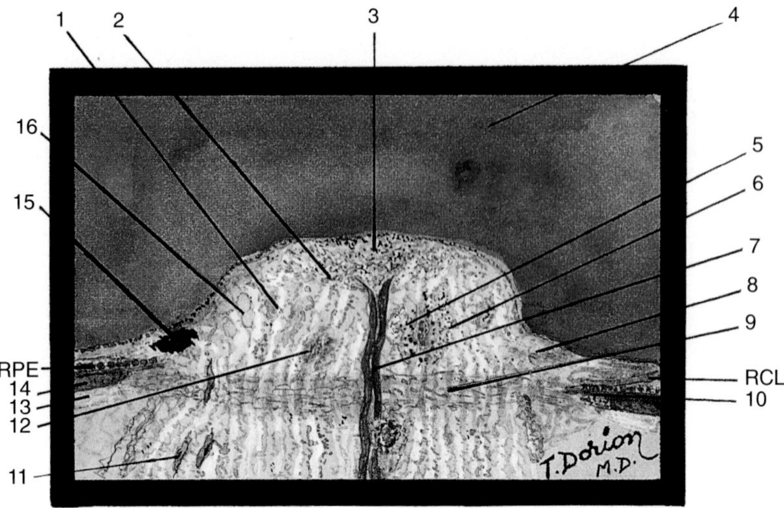

Figure 3-2. *Histopathologic findings in papilledema. (1) Swelling and separation of the neurofibrils. (2) Increased tissue mass in the optic nerve head. (3) Obliterated physiologic cup. (4) Vitreous. (5) Perivascular proliferation of the neuroglia. (6) Proliferation of the connective tissue. (7) Central retinal artery and vein. (8) Peripapillary intermediary tissue of Kuhnt. (9) Thickening of the lamina cribrosa. (10) Bruch's membrane. (11) Spindle-shaped cytoid bodies. (12) Dilated capillary plexus. (13) Sclera. (14) Choroid. (15) Peripapillary retinal hemorrhage. (16) Wallerian degeneration of the optic nerve fibers. (RPE, retinal pigment epithelium; RCL, rod and cone layer [photoreceptors].)*

Pseudopapilledema

Pseudopapilledema is a bilateral, congenital anomaly of the disc (Figure 3-3). It is not pathologic but simulates papilledema. It occurs in hypermetropia, astigmatism, or disc drusen.

In pseudopapilledema, the disc appears slightly elevated and full, with blurred margins; it peaks from the edges to the center. The disc often is red and usually is of normal size, but the physiologic cup is absent. The fullness of the disc may be due to drusen, buried or visible. Vessels exit on top of the disc and course over its surface, but they are not buried. Veins maintain their normal color, are sometimes slightly distended but not dilated, and remain at the retinal level. Occasionally, spontaneous venous pulsation continues. Such vascular abnormalities as multiple trifurcations of the arteries or an excessive number of major

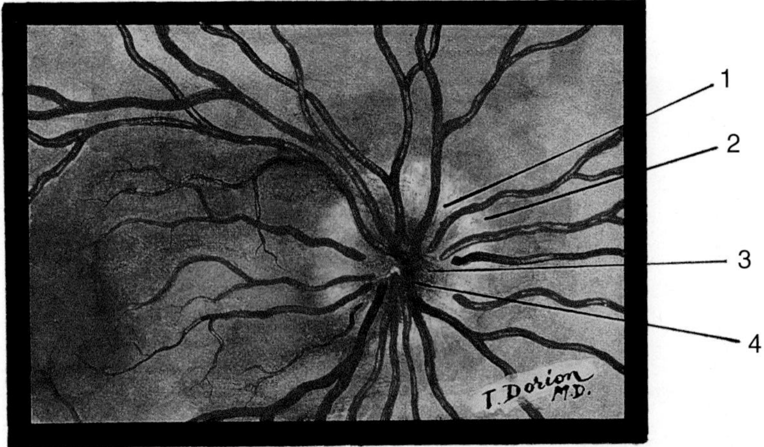

Figure 3-3. *Pseudopapilledema. (1) Elevated disc. (2) Blurred margins. (3) Absence of physiologic cup. (4) Vessels on top, not buried.*

vessels may be seen. Few disc drusen or even persistent hyaloid tissue on the surface of the disc may be present. Usually, no capillary dilatation, no hemorrhage, no infarctions, and no exudates are seen.

Diagnosis

The visual field examination is normal, revealing a normal blind spot. Intracranial pressure also is normal.

Differential Diagnosis

Conditions that should be considered in the differential diagnosis include papilledema, optic neuritis, drusen of the disc, hypermetropia, astigmatism, Bergmeister's papilla, myelinated nerve fibers, anomalous branching of retinal vessels, Wyburn-Mason syndrome, and tumors of the disc.

Histology

On histologic evaluation, the optic nerve structure appears normal; neural fibrils are not swollen or degenerated. The disc lies slightly above

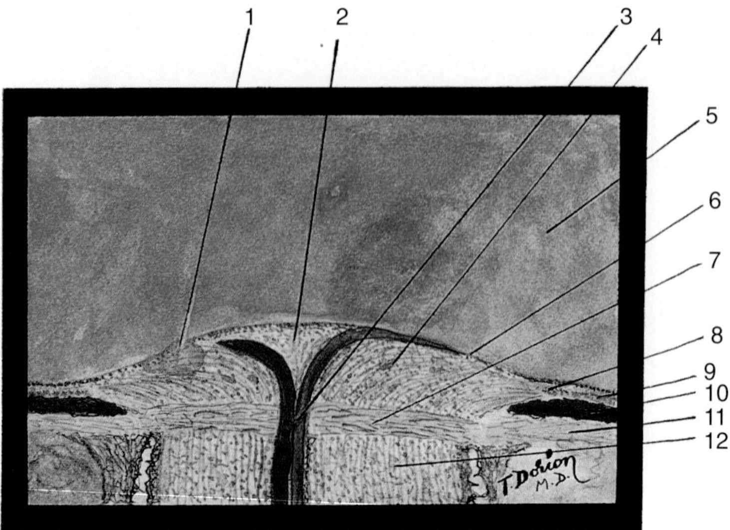

Figure 3-4. *Histologic findings in pseudopapilledema. (1) Drusen of the disc. (2) Absence of physiologic cup. (3) Central retinal vessels on top of disc, not buried. (4) No capillary dilatation. (5) Vitreous. (6) Slightly elevated disc, which peaks from the edges to the center. (7) Lamina cribrosa not thickened. (8) Clear nerve fiber layer. (9) Retina. (10) Choroid. (11) Sclera. (12) Normal optic nerve.*

the retinal level (Figure 3-4). Few disc drusen may be present. The retina is normal, and the nerve fiber layer is clear and does not obscure the vessels. The photoreceptor layer is not displaced, capillaries are not dilated, and the lamina cribrosa is not thickened. No intraretinal hemorrhages are present at the disc margin.

Anterior Ischemic Optic Neuropathy

AION also known as *optic disc infarction*, *pseudopapillitis*, and *capillary apoplexy*) is a noninflammatory neuropathy of the disc (Figure 3-5) that can occur as one of two types: nonarteritic and arteritic. It may be associated with systemic diseases such as periarteritis nodosa, Raynaud's disease, Burger's disease, Takayasu's disease, diabetes, and Graves' disease, or may appear after cataract surgery, ocular trauma, optic nerve compression, or in glaucoma.

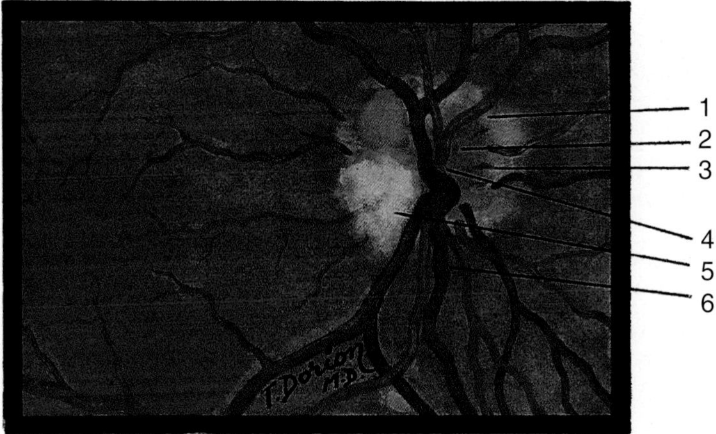

Figure 3-5. *Nonarteritic anterior ischemic optic neuropathy. (1) Mildly swollen disc, with blurred margin. (2) Disc hyperemia. (3) Flame-shaped hemorrhage. (4) Absent physiologic cup. (5) Segmental disc edema. (6) Engorged veins.*

AION may be caused by an occlusion of the short posterior ciliary artery, which supplies the optic nerve, producing an infarction of the disc and surrounding nerve fiber hemorrhage. Alternatively, it may be due to an autoimmune mechanism, which may play a role in some AIONs of younger patients with systemic lupus erythematosus or other collagenous diseases.

Nonarteritic (*arteriosclerotic* or *garden-variety*) **anterior ischemic optic neuropathy** occurs in arteriosclerotic patients older than 60 years. It appears usually as a unilateral, asymmetrically pale, somewhat enlarged disc, elevated approximately 1 dd, with segmental edema, hyperemia, and blurred margins. A few fine, superficial, linear, flame-shaped hemorrhages or subretinal hemorrhages may be present, more commonly at the nasal margin. Occasionally, an opacification of the nerve fibers is seen inferiorly. The physiologic cup may be filled with exudate or may be absent. At a later stage, the disc may become atrophic, the arteries narrowed, and the veins mildly engorged. There may be a **macular star** in the resolving stages.

Arteritic anterior ischemic optic neuropathy usually occurs in patients who have giant-cell arteritis (temporal arteritis). The neuropathy appears as bilateral, milky, pale discs, much paler than in the nonarteritic form, with papilledema that may extend some considerable distance into the retina. A **cherry-red spot** due to a central retinal artery occlusion may be seen. As the disease progresses, a choroidal ischemia with irregular streaks and pigmentary patches may develop. The optic disc may display an enlarged and deep cup, which may simulate glaucoma.

Symptoms

Vision loss is unilateral, sudden, and nonprogressive, but rapidly may become bilateral, to counting fingers or worse. Patients may have headache, jaw claudication, scalp tenderness, anorexia, weight loss, and fever. The temporal artery will be tender, nonpulsating, and palpable. A relative afferent pupillary defect (RAPD) is possible.

Diagnosis

Visual field examination may reveal a central scotoma and an altitudinal inferior field defect, which may be permanent. Fluorescein angiography may demonstrate impaired filling, with dilatation of retinal capillaries and leakage. Serum lipids may be elevated. Serologic tests for syphilis also may be positive. Blood will be abnormally viscous, with increased levels of hemoglobin and fibrinogen. The Westergren erythrocyte sedimentation rate will be markedly increased. Urgent temporal artery biopsy and ocular pneumoplethysmography can help to establish the diagnosis.

Differential Diagnosis

Neuropapillitis, optic nerve tumor, central retinal artery occlusion, and central retinal vein occlusion must be considered in the differential diagnosis.

Histopathology

Histologic evaluation reveals an optic disc edema of the noninflammatory type (Figure 3-6). Optic nerve infarction also is present. The optic nerve may be atrophic in its retinal layers, and atrophy and gliosis might be seen in its choroidal and scleral layers. Foamy, fat-laden histiocytes

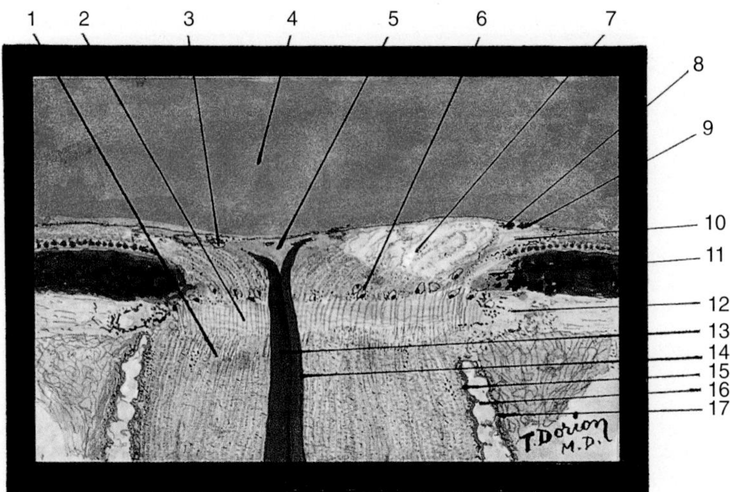

Figure 3-6. *Histopathologic findings in anterior ischemic optic neuropathy. (1) Optic nerve. (2) Lamina cribrosa. (3) Dilated capillaries on disc surface. (4) Vitreous. (5) Physiologic cup filled with exudate. (6) Foamy fat-laden histiocytes (glitter cells). (7) Segmental disc edema. (8) Nerve fiber layer lacerations. (9) Flame-shaped hemorrhages. (10) Optic nerve atrophy in retinal layer. (11) Optic nerve atrophy and gliosis in choroidal layer. (12) Optic nerve atrophy and gliosis in scleral layer. (13) Engorged central retinal vein. (14) Narrowed central retinal artery. (15) Pia mater. (16) Subarachnoid space. (17) Dura mater.*

(glitter cells) may be present in the scleral layer of the optic nerve. In the adventitia of the posterior ciliary arteries, there may be fragmented internal elastic lamina and inflammatory cells. Marked atrophy of the ganglion cell layer and of the nerve fiber layer at the macula is possible. Retinal capillaries on the disc surface may be dilated.

Treatment

Systemic corticosteroids are appropriate in giant-cell arteritis (prednisolone, 5 mg/day PO for several years). Anticoagulants (e.g., warfarin [Coumadin], 2.5–7.5 mg/day PO) should be administered for a few days. Such vasodilators as hydralazine, 25 mg PO twice per day;

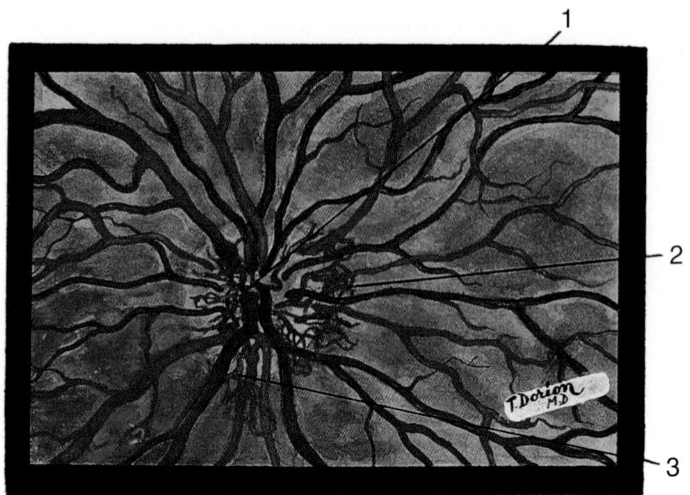

Figure 3-7. *Neovascularization of disc (NVD). (1) Epipapillary NVD. (2) Peripapillary NVD. (3) Papillovitreal NVD.*

captopril (Capoten), 50 mg/day PO 1 hour before meals; and nifedipine (Procardia), 20 mg sublingually PO three times per day, also are helpful. Vitamin supplementation may be added.

Neovascularization of the Disc

Neovascularization of the disc (NVD) is the term given to abnormal new vessels that arise from the optic disc or within 1 dd from the margin of the disc (Figure 3-7). *High-risk NVD* is neovascularization that is greater than or equal to one-fourth of the disc areas in eyes with a large optic disc or one-third of the disc area in eyes with a small optic disc, or neovascularization of any size that is associated with preretinal hemorrhage or vitreous hemorrhage.

NVD probably is caused by stimulation of an **angiogenic factor** released from a retinal ischemic zone.

Usually three clinical forms are recognized: (1) epipapillary, (2) peripapillary, and (3) papillovitreal.

Epipapillary Neovascularization of the Disc

Epipapillary NVD appears on the surface of the disc as a patch of fine, wispy, naked, flat, threadlike new vessels, of approximately 0.25–0.33 dd or less, radiating in a cartwheel pattern out from the center of the disc toward a circumferential peripheral vessel and protruding into the vitreous, probably along a detached posterior hyaloid membrane or anteriorly within Cloquet's canal. The new vessels may progress to further proliferation and formation of connective tissue. They may rupture, producing preretinal or vitreous hemorrhage, which then converts the condition to high-risk NVD. Occasionally, there may be exudative arteriolar sheathing.

Peripapillary Neovascularization of the Disc

Peripapillary NVD appears within 1 dd as a saucer of new vessels that extends centrifugally from the optic disc in a mesentericlike distribution, slightly elevated over the surrounding retina, the vascular arcades, and sometimes over the macula. The new vessels form delicate webs of multiple arterioles and venules.

Papillovitreal Neovascularization of the Disc

Papillovitreal NVD is seen as a massive amount of combined new vessels and glial tissue. It usually occurs after a branch retinal vein occlusion with capillary closure, which extends from the disc into the vitreous, occasionally producing a partial posterior vitreous detachment. As papillovitreal NVD progresses, the glial tissue becomes more prominent, and the vessels resolve. This type of neovascularization may appear in three clinical forms: (1) **columnar**, which extends along the posterior hyaloid membrane; (2) **arcuate**, which extends along the vascular arcades; and (3) **confluent**, which extends from the disc into the vitreous, without any lateral extensions or association with the vascular arcades.

Disc Hemorrhages

Disc hemorrhages are superficial, transient, and recurrent hemorrhages of the optic disc. They usually occur in acute infarction of the optic

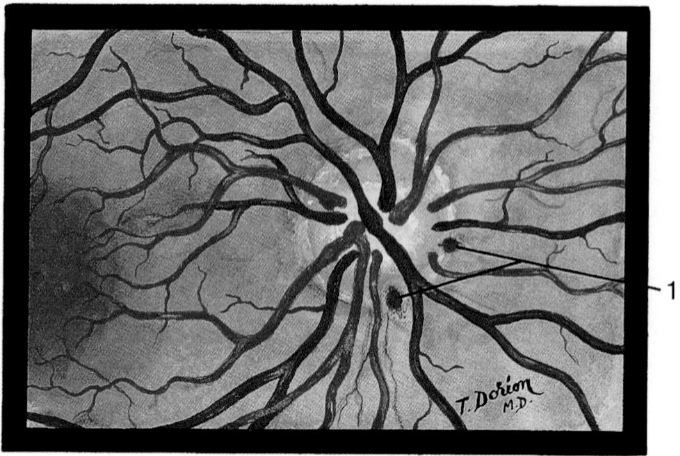

Figure 3-8. *Disc hemorrhages. (1) Superficial flame-shaped hemorrhages at edges of optic disc.*

nerve head, idiopathic optic neuritis, diabetes, or uncontrolled or low-tension glaucoma (Figure 3-8). These hemorrhages are caused by an insufficiency in the posterior ciliary artery circulation or by an occlusion of the peripapillary choroidal artery.

Disc hemorrhages are small, flame-shaped hemorrhages located at the disc edges, more commonly at the nasal margin inferiorly, and they cross the margins of the disc. They often are followed by an arterial attenuation, such as a reduction in central retinal artery caliber. They may resolve, generally incompletely, after several weeks or months.

Optic Neuritis

Optic neuritis (also known as *papillitis*, *neuroretinitis*, *Leber's hereditary optic neuropathy*, *Behr's syndrome*, *Wolfram's syndrome*, and *Kjer's syndrome*) is a hereditary, autosomal dominant or recessive, or acquired, usually unilateral disease, although the second eye may subsequently become involved. It may be *acute*, *subacute*, or *chronic*. It also may be *retrobulbar*. Optic neuritis occurs in arteriosclerosis, diabetes, Graves' disease, viral respiratory infections in children, aspergillosis, sarcoidosis, tuberculosis, syphilis, cryptococcosis, remote carcinoma, inflammatory bowel disease, acquired immunodeficiency syndrome (AIDS), Lyme disease, toxic amblyopia, tobacco or alcohol abuse, quinine poisoning, methyl alcohol poisoning, autointoxication (e.g., as occurs in massive burns), pregnancy, lactation, or menstrual disorders. It also may be seen in central nervous system diseases, infections, hematologic disorders, chronic nephrosis, orbital cellulitis, or intraocular inflammations.

Multiple etiologies have been implicated: infectious, viral, vascular, tumoral, nutritional, metabolic, parasitic, dystrophic, and idiopathic.

The disc appears hyperemic, with abnormal, dilated, tortuous retinal vessels, some circumpapillary telangiectatic microangiopathy, and mild swelling of the nerve fiber layer surrounding the disc (called *pseudopapilledema*). The margins of the disc may be blurred, and some splinter hemorrhages may be seen on the disc surface or surrounding it. The disc may be slightly opacified and grayish red but not glassy or transparent and not particularly enlarged. It may be moderately elevated (approximately 1–2 D), and the cup may be partially obliterated, absent, or filled with exudate. Retinal arteries may be narrowed, veins may be sheathed, and capillaries in the nerve fiber layer may be tortuous and dilated. Spontaneous venous pulsation may be absent. Cells might appear in the vitreous. **Neuroretinitis** describes involvement of the retina.

Forms of Optic Neuritis

There are a number of particular forms of optic neuritis. In **retrobulbar neuritis**, the disc is normal but occasionally pale, as a result of secondary optic atrophy. **Uveopapillitis** is characterized by a congested disc and retinal exudates in the macula. **Cuban optic neuropathy** is an endemic disease in which there is thinning or sometimes swelling of the retinal nerve fiber layer. This neuropathy may appear bilaterally as temporal optic nerve pallor and nerve fiber layer dropout in the papillomacular bundle. **Kjer's syndrome** is an autosomal dominant disease that appears as a wedge of temporal pallor of the disc.

Leber's hereditary optic neuropathy (Figure 3-9) or *maternal neuropathy* is a bilateral X-linked and autosomal dominant disease that is rapidly progressive and that occurs almost exclusively in men aged 20–40 years. It is commonly associated with cardiac conduction defects and dysrhythmia. Leber's neuropathy is produced by maternal transmission to 50% of sons and to only 10% of daughters, all of whom will become carriers. It may be caused by a nucleotide mutation at position 11778 of the mitochondrial DNA in ovum, which changes the coding

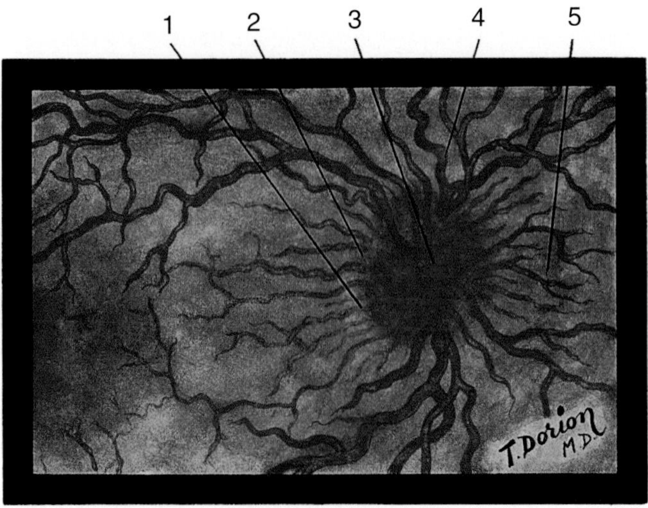

Figure 3-9. *Leber's hereditary optic neuropathy. (1) Peripapillary telangiectatic microangiopathy. (2) Pseudoedema. (3) Congested, hyperemic disc. (4) Prominent, tortuous, and dilated vessels. (5) Opacified retinal nerve fiber layer, usually nasally.*

for an amino acid in one of the proteins essential to the oxidative phosphorylation.

In the acute stage, Leber's neuropathy is evidenced as a hyperemic congested disc surrounded by dilated, tortuous vessels, called **peripapillary telangiectatic microangiopathy**. There is a circumpapillary, opacified swelling of the nerve fibers, called **pseudoedema**. Color vision testing may reveal a red-green defect. In the chronic stage, the disc is diffusely pale and atrophic, with sharp delineated margins. When Leber's neuropathy is associated with severe neurodeficits, it is called **Leber's plus disease**.

Behr's syndrome, or **infantile optic neuropathy**, is an autosomal recessive disease that appears as a diffuse optic atrophy.

Wolfram's syndrome is an autosomal recessive disease that also appears as a diffuse optic atrophy and that comprises *d*iabetes *i*nsipidus, *d*iabetes *m*ellitus, *o*ptic *a*trophy, and *d*eafness, or DIDMOAD.

Symptoms

Optic neuritis may be asymptomatic. However, severe decreased central vision at distance and near is possible, as is a sudden decrease in visual acuity, manifested as transient blurring of vision for minutes or hours (*amaurosis fugax*) or sometimes as overnight blindness. Pain or periocular discomfort that worsens with eye movement may occur. The patient might experience subjective visual disturbances, such as phosphenes, photopsia, and reduced perception of light intensity such that vision is better in scotopic illumination. A visual deficit called *Uhthoff's sign* might occur with exercise or increased body temperature. The patient may acquire color vision loss, specifically red, which appears desaturated. There may be a history of an antecedent viral syndrome. Vision loss may recover within several weeks.

Diagnosis

Visual field examination might reveal an absolute or relative centrocecal scotoma, nerve fiber bundle defects, an arcuate defect, or an altitudinal defect. Central nervous system symptoms and signs include episodic numbness, paresthesias, weakness, and incoordination of limbs. Vertigo, sphincter difficulties, trigeminal neuralgia, and psychiatric disorders also might be seen. Visual evoked responses may exhibit reduced amplitude, with marked delay of the waveform. An RAPD is possible.

The Snellen visual acuity chart and Pelli-Robson contrast sensitivity test are helpful in establishing the diagnosis. The Farnsworth-Munsell 100-hue (FM-100) test, a complete blood cell count, fasting blood sugar (FBS) test, erythrocyte sedimentation rate (ESR), chest roentgenograms, an antinuclear antibody (ANA) test, and serologic tests for syphilis (VDRL, rapid plasma reagin [RPR] test, fluorescent treponemal antibody absorption [FTA-ABS] test, microhemagglutination assay for *Treponema pallidum* [MHA-TP]) should be performed. Fluorescein angiography may reveal a mild hyperfluorescence and, in a late phase, deep staining of the disc. Ocular and parasellar CT scans with high resolution in axial and direct coronal views should be obtained. MRI may reveal white matter lesions on T2-weighted scans. Lumbar puncture for cerebrospinal fluid analysis should be performed, if possible.

Differential Diagnosis

Conditions that should be considered in the differential diagnosis include AION, multiple sclerosis, choroidal angioma, papilledema, pseudopapilledema, disc drusen, neuromyelitis optica, hypertension, and intracranial or orbital tumors.

Treatment

Optic neuritis may simply be observed. Corticosteroid therapy may be beneficial in hastening recovery but does not improve vision and may increase the recurrence rate of optic neuritis. If corticosteroids are used, a regimen of methylprednisolone, 250 mg IV four times per day for 3 days, followed by prednisone, 1 mg/kg/day PO for 10 days, and then tapered for 2 weeks is appropriate. Antiulcer medication (ranitidine, 150 mg PO twice per day) should be given during the period of corticosteroid therapy. Adrenocorticotropic hormone may be applied both intravenously and intraorbitally. Treatment of any underlying disease should be undertaken by an internist and a neurologist.

Optic Disc Anomalies

The optic disc may be anomalous in size and shape or in axial length. **Congenital disc anomalies of size and shape** include disc coloboma, morning-glory anomaly, optic pit, optic disc hypoplasia, optic disc aplasia, crescent, tilted disc, and pseudopapilledema. **Congenital disc anomalies of axial length** include hypermetropic or myopic disc, myelinated nerve fibers, drusen of the disc, anomalous blood vessels, situs inversus, prepapillary vascular loops, Bergmeister's papilla, and persistent hyaloid artery. A detailed description of each of these anomalies appears elsewhere in this book.

Disc Coloboma

Disc coloboma is a unilateral or bilateral congenital anomaly of the disc, usually inherited via an autosomal dominant route (Figure 3-10). It may be a part of **Pagon's syndrome** or CHARGE (*c*oloboma, *h*eart defects, *a*nal atresia, *r*etardation of growth, *g*enital and *e*ar defects).

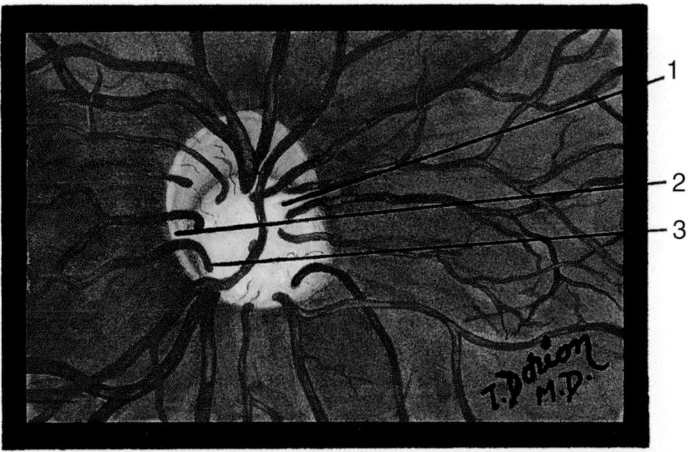

Figure 3-10. *Disc coloboma. (1) Excavation of the disc, inferiorly and nasally. (2) Thin neuroretinal rim. (3) Retinal vessels emanating from periphery of disc.*

Disc coloboma may be associated with chorioretinal coloboma, macular detachment, hypertelorism, central serous choroidopathy, retrobulbar cyst, retinal dysplasia, Aicardi's syndrome, Patau's syndrome (trisomy 13), Edward's syndrome (trisomy 18), Meckel-Gruber syndrome, Goldenhar's syndrome, persistent hyaloid artery, Gorlin-Golz focal hypoplasia, Lenz's microphthalmia, or Hallerman-Streiff syndrome. It may be *papillary* or *peripapillary*.

Disc coloboma may be caused by incomplete closure of the fetal fissure at the optic nerve, which becomes ectatic, or by aplasia of the primitive Bergmeister's papilla. The appearance is of a large excavation on the disc, up to 2 dd wide and 25 D deep, white-yellow, oval or round, sharply demarcated, usually located inferiorly and nasally, at the site of the fetal fissure. Retinal vessels course over, more frequently entering and exiting from the borders, but also from the depth of the coloboma, and they may coalesce at the base of the excavation. There may be peripapillary retinal pigment epithelium (RPE) atrophy, choroidal neovascularization, serous retinal detachment with striae radiating from disc to macula, or glial tissue at the center of the disc. The neuroretinal rim is thin.

Contractile disc coloboma is a rare form that, with every contraction of the excavation's floor, arises at about the level of the sur-

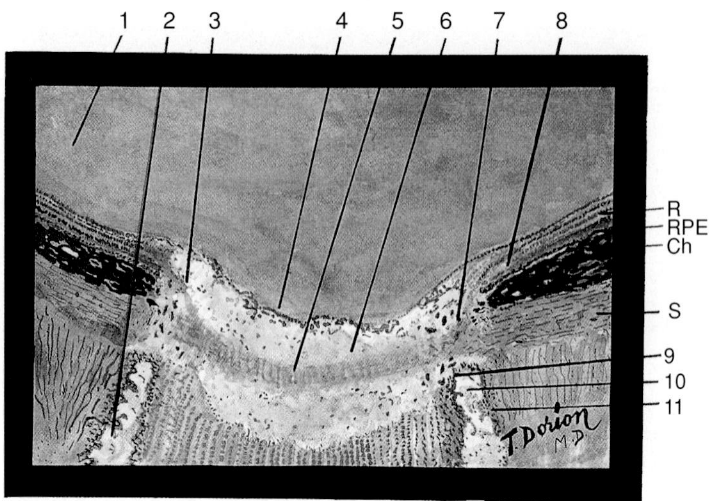

Figure 3-11. *Histopathologic findings in disc coloboma. (1) Vitreous. (2) Subarachnoid space. (3) Gliosis. (4) Large depression or defect at optic nerve head site, which involves retina, choroid, and sclera. (5) Lamina cribrosa. (6) Optic nerve atrophy. (7) Fusiform smooth-muscle cells, with spindle nuclei located centrally. (8) Retinal hypoplasia, which stops abruptly at the margin of the scleral defect. (9) Pia mater. (10) Arachnoid. (11) Dura mater. (R, retina; RPE, retinal pigment epithelium; Ch, choroid; S, sclera.)*

rounding retina so that its horizontal diameter is diminishing while the retinal vessels near the rim are becoming visible. During the relaxation, the coloboma borders appear more sharply. *The contractions of coloboma do not coincide with the respiration or the pulse.* They probably are due to a sphincterlike contracture of a heterotopic muscle around the optic disc.

Symptoms of disc coloboma include decreased visual acuity, often from 20/200 to hand motion.

Visual field examination may reveal a central scotoma or altitudinal defect. At the entrance of the optic nerve, a large depression and a defect are seen, which may involve the retina, the choroid, and the sclera (Figure 3-11). There is dysplasia or atrophy of the optic nerve, involving fusiform smooth-muscle cells with centrally located spindle nuclei. Gliosis is possible and may simulate a neoplasm. A peripapillary staphyloma may also be present.

Tilted Disc

Tilted disc is a nonhereditary congenital abnormality of the disc, a usually bilateral dysversion caused by oblique entrance of the optic nerve into the eye. This condition appears as a small, oval, hypoplastic disc of which the vertical axis is directed obliquely, inclined from its normal position in any direction. There is a disparity between the retinal opening and the scleral opening. A crescent, or congenital conus, that is hypopigmented may be located at the inferior side of the disc. A hypopigmented inferonasal fundus may be seen contiguous to the crescent. Retinal vessels usually emerge from the disc in an irregular vascular pattern, with a **situs inversus** of their origin, which causes the vessels of the right eye to resemble the vessels of the left eye. There may also be an **anomalous trifurcation** of the inferior central retinal artery. Inferior ectasia of the fundus is possible. Occasionally, retinal and choroidal segmental hypoplasia are seen. *No chorioretinal degeneration or lacquer cracks occur.*

Decreased visual acuity occurs as a result of a myopic astigmatism with an oblique axis.

Visual field examination may reveal bilateral depression, with superotemporal quadrantic defects that do not cross the vertical midline, unlike the visual defects from a chiasmal compression. Alternatively, there may be an altitudinal defect, or *refractive scotomas*, due to a marked astigmatism at an oblique axis, which may disappear with adequate correction. Myopia and chiasmal tumor should be considered in the differential diagnosis.

Correction of the oblique myopic astigmatism is appropriate.

Morning-Glory Anomaly

Morning-glory anomaly (also known as *central coloboma of the disc*, *peripapillary scleral staphyloma*, *axial coloboma*, and *scleral ectopia*) is a unilateral, nonhereditary congenital deformity of the optic nerve head that often is associated with astigmatism, basal encephalocele, absence of the corpus callosum, and hare lip and cleft palate (Figure 3-12). It probably is due to a developmental posterior displacement of the disc through a scleral ectasia.

Morning-glory anomaly features an enlarged excavation of a pale disc that lies posterior to the globe within a funnel-like optic nerve defect having a rough, irregular surface. A central core of a white-gray

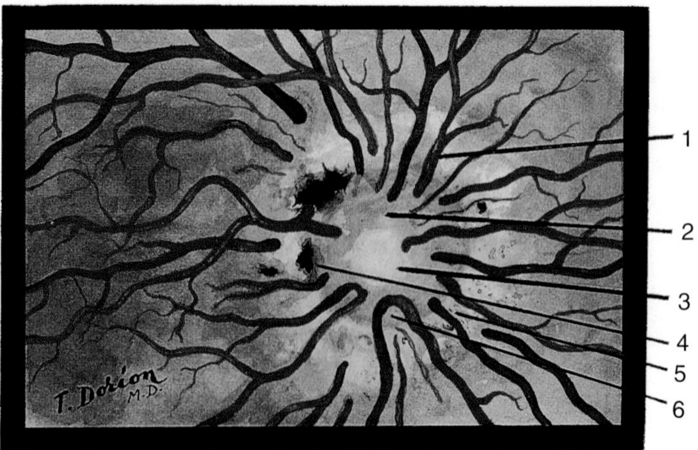

Figure 3-12. *Morning-glory anomaly. (1) Spokelike radiating vessels. (2) Large excavation of disc. (3) Fibroglial tissue mass. (4) Pigment deposition. (5) Peripapillary choroidal atrophy. (6) Arteriovenous communication.*

or greenish mass of fibroglial tissue is seen, surrounded by chorioretinal pigmentation and exhibiting spokelike radiating blood vessels at the periphery; this combination of features resembles a flower. A complete staphyloma may be present. Arteriovenous communications and persistent hyaloid artery within the anomaly's base may also be present. Sometimes a ring of peripapillary choroidal atrophy is seen. Rhegmatogenous retinal detachment occasionally occurs, whereas persistent hyperplastic primary vitreous is common.

Decreased vision and an RAPD are symptoms of morning-glory anomaly.

Histologically, mass proliferation of the glial tissue, a remnant of Bergmeister's papilla, and fat heterotopic tissue, are seen. Other histopathologic findings are scleral ectasia, peripapillary staphyloma, and optic nerve atrophy.

Diffuse Unilateral Subacute Neuroretinitis

Diffuse unilateral subacute neuroretinitis (*wipe-out syndrome*) is characterized by widespread destruction of the sensory retina, which occurs in healthy young persons in the Southeast and Midwest of the United States. It is caused by an inflammatory process from a living nematode in the eye.

In the early stages, multiple, small, yellow-white spots are located deep in the retina. Frequently, the background of the ocular fundus remains unchanged. There may be mild swelling of the disc, with peripapillary thinning and pigment accumulation. A mild hyalitis, in which few cells appear in the vitreous, may also be seen. Occasionally, a small worm (measuring 50 μm or more) in a coiled or uncoiled position may be seen migrating beneath a glistening sheen of the inner retina or in the vitreous. Its movements may be accelerated by bright light and slowed by red-free illumination. This nematode may disappear in several days or weeks. In the late, inactive stage, scattered patches of RPE atrophy and peripapillary fibrous proliferation may be present. Retinal vessels may be narrowed and attenuated, and the optic disc may become pale and atrophic.

As the lesion progresses, the patient suffers unilateral severe decreased visual acuity to 20/200 or more. Visual field examination may reveal central and peripheral scotomas. Fluorescein angiography may show hypofluorescent spots.

Laser photocoagulation of the nematode and vitrectomy are treatment options.

Myelinated Nerve Fibers

Myelinated nerve fibers (known also as *medullated nerve fibers* and *opaque nerve fibers*) consitute a benign, unilateral optic disc anomaly acquired shortly after birth and occurring primarily in male individuals. The condition is the result of postnatal continued myelinization of the optic nerve, which normally ceases at birth. This persistent myelinization does not stop at the lamina cribrosa but extends onto the nerve fibers surrounding the disc or elsewhere in the peripheral retina.

Myelinated nerve fibers appear as superficial, bright, yellow or pearl-white, opaque, glistening patches (Figure 3-13). They may be flame-shaped, arcuate or discoid, or hemispheric bundles, with shiny streaks or radiations and soft feathered edges, and they follow the course of the nerve fiber layer. These patches commonly are located at the margins of the disc, obscuring the retinal vessels, but *they do not extend beyond the second arterial bifurcation.* They may be located more peripherally, separated from the disc by a normal retina. Occasionally,

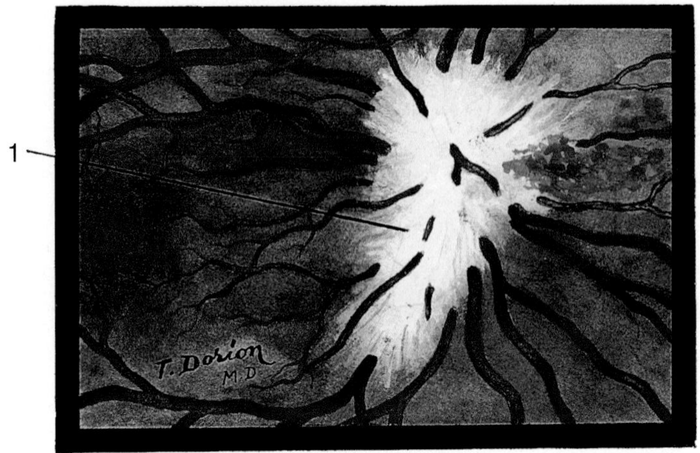

Figure 3-13. *Myelinated nerve fibers. (1) Pearly white radiating nerve fibers, with feathered edges.*

small islands of normal retina that simulate a hemorrhage may reside within these patches.

Visual field examination is normal. The condition is asymptomatic except when macula is involved, which may affect the vision.

Histopathologically, an accumulation of **myelin**, and possibly of oligodendrocytes, is seen in the inner layers of the sensory retina and in the ganglion cell axons of the nerve fiber layer but not at the lamina cribrosa. There is no pigment proliferation.

Optic Nerve Hypoplasia

Optic nerve hypoplasia is a unilateral or bilateral congenital anomaly of the disc, the origin of which is unknown. It usually is associated with abnormalities of the lamina cribrosa, physical underdevelopment, diabetes insipidus, deficiency of growth hormone, endocrine or central nervous system disorders, tetraploid-diploid mosaicism, microphthalmos, and hydrocephalus. Alternatively, it may be part of **de Morsier's syndrome** (septo-optic dysplasia), which consists of absence of the septum pellucidum, pituitary dwarfism, and optic nerve hypoplasia. It may also be associated with young maternal age, maternal diabetes, and drug use during pregnancy (e.g., quinine, antiepileptics, lysergic acid diethylamide [LSD]).

Optic nerve hypoplasia is caused by failure of the ganglion cell axons either to develop or to reach the optic disc. The disc appears small, pale, and often full and may be tilted or may have crowded nerve fibers that simulate a swollen disc. Often, there is a concentric choroid-RPE abnormal pigmentation that presents as two depigmented rings (called the *double-ring sign*) surrounding a peripapillary atrophy: The *inner ring*, which is yellow-white and in which pigmentation varies, represents termination of the retina and RPE, whereas *the outer ring* is depigmented and represents the junction between the sclera and the lamina cribrosa. Vessels may be normal or enlarged, and there may be an *abnormal trifurcation* of the inferior retinal artery. Occasionally, only a **segmental optic nerve hypoplasia** may occur.

Symptoms

Visual acuity may be normal or severely decreased to no light perception. Nystagmus, strabismus, and RAPD are possible.

Diagnosis

Visual field examination will reveal defects that cross the midline. MRI is useful in making the diagnosis.

Histopathology

On histopathologic evaluation, fewer axons than normal are seen entering the disc, and myelin is almost completely absent. There is a peripapillary atrophy, with two annular, concentric, depigmented areas. Termination of the RPE at the margin of the disc is irregular. Retinal vessels are normal or enlarged.

Treatment

Amblyopia therapy may be tried but usually is not satisfactory. Refractive errors should be corrected. Polycarbonate protective lenses are in order, as is consultation with an endocrinologist.

Optic Disc Aplasia

Optic disc aplasia is a rare, congenital condition in which the optic nerve head is absent. It usually is unilateral and can occur in otherwise healthy persons. It may be caused by failure of proper development of the ganglion cells, or it may result from an abnormal invagination of the ventral fissure.

The disc and retinal vessels are not seen, and there is no optic nerve. The retinal ganglion cell layer may be diminished and may contain undifferentiated cells that lack axons and dendrites, or it may be absent. The internal limiting membrane of the periphery may be thin, and vitreous filaments may line it. On the external limiting membrane, there may be adherent areas of Müller cells and photoreceptors in a single plane. The inner retina may appear to be disorganized, but the outer retina, including the photoreceptors, may be normal.

Optic Atrophy

Optic atrophy is a loss of nerve fibers at the disc, which may be *congenital* or *acquired*, *primary* or *secondary*, *ascending* or *descending* (Figure 3-14). It may be caused by a vascular process such as an infarction; by an abnormality such as demyelinization; by pressure such as glaucoma or tumor; or by inflammation, trauma, toxicity, or degeneration. These processes may produce poor perfusion, an *ischemic necrobiosis*, which ultimately may cause the death of the ganglion cells. The intensity of the pallor is attributable to the amount of nerve tissue and capillaries lost as well as to the amount of glial tissue present. Symptoms include loss of vision and loss of pupillary reaction.

Types of Optic Atrophy

Several types of optic atrophy may be seen. In **primary optic atrophy**, no evidence exists of any preceding inflammation or edema of the disc. The disc appears pale, totally or partially whitish, or porcelain-white, and displays sharp, delineated margins.

Secondary optic atrophy occurs usually after a papillitis, papilledema, choroidoretinopathy, pressure, vascular disease, loss of blood, or trauma. Retinal vessels may be displaced nasally, and the physiologic cup may be wide and deep.

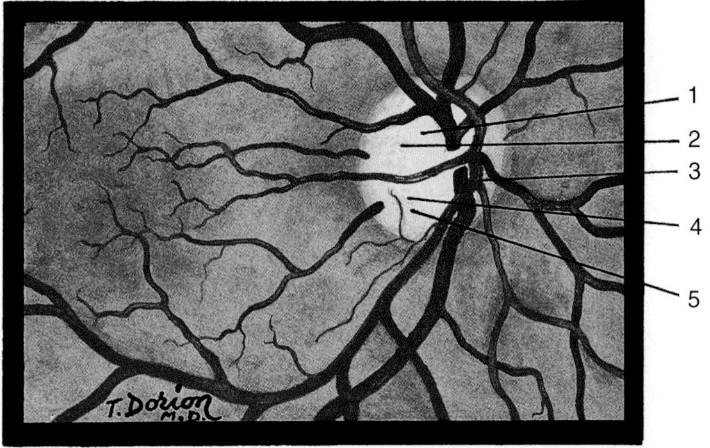

Figure 3-14. *Optic atrophy. (1) Pale disc. (2) Loss of nerve fibers. (3) Nasal displacement of vessels. (4) Avascularity or decreased capillary network. (5) Wide physiologic cup.*

Hereditary familial optic atrophy is a congenital, X-linked or autosomal recessive disease. It begins with an *acute stage*, in which the disc appears elevated, swollen, and hyperemic, and advances to a *late stage*, in which the swelling recedes and the disc flattens and exhibits a decreased papillary capillary network.

Consecutive optic atrophy is a noninflammatory optic atrophy that occurs in diseases that destroy the retinal ganglion cells. The disc appears pale with sharp margins.

Postneuritic optic atrophy occurs after a papillitis or papilledema. The disc usually appears white, has blurred margins, and often displays a glial proliferation on its surface, which is evidence of a pre-existing neuritis. The normal spongy structure of the disc is lost. Lamina cribrosa is not visible. Arteries are thinned and less numerous than normal and exhibit perivascular sheathing.

Retinochoroidal optic atrophy occurs after severe choroiditis or chorioretinitis, in retinitis pigmentosa, or in high myopia. The disc is pale, opaque, and shiny, with irregular, well-defined margins. Retinal vessels may be distorted or obscured by a scarring tissue.

Optic atrophy after blood loss occurs as a consequence of massive gastrointestinal hemorrhage, injuries, birth delivery, or abortion. The disc appears pale with blurred margins, but it is not elevated above the retina.

Traumatic optic atrophy occurs after fractures of the face or base of the skull, a gunshot wound, or intraorbital penetration by a sharp object. The disc usually appears chalky white and has well-defined margins.

In **ascending optic atrophy**, the primary lesion is in the disc and retina, whereas the secondary effects occur in the optic nerve and the brain. In contrast, in **descending optic atrophy**, the primary lesion is in the intracranial optic nerve and the white tracts of the brain, whereas the secondary effects appear in the disc and retina.

Symptoms

Loss of vision and pupillary reaction are usually the symptoms of optic atrophy.

Histopathology

A reduction or absence of the nerve fibers is seen on histologic examination, the fibers being replaced by a proliferation of astrocytes rearranged into dense parallel layers across the optic nerve head or by glial connective tissue. Myelin is lost from the axons of the nerve fibers. Ganglion cells are altered or absent. Choroidal vessels have thickened walls and narrowed lumina. The sensory retina may be reduced to a thin layer or replaced by glial tissue. The internal limiting membrane of the retina may be intact.

Treatment

Early treatment of the underlying cause is recommended, although it is rarely successful.

Crowded Nerve Fibers

Crowded nerve fibers is the term that designates a benign accumulation of optic nerve fibers on the disc surface, more commonly at its nasal side, simulating a papilledema. The condition occurs in optic disc hypoplasia and in hypermetropia, in which the eye usually is smaller than normal. It is due to a disparity between the size of the scleral opening, which is smaller, and that of the retinal opening, which is larger and allows a great number of axons to pass through the disc.

The condition results in a small disc with a diminished or absent physiologic cup. The disc is full of crowded nerve fibers, which gives the appearance of swelling or a *pseudopapilledema*. Retinal vessels are normal.

Nerve Fiber Layer Defect

Nerve fiber layer defect is a focal or diffuse loss of the retinal nerve fiber layer, occurring in glaucoma and occasionally in migraine. It is produced by infarction or edema of the nerve fiber layer, which may progress to a diffuse atrophy of this retinal layer. Four types are identified: *slit defect*, *wedge defect*, *diffuse atrophy*, and *total atrophy.*

Nerve fiber layer defect appears as an attenuated area of the retina along the ganglion cell axons that is pale, whitish, and located usually inferior and temporal to the disc. A few cotton-wool spots, flame-shaped hemorrhages, and dark spots may be present at the posterior pole. The physiologic cup may be deep and glaucomatous, with an *abnormal, even neuroretinal rim*. (Normally, the rim is uneven, the widest portion being inferior, the next widest portions being superior and nasal, and the narrowest portion located temporally.)

Histopathologic findings include edema of the nerve fiber layer, areas of bulbous swellings and infarcts, and distension and disruption of the axons, with inclusions that resemble the cell nucleus (called *cytoid bodies*). Marked diffuse atrophy of the nerve fiber layer also may be seen.

Leber's Idiopathic Stellate Neuropathy

Leber's idiopathic stellate neuropathy is a rare, unilateral optic disease of unknown etiology that occurs in adults who have frequent exposure to cats, such as veterinarians, or who may have incurred a cat-scratch lesion. The neuropathy may be due to a hyperpermeability of the disc vessels at the peripapillary area. A macular star exudate is noted, and the optic disc is mildly swollen, with blurred margins.

Symptoms of Leber's idiopathic stellate neuropathy include unilateral decreased vision, which may improve in several weeks, and scotoma.

Diagnostic aids include serologic tests for syphilis (FTA-ABS test, treponemal passive hemagglutination assay for syphilis [TPHA], VDRL), which may be positive. Blood culture may show a gram-negative bac-

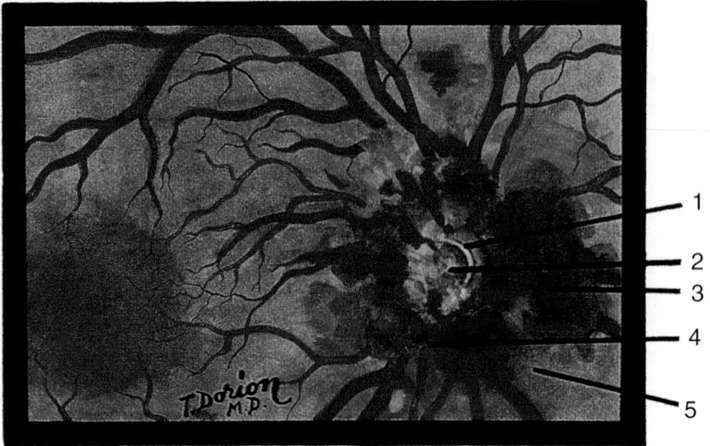

Figure 3-15. *Optic nerve avulsion. (1) Disinsertion of the optic nerve head. (2) Large papillary excavation. (3) Choroidal detachment. (4) Severed retinal vessels. (5) Liquefied vitreous.*

teria, *Bartonella henselae,* in serum. Fluorescein angiography may reveal fluorescence of the disc, leakage from the peripapillary capillaries, and venous engorgement, but *no perimacular leakage* is seen.

No effective treatment is known.

Optic Nerve Avulsion

Optic nerve avulsion is a traumatic disinsertion of the optic nerve head (Figure 3-15). It usually is produced by posterior orbital blunt trauma, which may leave the conjunctiva intact, or by a penetrating injury by a sharp object, such as an umbrella tip, a ski pole end, or a cow horn, which may enter tangentially and cause forced rotation of the globe, with brutal distortion and tearing of the nerve. Alternatively, optic nerve avulsion may be due to an acute increase of the IOP, which produces a separation of the nerve at the lamina cribrosa.

Optic nerve avulsion appears as a displacement of the optic nerve head, which may be disinserted, separated, or torn. The nerve fibers may be frayed temporally at the level of the papilla, where the nerve is narrower and resistance is diminished. Often, the lamina cribrosa is

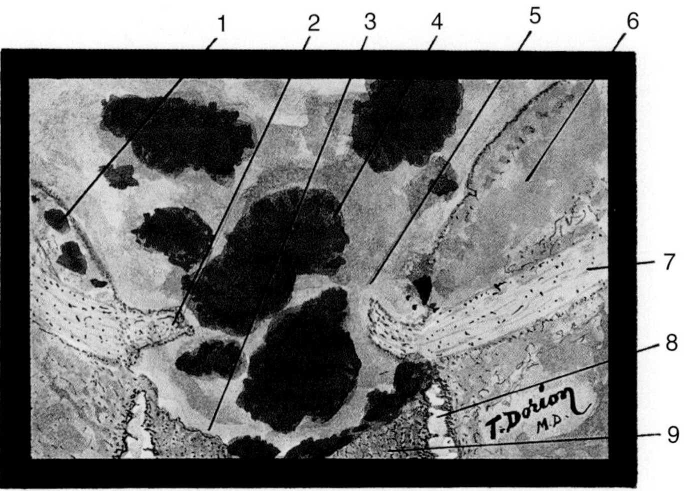

Figure 3-16. *Histopathologic findings in optic nerve avulsion. (1) Intraretinal hemorrhage. (2) Discontinuity of lamina cribrosa. (3) Displacement of optic nerve entrance. (4) Vitreal hemorrhage. (5) Liquefied vitreous. (6) Choroidal and retinal detachment. (7) Sclera. (8) Subarachnoid space. (9) Optic nerve tissue.*

ruptured and may appear as a pit or a hole surrounded by retinal and vitreal hemorrhage. After the hemorrhage resolves, a large papillary excavation without evidence of any nervous tissue or central retinal vessels is seen. In the peripapillary region, the retinal vessels are severed. There may be extensive choroidal or retinal detachment. Vitreous may also be detached or liquefied.

Unilateral sudden visual loss generally occurs after ocular trauma.

On histologic examination, the lamina cribrosa is seen to be discontinuous (Figure 3-16), and the optic nerve's entrance into the eye is displaced.

An effective treatment is not known.

Bergmeister's Papilla

Bergmeister's papilla (also known as *congenital prepapillary veil*) is a remnant of the fetal vasculature (in which glial tissue and periarterial sheathing are retained) at the optic disc, and of the intravitreal hyaloid

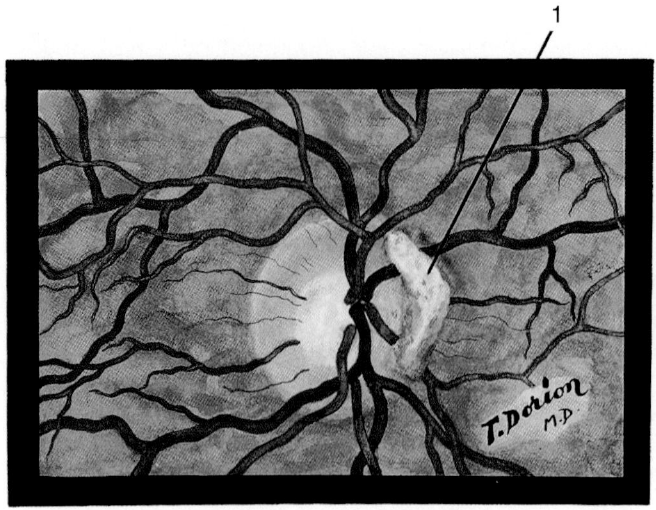

Figure 3-17. *Bergmeister's papilla. (1) Ragged strand of vascularized glial proliferation at the nasal side of the optic nerve head, extending into the vitreous.*

artery, which normally regresses at birth. It usually is associated with other optic disc abnormalities, such as prepapillary loops, morning-glory anomaly, or persistent hyperplastic primary vitreous.

Bergmeister's papilla appears as a stalklike vascularized tissue, a whitish mass of glial proliferation that extends into the vitreous from the optic nerve head as a ragged strand or as a membrane stretching over the disc, more often at its nasal side (Figure 3-17). The disc surface may be slightly elevated, determining in part the depth of the physiologic cup.

Suggested Reading

Avery R, Jabs DA, Wingard JR, et al. Optic disc edema after bone transplantation. Ophthalmology 1991;98:1294–1301.

Benson WE, Shakin J, Sarin LK. Blunt Trauma. In W Tasman, EA Jaeger, MM Parks, et al. (eds), Duane's Clinical Ophthalmology, vol 3. Philadelphia: Lippincott–Raven, 1996;31:1–12.

Brazikitos PD, Safran AB, Simona F, Zulauf M. Threshold perimetry in tilted disc syndrome. Arch Ophthalmol 1990;108:1698–1700.

Brodsky MC, Hoyt CS, Miller RN, Lamb BL. Atypical retinochoroidal coloboma in patients with dysplastic optic discs and transsphenoidal encephalocele. Arch Ophthalmol 1955;113:624–628.

Brown DM, Kimura AE, Ossoinig KC, Weiner GJ. Acute promyelocytic infiltration of the optic nerve treated by oral trans-retinoid acid. Ophthalmology 1992;99:1463–1467.

Collins ML, Traboulsi EI, Maumenee IH. Optic nerve swelling and optic atrophy in the systemic mucopolysaccharidoses. Ophthalmology 1990;97:1445–1449.

Corbett J. Diagnosis and management of idiopathic intracranial hypertension (pseudotumor cerebri). Focal Points 1989;3:1–12.

De Souza EC, Nakashima Y. Diffuse unilateral subacute neuroretinitis. Ophthalmology 1995;102:1183–1186.

Diehl DL, Quigley HA, Miller NR, et al. Prevalence and significance of optic disc hemorrhage in a longitudinal study of glaucoma. Arch Ophthalmol 1990;108:545–550.

Glaser JS, Teimory M, Schatz NJ. Optic nerve sheath fenestration for progressive ischemic optic neuropathy. Arch Ophthalmol 1994;112:1047–1050.

Hobbs H. Affections of the Optic Nerve. In A Sorsby (ed), Modern Ophthalmology, vol 4 (2nd ed). Philadelphia: Lippincott, 1972;763–781.

Jabs DA. Ocular Manifestations of Rheumatic Diseases. In W Tasman, EA Jaeger, MM Parks, et al. (eds), Duane's Clinical Ophthalmology, vol 5. Philadelphia: Lippincott–Raven, 1996;26:3–16.

Sadun AA. Epidemic optic neuropathy in Cuba. Arch Ophthalmol 1994;112: 696–698.

Schuman JS, Hee MR, Puliafito CA, et al. Quantification of nerve fiber thickness in normal and glaucomatous eye using optical coherence tomography. Arch Ophthalmol 1995;113:624–628.

Sedwick LA. Optic neuritis update. Focal Points 1988;12:1–12.

Sorsby A. Affections Manifest in Postnatal Life. In A Sorsby (ed), Modern Ophthalmology, vol 3 (2nd ed). Philadelphia: Lippincott, 1972;290–350.

Sorsby A. Congenital Malformations. In A Sorsby (ed), Modern Ophthalmology, vol 3 (2nd ed). Philadelphia: Lippincott, 1972;221–289.

Trobe JD. Managing optic neuritis: results of the optic neuritis treatment trial. Focal Points 1994;3:1–10.

Ulrich GC, Walker NJ, Meister SJ, et al. Cat scratch disease associated with neuroretinitis in a 6-year-old girl. Ophthalmology 1992;99:246–249.

Yedavally S, Frank RN. Peripapillary subretinal neovascularization associated with coloboma of the optic disc. Arch Ophthalmol 1993;111:552–553.

4

Vascular Retinopathy

Central Retinal Artery Occlusion

Central retinal artery occlusion (CRAO) is an acute unilateral retinal edema at the posterior pole involving the macula, affecting the vision gravely, and occurring mostly in elderly men (Figure 4-1). It may be preceded by a transient ischemic attack of blurred vision or blackout.

CRAO is caused by a blockage of the retrobulbar flow in the central retinal artery (an embolization) due to a thrombus, such as fat from an atheroma, calcium from heart valves, or platelets or fibrin that occludes the artery. The embolization may originate far from the eye in the left side of the heart or in the carotid artery. It may be caused also by an intimal arteriosclerosis at the lamina cribrosa or by hypertension; collagen diseases; giant-cell arteritis; oral contraceptives; sickle cell anemia; retrobulbar hemorrhage; endocrine hemophthalmos; mucormycosis of the orbit; a retinal vein occlusion; anterior ischemic optic neuropathy (AION); a severe increase in the intraocular pressure (IOP); a premacular, macular, or vitreous hemorrhage; or a vasospasm (as in migraine).

CRAO appears as a large area of milky, creamy, cloudy, or whitish gray opaque and slightly elevated retina at the posterior pole. The macula is edematous and ischemic, sometimes finely pigmented, and the foveal reflex is absent. In the foveola, however, where the retina is relatively thin, the normal choroid that is supplied by its own circulation is visible as a **cherry-red spot**. Retinal arteries are thin and attenuated—with caliber irregularities called *boxcarring vessels* or

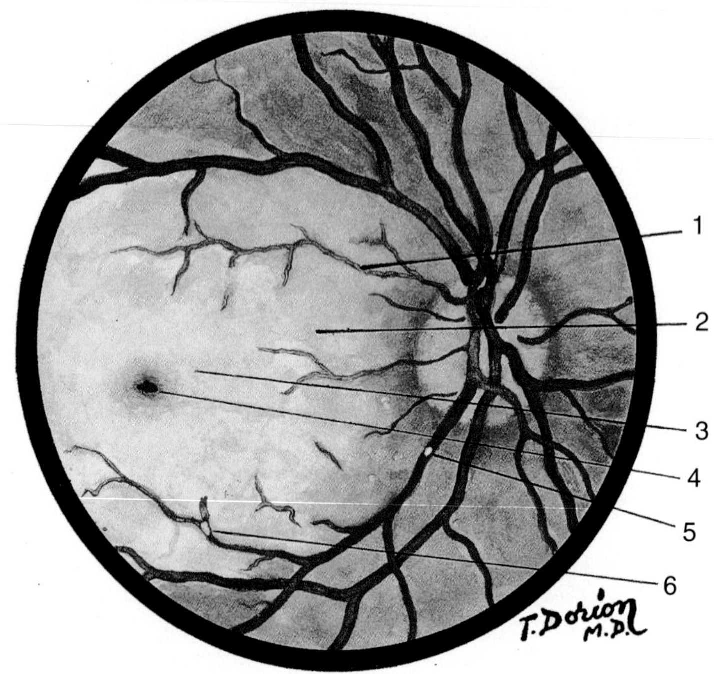

Figure 4-1. *Central retinal artery occlusion. (1) Thin and attenuated arteries. (2) Retinal edema. (3) Edematous and ischemic macula. (4) Cherry-red spot. (5) Calcium emboli. (6) Hollenhorst plaque.*

sludging segmentation called *cattle trucking*—or are collapsed. At the bifurcation of the arteries, there may be small glistening *cholesterol emboli*, called *Hollenhorst plaques*, originating from the carotid artery or the aortic arch.

Occasionally, large white *calcium emboli* emanating from the aortic valve may be present. When a **cilioretinal artery** is present, a darker horizontal area of normal retina may be seen in the area of distribution of that artery, and the central vision may be spared. Veins also are thinned and narrowed. Rarely, CRAO may be associated with a central retinal vein occlusion. The disc may show a diminution of the nerve fiber layer and some degree of optic atrophy.

Symptoms

CRAO symptoms include sudden, unilateral, painless, and severe loss of vision to 20/400 or even counting fingers or hand motion. Usually, vision loss is permanent. Relative afferent pupillary defect can occur.

Diagnosis

Fluorescein angiography may reveal an increased retinal arteriovenous (AV) transit limit, a delay or lack of retinal arterial filling, but the *filling of the choroid or of the cilioretinal artery usually is normal*; there may be a blockage in the macula, secondary to the overlying edema. Electroretinography (ERG) shows a diminution of the **b-wave** amplitude, which corresponds to a reduced function of Müller cells or of bipolar cells, and a normal **a-wave**, which reflects the intact function of the photoreceptors. Visual field examination may show remaining islands of vision, usually temporally. The erythrocyte sedimentation rate (ESR) may be elevated.

Histopathology

On histologic evaluation, there may be a retinal atrophy and an infarction of two-thirds of the inner retinal layers, but *the outer retinal layers are not affected*. There may be a homogeneous, diffuse acellular zone, retinal necrosis, foamy macrophages, and (in a late stage) an excessive hyalinization that replaces the inner plexiform layer, the ganglion layer, and the nerve fiber layer. The inner nuclear layer may be thin.

Treatment

CRAO is an emergency. It should be treated within the first 30–60 minutes (maximum, 2 hours) of onset to relieve the vascular spasm or to dislodge the embolus. Indicated treatment is inhalation of a mixture of 95% oxygen and 5% carbon dioxide for 15 minutes each hour. Digital massage is applied for 5 seconds, then is repeated. One 500-mg sustained-release capsule PO twice a day or one 500-mg vial IV of acetazolamide (Diamox sequels) should be administered. Methylprednisolone, 100 mg IV, also is helpful. Paracentesis of the anterior chamber can be performed with a No.

11 Bard-Parker blade or a 25-gauge needle with syringe, to decrease the IOP and to restore the blood flow in the central retinal artery. Anticoagulants such as heparin, 5 ml (25,000 IU) IV, can be used. Stellate ganglion block may be achieved with procaine 1% or lidocaine 1%. Systemic medications include vasodilators—nicotinic acid (Eupaverine forte), one vial IV; amyl nitrate tablets, one tablet sublingually as needed; isosorbide (Sorbitrate), 10-mg tablet PO three times a day; or fibrinolysin, one vial IV. Argon laser panretinal photocoagulation may be effective.

Branch Retinal Artery Occlusion

Branch retinal artery occlusion (BRAO) is an obstruction of a retinal artery, usually the temporal branch (Figure 4-2), which occurs as a result of diabetes, hypertension, collagen diseases, toxoplasmosis, arterial macroaneurysms, hemoglobinopathies, protein S deficiency, inflammatory bowel disease, giant-cell arteritis, atrial myxoma, rheumatic heart disease, myocardial infarction, Barlow's syndrome (mitral valve prolapse), oral contraceptive use, migraine, trauma, IV drug use, or pregnancy. It is due to an atheroma, a vascular spasm, or emboli from a distance.

BRAO is characterized by a superficial, opaque retinal whitening that is milky, creamy, or gray. A sharply delimited edema is located along the distribution of the obstructed artery, distal to the embolus. The arterial branch is extremely attenuated or may have segmental opacification and necrosis of its wall. **Boxcarring vessel** sludging of the blood may be present. The occlusion may affect the macula. Occasionally, bright **Hollenhorst plaques** of cholesterol, lodging at the arterial bifurcation, or microemboli in the artery may be seen. In time, the vessel recanalizes, the edema resolves, and the visual acuity may return to 20/40 or better, but *the visual field defect remains.*

BRAO may occur also as **cilioretinal artery occlusion** as one of three types: (1) isolated, (2) associated with central retinal vein obstruction, or (3) associated with AION.

Symptoms

BRAO results in unilateral, sudden, painless loss of visual acuity in a part of the visual field corresponding to the affected retina. Often, it is preceded by attacks of **amaurosis fugax**, a transient visual loss for minutes produced by a vascular spasm and usually caused by a *platelet-thrombin* aggregate.

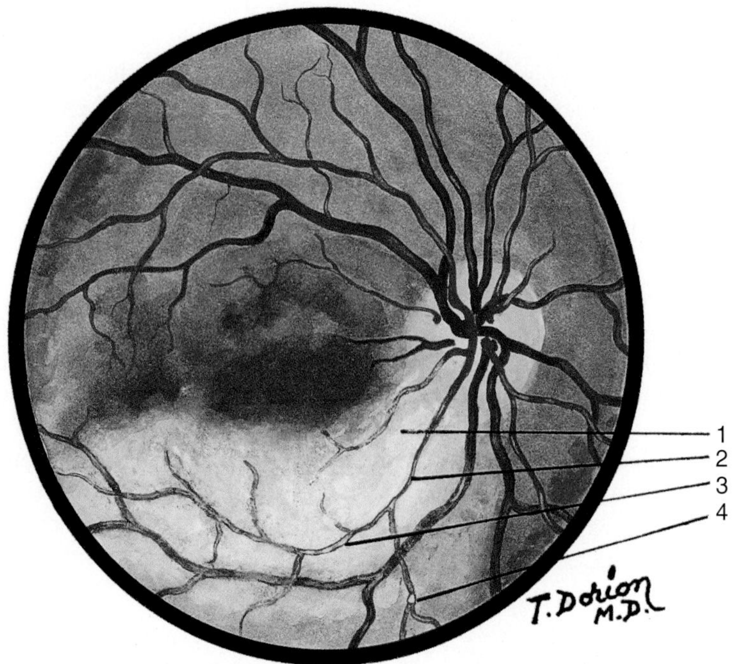

Figure 4-2. *Branch retinal artery occlusion. (1) Retinal edema. (2) Arterial attenuation. (3) Boxcarring vessel. (4) Hollenhorst plaque.*

Diagnosis

Visual field examination reveals a defect, usually altitudinal, in the area of the damaged retina. Fluorescein angiography may reveal a delayed perfusion or lack of fluorescein filling of the branch of the involved artery.

Histopathology

Histologic evaluation reveals an edema and a retinal infarction in the area of the obstructed artery. As the edema clears, the inner retinal layers become atrophic. Vessels are narrowed and tortuous, with focal constriction or plaquelike deposits on the arterial wall surface and at its bifurcation. The optic disc may become pale.

Treatment

Usually treatment is not necessary, owing to the relatively good prognosis. Ocular massage is beneficial, but treatment of the underlying disease is indicated.

Central Retinal Vein Occlusion

Central retinal vein occlusion (CRVO; also termed *central retinal vein thrombosis* and *retinal apoplexy*) usually is a local, unilateral, circulatory disturbance of the flow in the central retinal vein owing to an occlusion (Figure 4-3). It occurs mostly in men older than 60 years or as a result of an inflammation in the young. Usually, it is associated with cardiovascular diseases, hypertension, diabetes, angle-closure glaucoma, increased intraorbital pressure, sarcoidosis, Behçet's disease, drusen of optic nerve, syphilis, systemic lupus erythematosus, blood dyscrasias, hyperviscosity syndromes, or use of diuretics and oral contraceptives.

Clinical Types

CRVO occurs as one of three types: (1) *nonischemic*, (2) *ischemic*, and (3) *degenerative*.

Nonischemic CRVO (or *venous stasis retinopathy*) results from a reversible, complete occlusion of the central retinal vein by a thrombosis and *is not associated with any significant hypoxia*. It may be the result of an inflammatory process, such as papillophlebitis in the young after use of birth control pills or diuretics, or of an arteriosclerosis in the elderly, or it may be idiopathic. It appears as retinal hemorrhages, which may vary from a few flame-shaped or punctate hemorrhages to numerous, large intraretinal hemorrhages.

Ischemic CRVO (or *hemorrhagic retinopathy*) is caused by an occlusion of the central retinal vein at or anterior to the lamina cribrosa and *is associated with retinal ischemia and significant retinal hypoxia*. It may occur after a trauma, in tumor, or in primary open-angle glaucoma. It appears as extensive hemorrhage, which gives the fundus a **blood-and-thunder** picture.

Degenerative CRVO is caused by a degeneration of the venous endothelium. It occurs more frequently in hypertension, cardiac decompensation, and diabetes, and in systemic granulomatous dis-

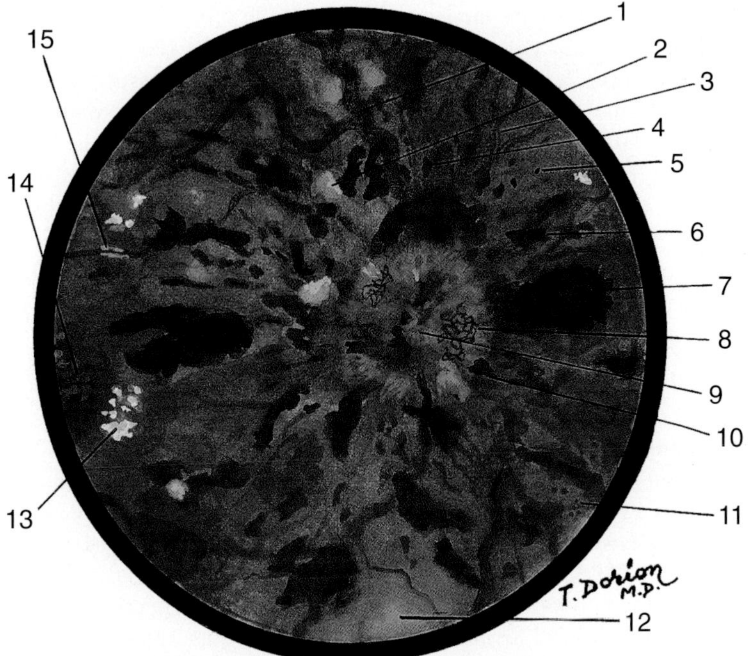

Figure 4-3. *Central retinal vein occlusion. (1) Tortuous, dilated, segmented veins. (2) Cotton-wool spots. (3) Narrowed arteries. (4) Flame-shaped hemorrhage. (5) Punctate hemorrhage. (6) Preretinal hemorrhage. (7) Dot-and-blot hemorrhage. (8) Neovascularization of the disc. (9) Filled cup. (10) Disc hemorrhage. (11) Microaneurysms. (12) Retinal edema. (13) Hard exudates. (14) Cystoid macular degeneration. (15) Parallel sheathing.*

eases. It appears as an intravascular detachment, as a proliferation, or as hydrops.

Mechanisms

CRVO is considered to be produced by three mechanisms: *compression*, *stasis*, and *degeneration*.

External compression of the vein results from an adjacent arteriosclerosis of the central retinal artery, from a connective tissue strand within the floor of the physiologic cup, or from a blockage at the lamina cribrosa. It may be facilitated by multiple crossings of the same artery or vein or by congenital loops or twists of the vein.

Venous stasis reduces the intravenous perfusion pressure, causing collapse of the vein and slowing of the blood column flow. Usually, it occurs in glaucoma, spasm of the retinal arteries, periphlebitis, blood dyscrasia, hyperviscosity syndromes, sudden reduction of the arterial blood pressure, cardiac decompensation, surgical or traumatic shock, or carotid artery occlusion.

Degeneration of the venous endothelium is the cause of CRVO, as discussed.

Clinical Appearance

CRVO appears as multiple hemorrhages in a variety of shapes at the posterior pole but also throughout the retina. These are superficial hemorrhages, as a rule triangular, *with the tip pointed toward the disc*. There may be flame-shaped or splinter hemorrhages parallel to the distribution of the nerve fibers, preretinal hemorrhages with horizontal level fluid, or dot-and-blot or punctate hemorrhages. There are also microaneurysms isolated or clustered around the small veins. Veins appear tortuous, engorged, and dilated (like sausages) or may reveal dark blue boxcarring vessel segmentation, and the veins may have parallel sheathing. *Spontaneous or induced venous pulse is absent.* Arteries are narrowed, segmented, or virtually invisible. Sometimes, the macula is edematous, with cystoid degeneration. The disc may appear hemorrhagic, discolored, and dirty, with blurred or obscured margins, hemorrhages, and edema. There may be neovascularization of the disc (NVD) or collateral communications on the disc surface or within the retina. Cotton-wool spots, hard exudates, and retinal edema also may be present.

Symptoms

CRVO may be asymptomatic or it may produce decreased visual acuity, sometimes severe, with possible complete recovery of vision.

Diagnosis

Analysis of the visual field may show a centrocecal scotoma. Fluorescein angiography may reveal capillary nonperfusion and areas of fluorescein masked by intraretinal hemorrhages. ERG may show a bright-flash, dark-adapted **b-wave–to–a-wave amplitude ratio.** A complete blood cell count (CBC), SMA 12, and ESR should be performed. Protein and lipid serum levels should be determined. A rapid plasma reagin test (RPR) and a fluorescent treponemal antibody absorption test for syphilis (FTA-ABS) are warranted, as is an antinuclear antibody test (ANA) for systemic lupus erythematosus.

Differential Diagnosis

Conditions that should be considered in the differential diagnosis include diabetes, hypertension, hyperviscosity syndromes, carotid artery occlusion, and papilledema.

Histopathology

Histologic evaluation confirms a thickening of the adventitia of the obstructed vein walls, occasionally with hydrops and endothelial detachment. In the vein lumen, thrombus formed by the proliferation of the endothelial cells may occur. Also, blood between the endothelium and the remaining vein wall may create a **dissecting aneurysm.** Inflammatory cells in the lumen and in the wall of the vein may be present, and recanalization of the occluded central retinal vein may be seen. A disorganization of the ganglion cell layer occurs, and hemorrhagic infarction may result in the nerve fiber layer. Intraretinal hemorrhages often are found between the internal limiting membrane and the nerve fiber layer, and blood pockets may occur in the outer plexiform layer, which may form dot-and-blot hemorrhages. Microaneurysms, retinal edema, retinal detachment, and hemorrhagic necrosis may be present in addition to hemosiderin-laden macrophages, retinal gliosis, and irregular cystic spaces within the retina. At the lamina cribrosa, a fibrous tissue encircling the common adventitia of both the artery and the vein may produce arteriosclerosis and phlebosclerosis. Fibrinous exudates also are found.

Treatment

No medical treatment is helpful. *Anticoagulants are contraindicated in occlusion secondary to periphlebitis.* Treatment of the underlying cause is appropriate. Diuretics and oral contraceptives should be discontin-

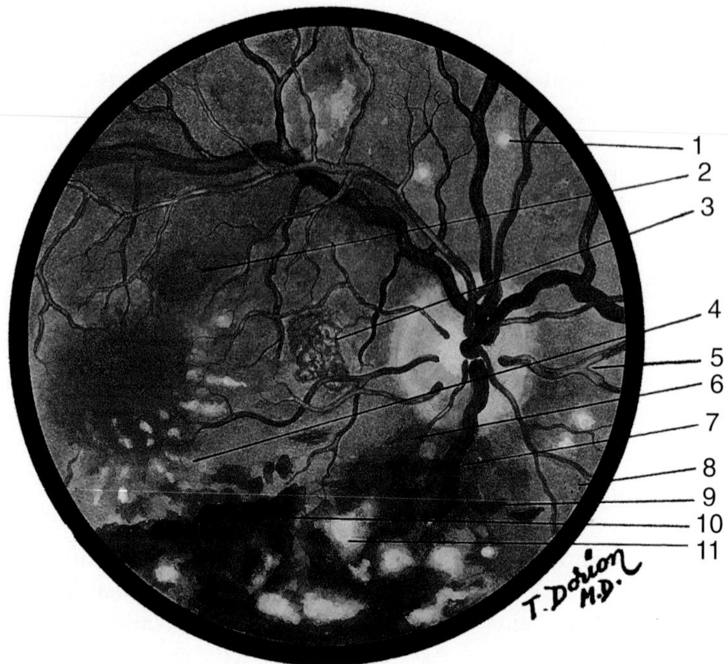

Figure 4-4. *Branch retinal vein occlusion. (1) Fatty infiltrates. (2) Vitreous bleeding. (3) Preretinal neovascularization. (4) Hard exudates. (5) Sheathed vessel. (6) Flame-shaped hemorrhage. (7) Dilated, tortuous vein. (8) Microaneurysms. (9) Preretinal hemorrhage. (10) Intraretinal hemorrhage. (11) Cotton-wool spots.*

ued, but aspirin, 60–360 mg/day PO, is beneficial. Early argon laser panretinal photocoagulation can be performed.

Branch Retinal Vein Occlusion

Branch retinal vein occlusion (BRVO) is a vascular retinopathy that consists of a blockage of the blood flow in a branch of the central retinal vein. It occurs frequently in the elderly with hypertension, diabetes, or arteriosclerosis (Figure 4-4).

BRVO usually is caused by a thrombus, an inflammation, or a degenerative process. It appears as an engorged, dilated, and markedly tortuous vein, distal to the occlusion, located more often at the AV crossing, at the edge of the disc, along the main vascular arcades, or peripherally and temporally. *The apex of the occlusion commonly is directed toward the AV crossing.* It results in multiple, superficial, flame-shaped striate hemorrhages or a deep intraretinal hemorrhage. The retina appears pie-shaped, with sharp delineation between the perfused and the nonperfused retina. Also seen are cotton-wool spots, fatty infiltrates, mild retinal edema, retinal fibrosis, vascular sheathing and sclerosis, circinate maculopathy or macular scars, and telangiectasia. Additionally, venous collaterals sometimes may be observed in the papillomacular bundle. In the late stage, a preretinal neovascularization may develop at the border of the involved and uninvolved retina, which may lead to vitreous bleeding. Occasionally, the vein may be prominent at its proximal segment, with subretinal hemorrhage, obliteration at the common sheath with the artery at the AV crossing, and mild retinal edema, which constitutes **prethrombotic Bonnet's sign**.

Ocular Ischemic Syndrome

Ocular ischemic syndrome (also termed *carotid occlusive disease*, *venous stasis retinopathy*, *hypoperfusion retinopathy*, or *hypotensive retinopathy*) is an occlusive vasculopathy, usually unilateral, which occurs more frequently in men aged 50–80 years (Figure 4-5). It is associated with hypertension, arteriosclerosis, previous cerebrovascular accidents, peripheral vascular disease, diabetes, giant-cell arteritis, or Eisenmenger's syndrome (ventriculoseptal defect with pulmonary hypertension and cyanosis).

Ocular ischemic syndrome is caused by a hypoperfusion of the retina owing to a severe carotid stenosis, at least 90% *critical stenosis* of the common or internal carotid artery in its extracranial portion, or by a choroidal perfusion defect.

The defect appears as retinal hemorrhages in the midperiphery (usually dot-and-blot hemorrhages), cotton-wool spots, microaneurysms, NVD, neovascularization elsewhere (NVE), and vitreous hemorrhage. Rarely, cherry-red spots may be present. Arteries are irregular and narrowed and, occasionally, there may be a *spontaneous pulsation of the arteries which, when present, is always pathologic.* Veins are dilated but *without tortuosity* and reveal sludged venous blood, venous beading, sheathing, and obliteration. AV anastomoses may be present, and the spontaneous venous pulse may be diminished or absent. Macular edema may occur, and the optic disc may show an AION. Occasionally, IOP is increased. Also, two types of microemboli are present. One is a bright, orange cholesterol embolus, slightly larger than the blood

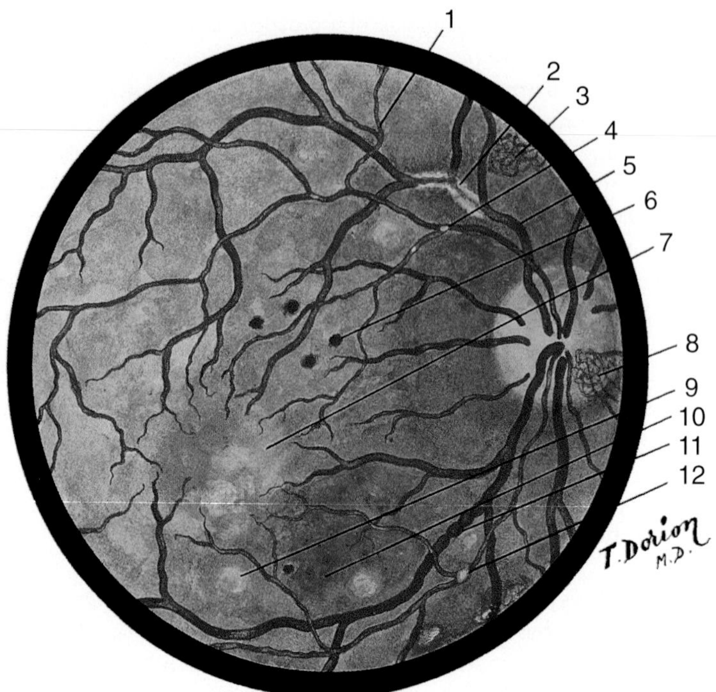

Figure 4-5. *Ocular ischemic syndrome. (1) Irregular, narrowed arteries. (2) Venous sheathing. (3) Neovascularization elsewhere (not in disc). (4) Platelet-fibrin embolus of approximately same size as the blood column. (5) Dilated but not tortuous veins. (6) Dot-and-blot hemorrhages. (7) Macular edema. (8) Neovascularization of the disc. (9) Cotton-wool spots. (10) Microaneurysms. (11) Venous beading. (12) Hollenhorst plaque, a cholesterol embolus larger than the blood column.*

column. It is located at or near the bifurcation of the artery and is called *Hollenhorst's plaque*. The other, a **platelet-fibrin embolus**, is gray-white, amorphous in structure, approximately the same size as the blood column, and mobile from one bifurcation to another.

Symptoms

The primary symptom of ocular ischemic syndrome is decreased visual acuity over a period of weeks or months, with an increased recovery time after exposure to bright light. Vision is blurred on going from a darkened area to a bright area. Additional symptoms include amaurosis fugax, afterimages, ocular and periocular aching pain, or ocular discomfort.

Diagnosis

Fluorescein angiography may reveal a delay in the retinal perfusion. In addition, it may confirm choroidal perfusion, capillary nonperfusion, microaneurysms, a slow arm-to-retina or -AV transit time, a late staining of the retinal vessels (especially the arteries), and (sometimes) a marked macular edema. Auscultation over the supraclavicular area may reveal a bruit. Periorbital and carotid Doppler ultrasonography may detect blood flow velocity changes. Duplex ultrasonography, with two techniques—a *pulse echo* or *b-mode ultrasonography*, which may give the anatomic image of the vessel, and a *pulsed Doppler ultrasonography*—may assess the changes in the blood flow. ERG shows diminution or a marked reduction of *a-* and *b-waves*.

Ophthalmodynamometry may show a reduction in the systolic pressure of the ophthalmic artery on the side of the carotid occlusion. Further confirmation can be obtained by oculoplethysmography and oculopneumoplethysmography and by carotid arteriography if surgery is planned.

Differential Diagnosis

Conditions that should be considered in the differential diagnosis are CRVO, diabetes, arteriosclerosis, hypertension, aortic arch syndrome, syphilis, and Takayasu's disease.

Histopathology

Histologic analysis shows microinfarctions in the nerve fiber layer and ganglion cell layer. Blood pockets in the inner nuclear layer and the outer plexiform layer are present. Spaces with fluid and cell debris may be found in the outer plexiform layer of the macula. Calcium or platelet-fibrin deposits occluding the lumen of the arteries may be present. There may be a decreased *pericyte-to–endothelial cell ratio* (normal, 1:1).

Treatment

Usually, treatment is not helpful. Carotid endarterectomy may be performed. Treatment may include extracranial-to-intracranial bypass, such as a superficial temporal artery to the middle cerebral artery. Platelet antiaggregation agents, such as aspirin, may be used. For treatment of neovascular glaucoma, panretinal photocoagulation can be combined with cryotherapy. Treatment of diabetes, hypertension, and hypercholesterolemia should be determined by the internist.

Carotid-Cavernous Fistula

The carotid-cavernous fistula is a communication between the internal or external carotid artery and the cavernous sinus. Usually, it is stationary and causes a shunt of the arterial blood to the orbital veins and raises the orbital and episcleral venous pressure.

Carotid-cavernous fistula may occur *spontaneously* in middle-aged or elderly women, owing to a rupture of the internal carotid artery, of an infraclinoid aneurysm, or of an arteriosclerotic artery onto the cavernous sinus. The condition also may occur after a cerebral *trauma*, usually in a younger age group, with severe fracture of the base of the skull, particularly basilotemporal fracture, as in motor vehicle accidents; or in penetrating orbitocranial wounds, including knife injuries; or from excessive straining during childbirth. Alternatively, it may be iatrogenic after transsphenoidal pituitary surgery, internal carotid endarterectomy, ethmoidal sinus surgery, or percutaneous gasserian procedure.

It may be *direct* or *indirect* (as a dural shunt) or *acute* or *chronic*, with *high flow* or *low flow.* It may close spontaneously within 3–18 months.

Barrow's Classification

The Barrow's classification describes four angiographic types. **Type A** is a direct shunt between the internal carotid artery and the cavernous sinus, with high venous pressure and flow. **Type B** represents a dural shunt between meningeal branches of the internal carotid artery and the cavernous sinus. **Type C** is characterized by a dural shunt between meningeal branches of the external carotid artery and the cavernous sinus. **Type D** delineates a dural shunt between both the internal and the external carotid arteries and the cavernous sinus.

Mechanisms and Clinical Appearance

Carotid-cavernous fistula is caused by an increased orbital and episcleral venous pressure, consequently producing orbital and ocular hypoxia that may result in a secondary glaucoma and rubeosis iridis. The defect appears as numerous intraretinal hemorrhages scattered throughout the fundus. Retinal vessels are tortuous and irregularly dilated. Spontaneous venous pulsation usually is absent. Occasionally, there may be protein flare and cells in the vitreous. Stasis retinopathy, such as in the ocular ischemic syndrome, may be present. Often, there is an optic nerve ischemia or a papilledema.

Symptoms

A *high-flow shunt* is characterized by an acute asymmetric proptosis, which may be pulsating and which may improve on one side only to increase on the opposite side, contralateral to the fistula. Dilatation and arterialization of the conjunctival vessels occur in a corkscrew pattern. Marked conjunctival chemosis may be observed, as is eyelid swelling. Also noticeable are rubeosis iridis and ophthalmoplegia. Trill and ocular or cephalic bruit is synchronous with the pulse, is audible by both examiner and patient, and is likened to the buzz of a bluebottle fly within a paper bag. It is abolished by ipsilateral carotid compression. The defect may also produce decreased vision, diplopia, headache, and pain.

A *low-flow shunt* results in dilated conjunctival vessels. Secondary glaucoma, abducens (sixth) cranial nerve palsy, and (less commonly) third, fourth, and seventh nerve palsies occur. Additional effects include small abduction defect and chronic unilateral redness. A low-flow shunt may precipitate rapidly progressive cataract.

Diagnosis

A computed tomography (CT) scan may show a prominent dilatation of the superior ophthalmic vein and, less frequently, moderate enlargement of the horizontal recti muscles, especially the medial rectus, and lateral bulging of the cavernous sinus. A-scan ultrasonography may reveal a dilated superior ophthalmic vein that has very low reflectivity, extending from the superior nasal aspect of the orbit posteriorly to the superior orbital fissure, with blurred spikes within the dilated vessel, indicating an increased blood flow.

B-scan ultrasonography may reveal a large, dilated superior ophthalmic vein, coursing from the superonasal orbit toward the orbital apex. Carotid angiography may reveal an opacification of the cavernous sinus and extensive filling of dural venous channels and orbital veins.

Differential Diagnosis

The conditions of CRVO and thyroid orbitopathy are possible diagnoses.

Treatment

Observation is the standard of treatment. Two procedures are possible to relieve the visual deterioration. First, surgical repair may be effected by intravascular closure using detachable balloon microcatheterization. Second, embolization with isobutyl-2-cryoacrylate or polyvinyl alcohol particles may be performed. Additionally, arterial ligature, trapping procedures, and direct intracranial attack may be used. Treatment of glaucoma includes administration of beta-blockers (timolol [Timoptic] 0.5%, 1 drop OU twice a day; levobunolol [Betagan] 0.5%, 1 drop OU twice a day; or carteolol [Ocupress] 1%, 1 drop OU twice a day), alpha-selective agonists (apraclonidine [Iopidine] 0.5%, 1 drop OU twice a day, or epinephrine [Glaucon] 2%, 1 drop OU three times a day), prostaglandins (lanatoprost [Xalatan] 0.005%, 1 drop OU once a day), or carbon anhydrase inhibitors (acetazolamide [Diamox sequels], one 500-mg sustained-release capsule PO twice a day). Filtering surgery often is used.

Cilioretinal Artery Occlusion

Cilioretinal artery occlusion is an infarcted retinal zone in the area supplied by the cilioretinal artery. The artery is a normal variation of the fundus arising from the vascular circle of Zinn behind the optic disc in the sclera and from the short posterior ciliary arteries, and it represents anastomosis between the choroidal and retinal circulation. It is present in some 20% of eyes. Cilioretinal artery occlusion may occur either in isolation or in association with CRVO or AION. It consists of two types, *arteritic* and *nonarteritic*.

Cilioretinal artery occlusion is caused by an ischemia or an inflammation (due probably to an occlusion of the short posterior ciliary artery), by an embolus from a carotid artery disease (e.g., Hollenhorst plaque), by heart disease (calcified valves, subacute bacterial endocarditis, left atrium thrombus, atrial myxoma), or by an autoimmune mechanism.

The defect appears as a pale whitening of the retina with cloudy swelling and is located superotemporal to the disc and above the macula, in the area of distribution of the cilioretinal artery. Occasionally, there may be a clumping of the blood column of the artery (*cattle trucking*). Conversely, the artery may appear as a hook that emerges from the temporal margin of the disc separate from the central retinal artery. In cilioretinal artery occlusion, the central retinal artery often is shunted.

The macula commonly is spared. Veins may be dilated and tortuous, and retinal hemorrhages may be present in the area. The disc is pale in the arteritic form and is hyperemic in the nonarteritic form. *A patency of the ciliary artery in cases of CRAO may allow a maintenance of vision*, by sparing a small area of the retina in the papillomacular bundle.

Diagnosis

Fluorescein angiography may reveal nonfilling of the cilioretinal artery superotemporal to the disc above the macula or may show only partial filling in the later AV phase.

Histopathology

Histologic examination reveals that there is an infarction in the retinal nerve fiber layer and ganglion cell layer. The macular region is normal, because it is devoid of these two layers.

Hypertensive Retinopathy

Hypertensive retinopathy is a vascular retinopathy that may occur in any stage of hypertension. The disease is classified into several groups: Keith-Wagener-Barker, Sheie's, Leishman's, Wagener-Clay-Gipner, and Thiel's.

Keith-Wagener-Barker Classification

In the Keith-Wagener-Barker classification, hypertension has four grades. **Grade 1** exhibits brightened arterial light reflex, moderate arterial attenuation, and focal arterial narrowing. *Arterial attenuation* is a focal or generalized constriction of the artery appearing as a thin red thread beyond the second bifurcation.

Grade 2 includes copper-wire reflex, silver-wire reflex, hard exudates, flame-shaped hemorrhages, Gunn's sign, and Salus' sign. *Copper-wire reflex* is a brighter arterial reflex: a burnished, metallic, copperlike streak that may occupy most of the vessel width. *Silver-wire reflex* is an increased arterial reflex in which the artery appears as a whitish tube containing a red fluid. *Hard exudates* are small, whitish yellow deposits of **lipoprotein**. They are waxy, refractile, and sharply delineated and are scattered throughout the fundus and located deep in the retinal outer plexiform layer or in the inner nuclear layer. *Flame-shaped hemorrhages* (*linear*, *streak*, or *splinter hemorrhages*) are superficial hemorrhages located in the nerve fiber layer. *Gunn's sign* is a deviation of a vein downward and laterally at the AV crossing. *Salus' sign* is deviation of a vein at a right angle, as an S or a Z, at the AV crossing, where the vein gradually becomes smaller and thinner, such that a segment of it is concealed.

Grade 3 contains marked arterial attenuation, cotton-wool spots, dot-and-blot hemorrhages, and retinal edema. *Cotton-wool spots* are microinfarcts located in the nerve fiber layer. *Dot-and-blot hemorrhages* are retinal hemorrhages located in the inner nuclear layer and in the outer plexiform layer. *Retinal edema* is a milky opacity of the retina, due usually to a sudden complete occlusion of an artery. It renders the fundus details indistinct, whereas the reflexes are more numerous, heightened, and irregular.

Grade 4 designates all the preceding characteristics and includes Elschnig's spots, Siegrist's streaks, tortuosity, sheathing, chorioretinal atrophy, and papilledema (Figure 4-6). *Elschnig's spots* are isolated yellow-gray, round spots with pigmented centers surrounded by a yellow or red halo. *Siegrist's streaks* are fine pigmented flecks or clusters and yellow-white streaks arranged linearly as chains along the sclerosed choroidal vessels. *Papilledema* is a swelling of the optic nerve head usually associated with other retinopathies. It contrasts with the **plerocephalic papilledema** of increased intracranial pressure, which is confined to the disc and usually lacks any other signs of retinal vascular disease.

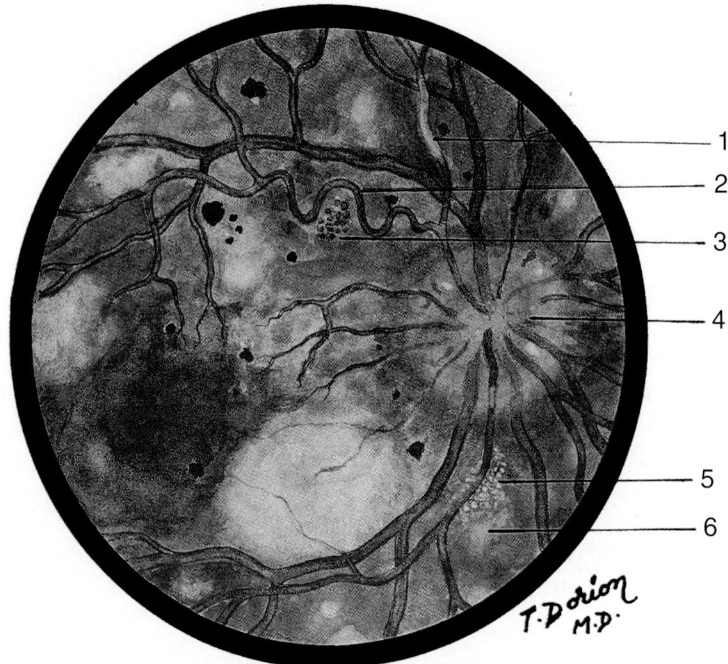

Figure 4-6. *Hypertensive retinopathy, grade IV, according to the Keith-Wagener-Barker classification. All changes seen in grade III occur—arterial attenuation, cotton-wool spots, hemorrhages, and retinal edema—plus (1) arterial sheathing, (2) arterial tortuosity, (3) Elschnig's spots, (4) papilledema, (5) Siegrist's streaks, and (6) chorioretinal atrophy.*

Scheie's Classification

Scheie's classification is based on the correlation between the changes in hypertension and the degree of retinal arteriosclerosis. It also has four grades. **Grade 1** represents slight, generalized arterial attenuation, arterial narrowing in secondary branches, and a broadened light reflex. **Grade 2** includes focal arterial attenuation, more arterial narrowing, and minimal AV changes. **Grade 3** embodies severe arterial attenuation, cotton-wool spots, and hemorrhages, copper-wire reflex, and more AV changes. **Grade 4** is composed of all the foregoing characteristics and silver-wire reflex, severe AV changes, and papilledema.

Leishman's Classification

The basis of the Leishman classification is correlation of the fundus picture with elevation of the blood pressure, age, and degree of involutional sclerosis of the patient.

Wagener-Clay-Gipner Classification

The Wagener-Clay-Gipner classification divides hypertension into five stages: (1) **neurogenic** (no ocular fundus pathologic findings); (2) **acute angiospastic** (generalized arterial narrowing, focal arterial constriction, retinal edema, cotton-wool spots, papilledema); (3) **benign chronic nonprogressive** (mild generalized arteriosclerosis, ischemic or hemorrhagic infarctions); (4) **benign chronic progressive** (generalized arteriolar narrowing, focal arterial constriction, arteriosclerosis, cotton-wool spots, hemorrhages); and (5) **terminal malignant** (generalized arteriosclerosis and arterial narrowing, focal arterial constriction, papilledema, retinal edema, macular star, cotton-wool spots).

Thiel's Classification

By Thiel's classification, hypertension represents four stages. **Stage 1** includes *early-stage hypertension*: deep red fundus reflex, distension and tortuosity of the arteries, copper-wire reflex, and early AV crossing signs. **Stage 2** is typified by *benign, late-stage hypertension* or *hypertension with sclerosis*: arterial thickening with segmental variation in vessel diameter and marked AV crossing signs. The stage includes few hard exudates and hemorrhages and maintains a normal optic disc. **Stage 3** designates *early angiospastic retinopathy*: arterial narrowing, nicking at AV crossings, cotton-wool spots, flame-shaped hemorrhages, and mild papilledema. **Stage 4** represents *late angiospastic retinopathy*: pale fundus, arterial segmentation, venous beading, silver-wire reflex, cotton-wool spots, macular star, and papilledema.

Clinical Types

Clinically, there may be four forms of hypertension: (1) *early* hypertension, (2) *fulminating* or *accelerated* hypertension, (3) *severe* hypertension, and (4) *malignant* hypertension. In **early hypertension**, the fundus background may appear normal, or it may appear as arterial narrowing, which usually first affects the nasal branches. The arterial reflex is increased and then may become narrower, glistening, and harder. Arteries branch at an increased angle, with **omega formation** at times, in a whiplike or corkscrew tortuosity with a firm filling. There is a **copper-wire reflex**—a burnished metallic reflex—due to a compensatory thickening of the arterial wall. A **Gunn's sign** is evident, a compression of a vein by an artery, as is a **Salus' sign**, a deflection of the course of a vein beneath the artery. Focal, localized, symmetric constriction of the arteries occurs, the artery abruptly changing from normal to constricted and then back to normal caliber. There is venous beading and some venous stasis with vein congestion distal to the AV crossing but *no vein concealment*. Hard exudates may be arranged in a circular garland pattern in the macula, forming a **circinate maculopathy**. At the periphery, some punched-out, depigmented areas may be present.

Fulminant or **accelerated hypertension** produces flame-shaped hemorrhages (also called *streak hemorrhages*), cotton-wool spots, and hard exudates as a **macular star**, retinal edema, microaneurysms, marked arterial attenuation and narrowing, tortuosity, parallel sheathing, and papilledema. *There is no arterial fibrosis.*

In **severe hypertension**, there is arterial fibrosis, hypertonia, and hyperplasia of the arteries. Veins are congested and humping, with banking at the AV crossing. Superficial and deep hemorrhages and spontaneous vitreous hemorrhages occur.

Malignant hypertension results in a generalized arterial narrowing, flame-shaped hemorrhages, cotton-wool spots, hard exudates as a macular star, choroidal sclerosis, arteriosclerosis, chorioretinal atrophy, Elschnig's spots, and Siegrist's streaks.

Histopathology

In *early hypertension*, histologic examination reveals that the artery wall is not thickened and portions of the vessel are collagenous with scant nuclei, but otherwise the wall is normal. Occasionally, elastic fibers may be absent, but no swelling or proliferation of the artery endothelium is seen. Capillaries are circular and patent, of uniform diameter just wider than the red blood cells. There may be a disturbance of retinal pigmentation and drusen in the Bruch's membrane.

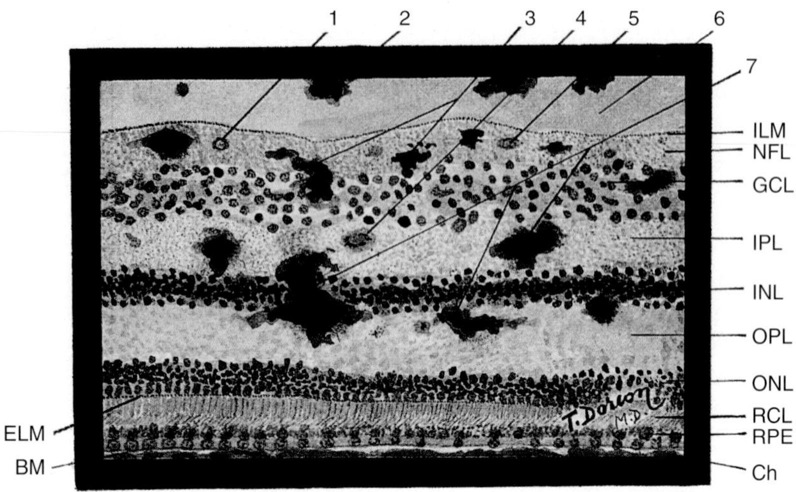

Figure 4-7. *Histopathologic findings in severe hypertension. (1) Hypertonic arterial segment. (2) Vitreous hemorrhages. (3) Superficial retinal hemorrhages in the nerve fiber layer. (4) Fibrotic arterial segment. (5) Hyperplastic arterial segment. (6) Vitreous. (7) Deep intraretinal hemorrhages in the inner plexiform layer, inner nuclear layer, and outer plexiform layer. (ILM, internal limiting membrane; NFL, nerve fiber layer; GCL, ganglion cell layer; IPL, inner plexiform layer; INL, inner nuclear layer; OPL, outer plexiform layer; ONL, outer nuclear layer; RCL, rod and cone layer [photoreceptors]; RPE, retinal pigment epithelium; Ch, choroid; BM, Bruch's membrane; ELM, external limiting membrane.)*

In *fulminant* or *accelerated hypertension*, hemorrhages and microinfarcts are observed in the nerve fiber layer. Hard exudates accumulate deep into the retina, underneath the vessels, or as a macular star in a radial distribution in the outer plexiform layer of Henle. Swelling of the optic disc may be present. Retinal edema with arterial occlusion also may be present. *Usually, arterial fibrosis is absent.*

In *benign chronic hypertension*, a hyaline degeneration of the walls is seen, which starts with a subendothelial deposition of lipohyaline material, continues with a gradual conversion into a homogeneous hyaline tube with a narrow lumen, and ends in hyperplastic sclerosis.

Severe hypertension (Figure 4-7) reveals fibrosis, hyperplasia, and hypertonia of different portions of the arteries. Vitreous hemorrhages and superficial and deep retinal hemorrhages also may be present. Two conditions characterize *hypertension with reactive sclerosis*. In the **fibrotic segment**, the artery has a wide lumen and a relatively thin wall and is acellular and collagenous, with numerous elastic fibers. The **hyperplastic segment** reveals a narrow lumen, and the wall is thickened. Numerous cell nuclei and new elastic fibers are seen. In the **hypertonic segment**, the wall has normal thickness but the elastic fibers are present even in small arteries. This condition is called *elastosis*.

Symptoms

Usually, hypertensive retinopathy is asymptomatic. Occasionally, it results in decreased visual acuity.

Diagnosis

Fluorescein angiography shows arteriolar constriction, with microaneurysms, capillary nonperfusion, and increased permeability. Diagnosis can be confirmed with blood pressure testing.

Differential Diagnosis

In the differential diagnosis, consideration should be given to the possibility that anemia, collagen vascular disease, diabetes, CRVO, or radiation retinopathy is present.

Treatment

Treatment of hypertensive retinopathy should be determined and performed by the internist.

Arteriosclerosis and Atherosclerosis

Arteriosclerosis is a diffuse hardening and stiffening of the smaller arteries (less than 300 μm) and of arterioles less than 30 μm (Figure 4-8). It occurs in hypertensive or obese patients or in the elderly as a result of the natural aging process. Arteriosclerosis is due to fibrosis and

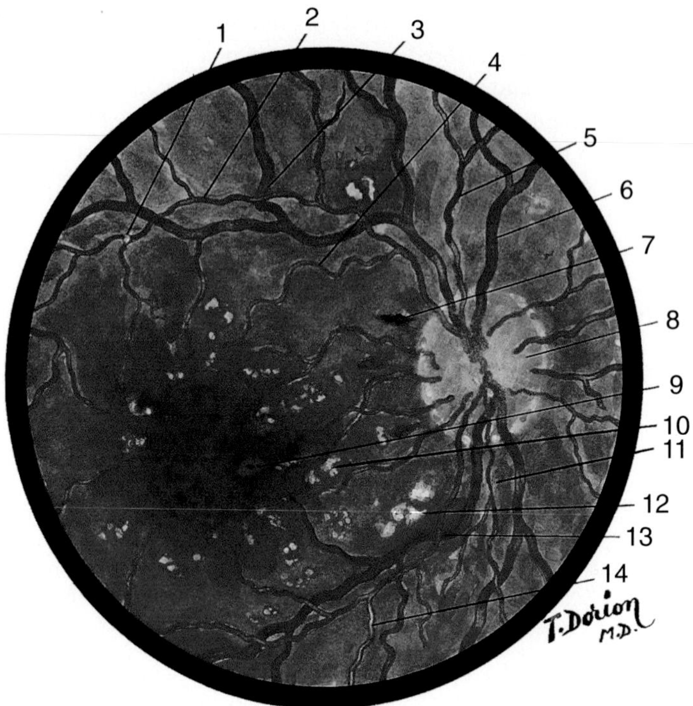

Figure 4-8. *Arteriosclerosis and atherosclerosis. (1) Hollenhorst plaque. (2) Narrowed arteries, of irregular caliber. (3) Salus' sign. (4) Tortuosities of the arteries. (5) Copper-wire reflex. (6) Dilated veins. (7) Flame-shaped hemorrhages. (8) Ischemic papillary edema. (9) Cherry-red spot. (10) Circinate maculopathy. (11) Perivascular sheathing. (12) Hard exudates. (13) Gunn's sign. (14) Silver-wire reflex.*

hyalinization of the arterial walls, which may cause a permanent increase of their rigidity, with a consequent diminution in both distensibility and resiliency, and which have a generalized hypertonus that increases the peripheral resistance.

In the early stage, arteriosclerosis appears as an enhanced yellow, refractile, thin light reflex, perhaps one-fifth the width of the blood column. Vessels are focally attenuated and are irregular in caliber. As the arteriosclerosis progresses, the blood column appears wider than normal, and the light reflex becomes broader. The vessel's wall loses its transparency, becomes visible, and assumes a metallic, rusty color owing to the blending of the yellow lipid and red blood. This condition is called *copper-wire reflex*.

In a later stage, the vessel assumes a whitish, pipe-stem appearance, called *silver-wire reflex*, as evidence of a severe arteriosclerosis. There may be marked tortuosity of the arteries, capillary exudates, and hard exudates, or even an occlusion of a retinal arterial branch. At the AV crossing, the vein is deviated, pushed downward and laterally, and is narrowed, with banking of the blood distally (*Gunn's sign*). There may be an arcuate vein deviated at a right angle at the AV crossing, where it gradually becomes smaller and thinner under the artery, concealing a segment of the vein (*Salus' sign*). The disc may be normal, ischemic, swollen, or even atrophic.

According to **Scheie's classification**, arteriosclerosis can be categorized into four grades. **Grade 1** represents increase or broadening of the light reflex, with minimal AV compression and vein concealment. **Grade 2** includes grade 1 plus a deflection of the vein at the AV crossing (Salus' sign). **Grade 3** encompasses grade 2, more AV compression, and copper-wire reflex. **Grade 4** includes grade 3, severe AV crossing changes, and silver-wire reflex.

Atherosclerosis is a progressive degenerative, localized hardening of the arteries. It is characterized by **atheroma**—a patchy accumulation of lipid and fibrosis in larger and medium-sized retinal arteries (more than 300 μm), such as the central retinal artery. Some probable contributing factors are hyperlipemia, obesity, hypertension, diabetes, and heredity. Alternatively, it may be a part of an *atherosclerotic disease* involving the internal carotid artery.

The condition is due to a fatty infiltration of the arterial walls and is associated with fibrosis. Sometimes, it may form a plug that interrupts the blood column, completely occluding the lumen in a wide portion of the artery and producing a retinal ischemia or edema.

Atherosclerosis appears as retinal arteries with caliber variation and rigid walls, because the lumen remains wide distal to the lesion. Initially, there may be an intermittent and localized spasm of the narrowed arteries, and the retina may appear opalescent from edema. The arterial blood column takes a straight course, and its color becomes darker, similar to the venous blood. The artery may be seen to empty and to refill with changes of posture. An atheroma usually is located in that portion of the central retinal artery that lies within the optic nerve, where the artery penetrates the dural sheath, and at the lamina cribrosa. The blood column appears normal proximal to the occlusion.

After several weeks, white, straight, parallel sheathing and diffuse arteriosclerosis may occur. An opaque white mass occasionally erodes, or even obscures, part of the blood column. Often, there may be glistening, refractile, yellow spots or plaques (*Hollenhorst plaques*) that arise from the atheroma and consist of emboli of cholesterol or fibrin. They usually lodge at the bifurcation of the arteries and may be larger than the vessel. Veins may appear dilated, with normal spontaneous central retinal vein pulsation. Capillaries may be varicose or may even rupture. Superficial, flame-shaped hemorrhages may be present. The retina may appear opaque and milky, with an ischemic edema that may cross the disc borders. At the macula, where the superficial retinal layers are thin, there may be a red area (*cherry-red spot*) in which the choroid is visible. Also visible may be macular exudates, macular degeneration, or circinate maculopathy. Sometimes, hard exudates may be seen. The disc may be pale, with sharply delineated margins, or occasionally an ischemic papillary edema may be present.

Symptoms

Arteriosclerosis and atherosclerosis may be asymptomatic. However, they may result in decreased vision.

Diagnosis

Diagnosis by fluorescein angiography may reveal arteriolar narrowing and focal areas of capillary obliteration. Carotid artery angiography may show a markedly narrowed lumen of the internal carotid artery or a concave pooling of the radio-opaque contrast dye in an area of the ulceration.

Histopathology

On histologic examination of atherosclerosis, a fibrosis in the media and adventitia of the central retinal artery is observed. The endothelium may be hyperplastic, the media may be hypertrophic, and the intima may be hyalinized. There is a subendothelial deposition of fat and fibrosis. The arterial wall is thickened and may have lipid streaks that progress to a fibrous plaque. The atheroma reveals an excessive amount of collagen elastic tissue and cellular infiltration.

Arteriosclerosis is characterized by focal necrosis, thickening of the intima, and hyperplastic and degenerative changes, especially in the muscular coat and in the internal elastic lamina. There may be ulceration, hemorrhage, thrombosis, and calcification, as well as organization and canalization within the lesion. There may be destruction of the elastic and muscular tissue of the media, which may produce ectasia and vessel ruptures. Cellular concentration may occur in some portions of the vein's wall and in the optic nerve in an area between the hyperplastic site and the arterial lesion.

Neovascularization Elsewhere

NVE describes new vessels that develop anywhere in the retina (Figure 4-9)—including the macula or the choroid, adjacent to an area of capillary closure—*except on the optic disc or within 1 dd of it.* NVE occurs after a BRVO, in retinopathy of prematurity (ROP), sickle cell anemia, diabetes, hemoglobinopathies, beta-thalassemia, Eales' disease, hyperviscosity syndromes, leukemia, age-related macular degeneration, disciform macular degeneration, familial exudative vitreoretinopathy, toxoplasmosis, sarcoidosis, histoplasmosis, myopia, angioid streaks, choroidal melanoma, choroidal rupture, toxemia of pregnancy, and multiple sclerosis, in IV drug abusers, or as a complication of laser photocoagulation. NVE may be caused by *angiogenic factors*, either *mitogenic* or *chemotoxic*, that are secreted from a zone of retinal ischemia, where a retinal capillary closure is a precursor of the retinal neovascularization.

NVE may be **classic** or **occult**. Three types—retinal, subretinal, and choroidal neovascularization—are recognized. **Retinal neovascularization** appears as new vessels on the surface of the retina, *not within the retina*, initially forming a flat area of superficial fine blood vessels, each with saccular and dilated tips that often are two to four times larger than the vessel's caliber. These vessels later arborize and cluster. They may extend into the vitreous and may bleed. At a later stage, the vessels appear as fibrotic fronds. In stage I of ROP, neovascularization usually develops at the periphery, at the junction between the vascularized and nonvascularized retina, where a *demarcation line* may be present. This line may signify the onset of the disease. There are cotton-wool spots and microaneurysms.

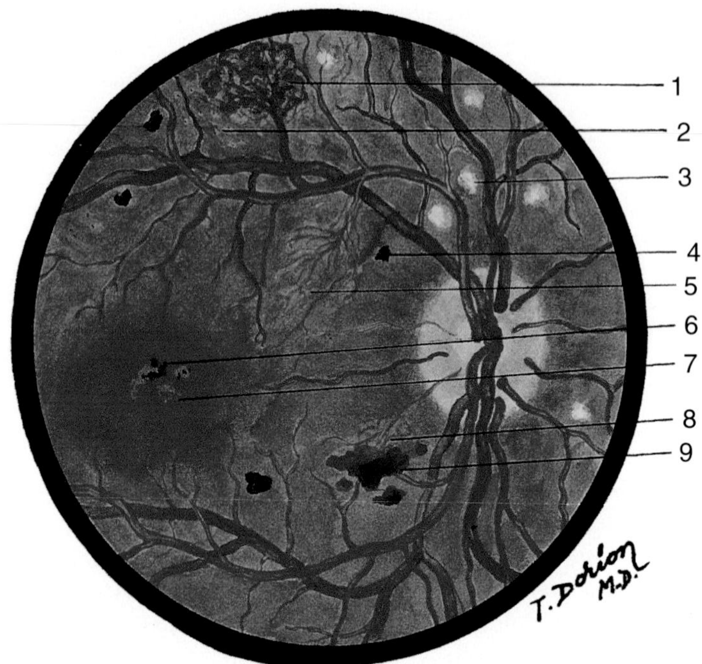

Figure 4-9. *Neovascularization elsewhere (other than in the disc). (1) Retinal neovascularization. (2) Microaneurysms. (3) Cotton-wool spots. (4) Pigment clumping. (5) Choroidal neovascularization. (6) Pigment dispersion. (7) Macular neovascularization. (8) Subretinal neovascularization. (9) Retinal hemorrhage.*

Subretinal neovascularization is characterized by new vessels beneath the retina, often obscured by hemorrhage, turbid serous fluid, excessive pigment clumping, or even retinal pigment epithelium (RPE) detachment. In the latter cases, the condition is called *occult subretinal neovascularization.* It may be associated with sensory retinal detachment, exudates, choroidal folds, or RPE tears.

Choroidal neovascularization features new vessels beneath the RPE, which usually arise adjacent to a vein as a dirty gray area of discoloration or as a membrane with an encircling pigment ring, called a *choroidal neovascular membrane.*

Symptoms

Blurred vision occurs, and edges or straight lines appear distorted.

Diagnosis

In an early phase, fluorescein angiography may reveal a hyperfluorescent, intense, bright filling with demarcated borders and retinal capillary nonperfusion adjacent to the new vessels. In a later stage, considerable accumulation of fluorescein leakage may be seen in the subsensory space. Digital indocyanine green videoangiography may help to establish the diagnosis. Visual field examination may reveal a cecoparacentral scotoma.

Histopathology

On histologic evaluation, new vessels are seen to arise from the choroid and to pass through pre-existing breaks in the Bruch's membrane or to produce such breaks and are located beneath the RPE or in the subsensory retinal spaces. Often, small cysts are present in the overlying retina. Anastomoses between the choroidal vessels and the retinal vessels occur frequently. In time, the fibrous tissue may proliferate and become dominant, after which a scar forms, and new vessels intermittently bleed at its edges.

Treatment

Argon laser photocoagulation sometimes is effective for extrafoveolar, juxtafoveolar, or subfoveolar neovascularization, especially if the neovascularization is located at least 200 µm from the foveolar avascular zone (FAZ). Application of 200-µm spots with 0.2- to 0.5-second duration for full coverage, using a red, green, or yellow wavelength, is appropriate. Antiangiogenic drugs also are appropriate.

Eales' Disease

Eales' disease (also known as *primary retinal perivasculitis*, *periphlebitis retinae*, and *peripheral idiopathic retinal vascular occlusive disease*) is

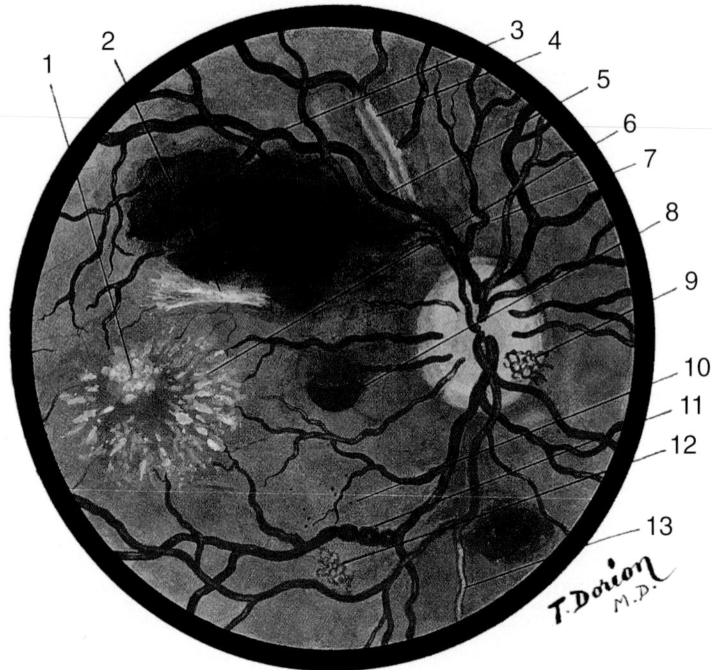

Figure 4-10. *Eales' disease. (1) Cystoid macular edema. (2) Retinitis proliferans. (3) Dilated vessels. (4) Perivenous exudate sheathing. (5) Vitreous hemorrhage. (6) Macular star. (7) Tortuous vessels. (8) Preretinal hemorrhage. (9) Neovascularization of the disc. (10) Microaneurysms. (11) Venous beading. (12) Neovascularization elsewhere (other than in the disc). (13) Ghost vessel.*

a bilateral, chronic, slowly progressive, obliterative retinal vasculopathy of unknown etiology that occurs more frequently in young men aged 20–40 years (Figure 4-10). It is usually associated with sarcoidosis, diabetes, systemic lupus erythematosus, sickle cell anemia, and collagen vascular disease. It may be due to a progressive ischemic process in the peripheral retina, and a vasculitis of the retinal veins, associated with recurrent vitreous hemorrhages and neovascular proliferation.

The disease appears as an irregular, creamy white, fluffy, perivenous cuffing or as patchy exudation of peripheral vessels, especially around the equatorial retinal veins (**periphlebitis**). There may also be segmental *parallel sheathing* of the veins, evidenced as white lines on both sides of the blood column or as a thick, heavy exudate, sometimes completely concealing the blood column or obscuring it in a thin haze. Peripheral veins and arteries may be dilated, markedly tortuous, or obliterated, often appearing as white lines of **ghost vessels**. There may be microaneurysms, arteriovenous anastomoses, and venous beading. Cystoid macular edema, circinate retinopathy, epiretinal membranes, or macular holes also may be seen. Often, NVD, NVE, an extensive fibrovascular proliferation, and fibrosis may occur. Sometimes preretinal hemorrhages extend into the vitreous. Retinal and vitreous hemorrhages recur every few months over a period of several years but then may clear completely, leading to a fibrous tissue formation called *retinitis proliferans*. Occasionally, retinal detachment or even secondary glaucoma may develop.

Symptoms

Eales' disease is marked by sudden loss of vision and the appearance of black spots with flashing lights.

Diagnosis

Fluorescein angiography may reveal segmental leakage around the retinal veins, hyperfluorescence and abnormal staining in the areas of excessive arteriolar sheathing, and peripheral capillary nonperfusion, particularly temporal, that is confluent with and sharply demarcated from the posterior perfused retina, with vascular abnormalities at the junction.

Histopathology

Histopathologic evaluation reveals perivascular lymphocytic infiltration with plasma cells and small granulomas, located perivascularly in the vessel wall and in the lumen. Veins may be occluded. Pockets of blood in the vitreous or preretinally are usually present.

Treatment

New vessels can be photocoagulated. Vitrectomy also is effective.

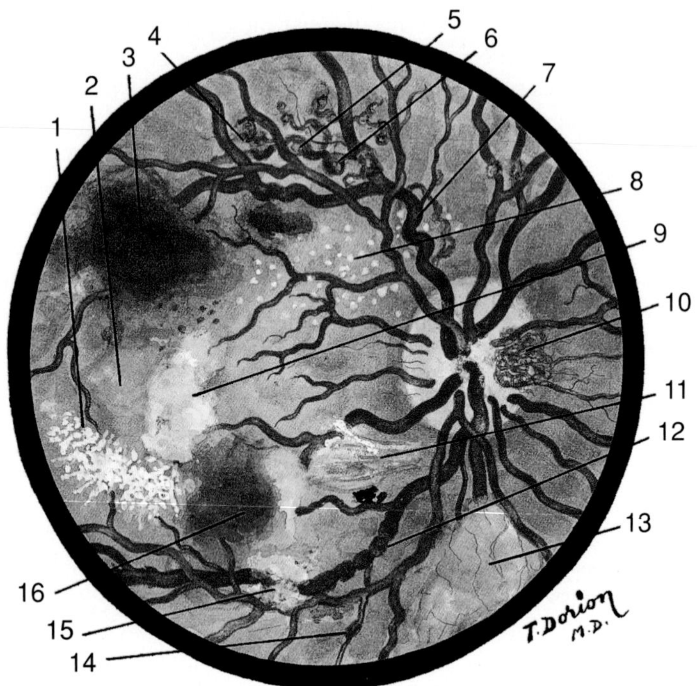

Figure 4-11. *Coats' disease. (1) Paramacular hard exudates, sometimes as circinate maculopathy or macular star. (2) Macular edema. (3) Vitreous hemorrhage. (4) Peripheral telangiectasia of arteries and veins. (5) Vessel anomalies. (6) Macroaneurysms. (7) Tortuous vessels, irregular in caliber. (8) Refractile cholesterol deposits (crystalline bodies). (9) Massive yellowish white exudate beneath the retinal vessels, located usually inferotemporally. (10) Neovascularization of the disc. (11) Proliferative retinopathy. (12) Venous beading. (13) Exudative retinal detachment. (14) Fusiform dilatations of peripheral vessels ("lightbulbs"). (15) Perivascular hard exudates. (16) Retinal hemorrhage.*

Coats' Disease

Coats' disease (also known as *congenital retinal telangiectasia*, *exudative retinitis*, and *hemorrhagic retinitis*) is a congenital, nonhereditary, usually unilateral anomaly of the retinal vessels, a chronic, slowly progressive retinal telangiectasia (Figure 4-11) of unknown etiology, probably of developmental origin, that occurs primarily in boys and men from 2 to 25 years of age. Coats' disease, together with Leber's miliary aneurysms and idiopathic perifoveal retinal telangiectasia may constitute a single primary vascular disease.

Coats' disease may be caused by a breakdown of the blood-retina barrier at the level of the retinal vascular endothelium, with leakage of plasma constituents and lipoprotein exudates into the retina and in the subretinal space through abnormally permeable vessels. Capillary toxins may play a role by producing severe capillary damage.

Massive, white-gray or yellow-white exudates are seen beneath the retinal vessels and located anywhere in the fundus. These exudates may simulate a tumor, such as retinoblastoma or pseudoglioma. Some of them are waxy and disappear in one area only to occur in another. Also seen is macular edema or lipid exudation arranged in the juxtafoveolar region as a **macular star**. Vessels are tortuous and irregular in caliber, with thickened walls, and there is telangiectasis of the arteries and veins, involving both the superficial and the deep capillary plexus, usually in a juxtafoveolar location. There may also be localized fusiform dilatation in the peripheral retina that resembles tiny red **lightbulbs**, venous loops, venous beading, neovascularization, focal or segmental capillary dilatation, and miliary aneurysms. Occasionally, a vascular network similar to that of the kidney glomerulus is seen, formed by division of an artery and a vein into a large number of smaller veins that subsequently reunite into a single vein, called *rete mirabile*. Subretinal hemorrhages may produce mounds of exudate and may regress spontaneously. In addition, numerous glistening **cholesterol** deposits, called *crystalline bodies*, may be seen in the subretinal space. Vitreal hemorrhages may occur and incite subsequent proliferative retinopathy. There may be retinal edema, hard exudates, and retinal detachment.

Symptoms

The patient may experience unilateral loss of central and peripheral vision, strabismus, leukokoria, and glaucoma.

Diagnosis

Fluorescein angiography reveals a lack of tight junctions, with fluorescein leakage and progressive staining of the vitreous; irregular saccular and beadlike lightbulb dilatations of vessels; aneurysms; coarse capillary dilatation in the early phase and capillary nonperfusion in the late phase of disease; a disciform area of chorioretinal atrophy in the macula; and AV collateral channels. Indocyanine-green videoangiography may demonstrate a subretinal neovascular membrane beneath the macula. CT scanning and magnetic resonance imaging (MRI) are useful for establishing the diagnosis.

Differential Diagnosis

Retinoblastoma, angiomatosis retinae, cavernous hemangioma, toxocariasis, persistent primary hyperplastic vitreous, ROP, and familial exudative retinopathy should be considered in the differential diagnosis.

Histopathology

Telangiectatic vessels are seen histopathologically in the inner retinal layers. Vessel walls are thickened by the deposit of material derived from plasma that stains positively with periodic acid–Schiff (PAS). Foamy macrophages appear in the area of retinal detachment, and fat-laden cells (bladder cells) and cholesterol crystals are present.

Treatment

Treatment frequently is ineffective. Obliteration of abnormal vessels by cryotherapy and argon laser photocoagulation has been used, as has vitrectomy. External drainage and scleral buckling are performed for retinal detachment.

Ophthalmic Artery Obstruction

Ophthalmic artery obstruction is an interruption of the blood flow in the ophthalmic artery, which is a branch of the internal carotid artery. It may be secondary to giant-cell arteritis and can occur as one of two types: acute and chronic.

Acute ophthalmic artery obstruction occurs suddenly and results in a severe visual loss. It may be produced by compression, a large embolus, trauma, or inflammation. The obstruction may be located distal or proximal to the origin of the posterior ciliary arteries.

Distal obstruction is nearly identical to CRAO, in which the inner and outer retina are markedly opacified and a **cherry-red spot** is seen. *Proximal obstruction* appears as a diffuse but homogeneous whitening of the retina, which corresponds to a retinal as well as to a choroidal ischemia. Vessels are markedly narrowed, with slow circulation and segmentation of blood flow. Both circulations, retinal and choroidal, are affected. A *cherry-red spot is not present*, because the choroidal circulation to the macula is not preserved. There may by diffuse pigmentary changes, a pale papilledema, or optic atrophy.

Chronic ophthalmic artery obstruction occurs slowly, due to chronic hypoperfusion caused by progressive stenosis of the ipsilateral internal carotid artery or of the common carotid artery, a condition called *venous stasis retinopathy.*

Ophthalmic artery obstruction appears as a reddish brown retina in the macular region, with some perimacular retinal whitening. Dot-and-blot hemorrhages are seen in the midperiphery of the fundus, usually sparing the posterior pole. Also present are tortuous veins, decreased retinal vascular caliber, sheathing, microaneurysms, and capillary nonperfusion. Macular edema may be seen. When the obstruction is bilateral, the collateral blood flow may be inadequate, leading to an **ocular ischemic syndrome** that may be accompanied by NVD, with compensatory connections between the retinal and ciliary circulation. Possible complications include general ocular ischemia with NVE in the retina, rubeosis iridis, iris necrosis, and cataract.

Symptoms

Patients will experience severe decreased visual acuity, often to no light perception.

Diagnosis

Fluorescein angiography may reveal a delay in the perfusion of the choroidal and retinal circulation. The ESR may be elevated. Visual field examination may reveal field defects.

Treatment

Treatment usually is not helpful. The potential for treatment efficacy depends on immediate care, within the first 90 minutes of obstruction. The globe is massaged digitally, and anterior chamber paracentesis is undertaken to reduce the IOP. Carbogen (a mixture of 95% oxygen and 5% carbon dioxide) should be inhaled for 10 minutes, every 2 hours for 48 hours. Oral vasodilators such as isosorbide (Sorbitrate), 10 mg PO three times a day, may be useful. Systemic anticoagulants—heparin, 5 ml/day (25,000 IU) IV, or acetazolamide, 500 mg/day IV—may be given. Topical beta-blockers—timolol (Timoptic) 0.5%, 1 drop twice a day, levobunolol (Betagan) 0.5%, one drop twice a day, or carteolol (Ocupress) 1%, one drop twice a day—also may be administered. Methylprednisolone, 100 mg/day IV, is prescribed for possible temporal arteritis. Argon laser panretinal photocoagulation might be attempted.

Takayasu's Syndrome

Takayasu's syndrome (also known as *pulseless disease* and *aortic arch syndrome*) is a giant-cell arteritis of the aorta, a granulomatous inflammation of large- and medium-caliber retinal arteries, of unknown etiology that occurs in children and young women, mainly in Japan. It is associated with rheumatoid arthritis, syphilis, and atherosclerosis.

Takayasu's syndrome may be due to a vascular insufficiency, which damages the large extraocular vessels, particularly the branches of the aorta, the elastic arteries, and the muscular arteries, but *not the retinal vessels directly.* The carotid and vertebral arteries are narrowed, producing a retinal ischemia and, consequently, a chronic hypoxia of the ocular tissues, reducing the blood flow and causing an abnormal filling of the arteries, with some congestion of the veins.

In the early stage, the syndrome is manifested as a dilatation of small vessels and microaneurysms. In a late stage, due to long-standing ischemia, there may be peripheral neovascularization and, consequently, vitreous hemorrhage. Retinal AV anastomoses, which are characteristic of Takayasu's syndrome, may be seen around the disc and in the midperiphery. Granularity of the blood column, pigment disturbances, exudates, retinitis proliferans, and retinal detachment may be seen. The disc may become pale, often displaying papilledema or optic atrophy. The fundus background also may develop pallor. CRVO may occur.

Symptoms

Transient position-dependent vision loss occurs. Syncope and absence of the radial pulse and pulsation in the upper extremities also are symptoms of Takayasu's syndrome.

Diagnosis

Ophthalmodynamometry reveals a decreased carotid flow on one or both sides.

Histopathology

Takayasu's syndrome is a granulomatous vascular inflammation with few giant cells in the active phase and sclerosing fibrosis in the chronic stage. There is a vascular wall dissection, with segmental aneurysmal dilatation. The intima is thickened, with proliferation and obstruction of the lumen. The media is heavily infiltrated with cells. The elastic coat is fragmented but does not exhibit fibrinoid necrosis. Like the intima, the adventitia is thickened, with giant-cell infiltration.

Persistent Hyaloid Artery

Persistent hyaloid artery (also known in various forms as *Cloquet's canal*, *Mittendorf's dot*, and *Bergmeister's papilla*) is incomplete regression of the hyaloid artery (Figure 4-12), which provides most of the blood supply to the posterior segment of the eye and to the lens, entering the embryonic tissue at the 5-mm stage of development and normally disappearing totally by the eighth month of gestation. It occurs usually in premature infants or in persistent hyperplastic primary vitreous.

Persistent hyaloid artery appears as a single, thin, threadlike artery or as a prepapillary loop emanating from the disc and coursing through the vitreous to insert on the posterior lens capsule. Sometimes, the artery is blood-filled; alternatively, it may appear as a thick, opaque cord. There may be dilatations in the mesodermal tissue that surrounds the artery, forming a cyst at the disc or in the vitreous. Occasionally, a glial sheath may extend into the vitreous as a falciform structure.

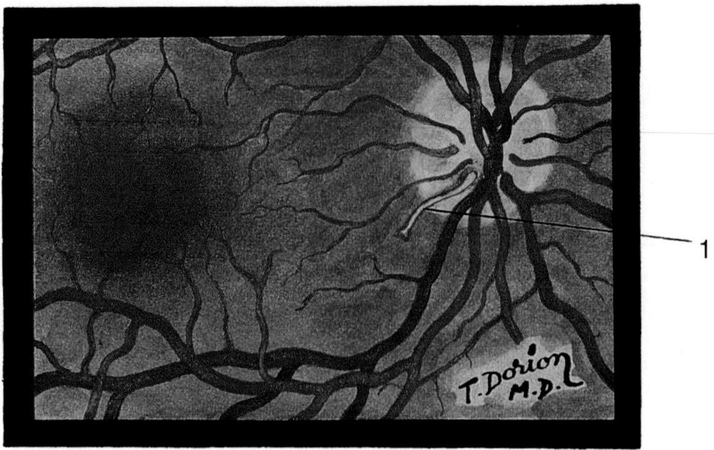

Figure 4-12. *Persistent hyaloid artery. (1) Glial sheath, remnant of the primitive hyaloid artery.*

Mittendorf's dot is a small, circular opacity of the posterior capsule of the lens that represents a remnant of the hyaloid artery *only at its anterior lens insertion.*

Bergmeister's papilla is an occluded remnant of the posterior portion of the hyaloid artery, a small fibroglial tuft of tissue that extends into the vitreous at the margin of the disc.

Emboli

Emboli are intravascular obstructive plugs of various origin located in the retina, choroid, or optic disc (Figure 4-13). They may be composed of fat, cholesterol, air, calcium, fibrin and platelets, medication, septic material starch, or particles.

Fat emboli occur from atheromatous plaques or after crush injuries such as fractures of long bones of the lower limb, bypass cardiac surgery, or external closed chest cardiac massage. These emboli are seen as a few or multiple discrete, white, soft exudates or cotton-wool spots, occasionally as large as 1 dd. They are scattered over large areas of the posterior pole, intravascularly in the retina, choroid, or disc. Often, they are lodged at the bifurcation of a major retinal artery and are visible as a marked yellowish white sheathing of the vessel called *trouser leg*. Reti-

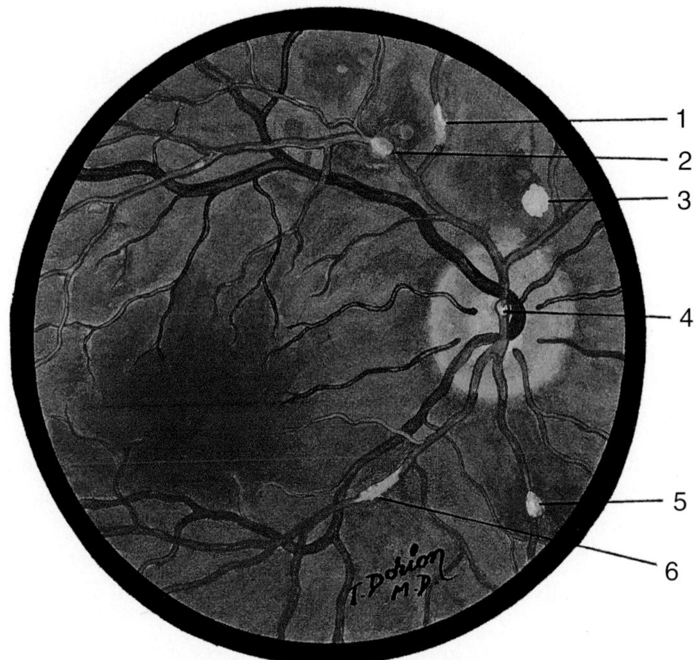

Figure 4-13. *Emboli. (1) Fibrin-platelet embolus. (2) Septic embolus. (3) Fat embolus in the retina. (4) Calcium embolus in the disc, from an aortic valve. (5) Cholesterol embolus or Hollenhorst plaque, from a carotid atheroma. (6) Lipid embolus.*

nal microinfarcts, retinal ischemia consequent to the arterial occlusion, preretinal and intraretinal hemorrhages, and collateral vessels may be present. Sometimes, a transient grayish white macular edema with a foveolar cherry-red spot may be seen.

Histopathologically, fat emboli are characterized by lipid deposition in the retinal vessels. The artery may appear thin, attenuated, or fibrotic. Intracellular swelling of the axons may occur, especially in the inner retinal layers.

Cholesterol emboli, called **Hollenhorst plaques**, result from the dislodging of cholesterol from an atheromatous plaque in the carotid artery. They are seen as intra-arterial, refractile, white, glistening, flat crystals, often located at the bifurcation of the retinal arteries, and may appear larger than the vessel that contains them.

Air emboli occur after surgery of or trauma to the chest or lungs. They appear as pale, silvery segments in the retinal arteries that alternate with the blood column.

Calcium emboli originate from a stenosed aortic valve or the ascending aorta. They appear as white, solid, calcified plugs in the arteries and may produce complete obstruction of the vessel and infarction of the distal retina.

Fibrin-platelet emboli occur from an ulcerative atheromatous plaque in the carotid artery or from a damaged heart valve or other cardiac lesions. They appear as dull or yellow, porridgy plugs with ill-defined margins, deposited within arteries. They usually are not lodged at a vessel's bifurcation.

Medication emboli occur more commonly after cortisone injections in the paranasal sinuses. They appear as small, white spots within arteries over the entire fundus.

Septic emboli occur in systemic infectious diseases. They appear as **Roth's spots** scattered throughout the posterior pole and at the peripheral retina.

Starch emboli occur in drug addicts after intravenous injections of crushed methylphenidate hydrochloride tablets. The emboli appear as glistening crystals, mainly in the small vessels around the macula.

Particle emboli usually result from therapy for embolization of dural fistulas. Such therapy generally uses nonabsorbable material such as beads of silicone, stainless steel, lead, and isobutyl-3-cyanoacrylate, and polyvinyl alcohol foam. Mildly attenuated arteries, nerve fiber layer edema of the posterior pole, and a faint **choroidal blush** appearance of the fundus are seen.

Retinopathy of Prematurity

Retinopathy of prematurity (also known as *retrolental fibroplasia*) is a bilateral and symmetric proliferative vascular disease that occurs soon after birth in low-birth-weight (<1,500 g [3 lb, 5 oz]) and premature infants in whom the retinal vasculature is not fully developed. It may be caused by exposure to a high oxygen concentration or to acidosis in the early neonatal period that leads to inactivation of specific enzymes by the hyperoxia, a disturbance of the metabolism, and a permanent hypoxia. The result is a primary retinal vasoconstriction with endothe-

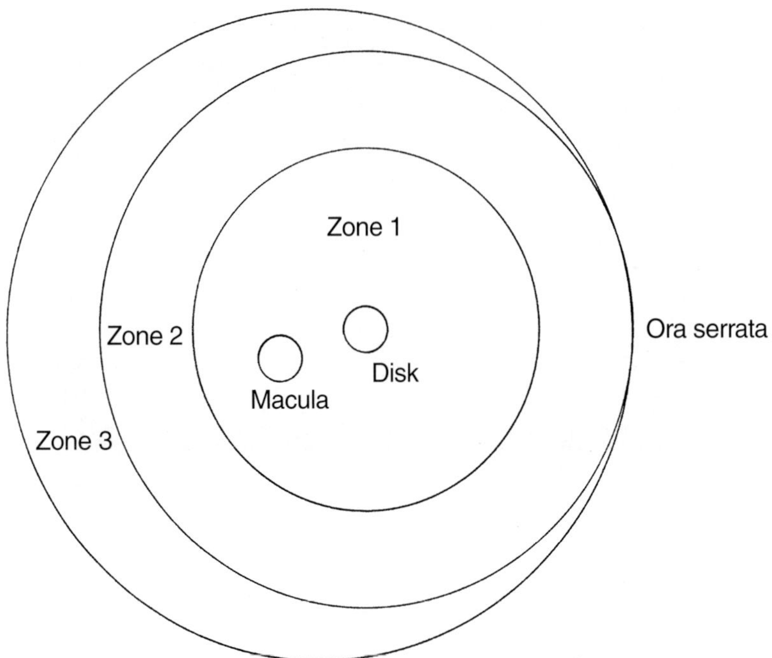

Figure 4-14. *Zoning of retinopathy of prematurity (ROP) according to the international classification of ROP. Zone 1 is a central zone having a radius twice the distance from disc to macula. Zone 2 describes the area from zone 1 to the nasal ora serrata. Zone 3 defines the crescent composed of the remaining superior, inferior, and temporal regions.*

lial necrosis, followed by a secondary retinal vasoproliferation and vaso-obliteration and suppression of normal retinal vascularization.

Classification

The **international classification of retinopathy of prematurity (ICROP)** (Figure 4-14) is based on the *degree* of the disease in relation to three retinal zones centered on the optic disc and on the *severity* of the disease expressed in five stages. **Zone 1** is a circular zone having the disc in its center and a radius that subtends an angle of 30 degrees (or double the distance from the disc to the macula). **Zone 2** extends from the

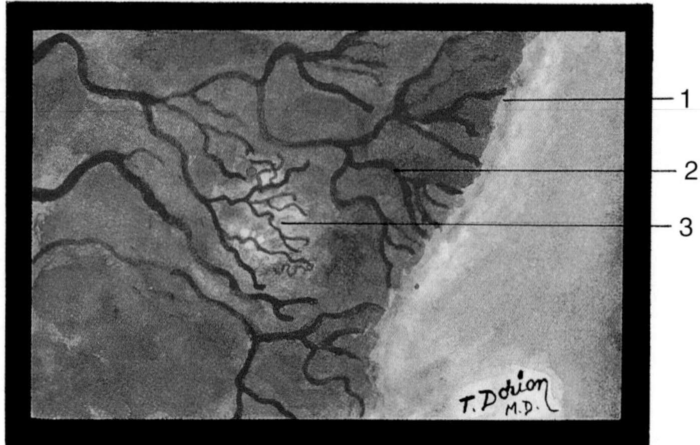

Figure 4-15. *Retinopathy of prematurity, stage II. (1) Ragged peripheral ridge of fibrovascular proliferation. (2) Dilatation and tortuosity of retinal vessels. (3) Neovascularization posterior to the ridge* (popcorn proliferation).

margin of zone 1 to a point tangential to the nasal ora serrata. **Zone 3** is the zone represented by the crescent of the remaining superior, inferior, and temporal regions.

ROP may occur in two major phases: **retinal** and **vitreoretinal**, each of which may be subdivided into *acute* and *cicatricial* phases. The **acute** or **active phase** is characterized by cessation of the normal vasogenesis, which actually starts from the optic disc at 16 weeks' gestation and is completed in the nasal retina at 36 weeks and in the temporal retina at term. It occurs in five stages.

Stage 1, the **demarcation line**, is a thin, flat, white structure within the plane of the retina that separates the *anterior vascular retina* from the *posterior avascular retina*. It is located at the junction between the end of retinal vessels and the immature peripheral retina and signifies the onset of the disease. Abnormal branching vessels or arcading vessels leading up to the line or functioning AV collaterals may be present.

Stage 2, the **ridge**, is a pinkish white, ragged, peripherally elevated ridge of fibrous, vascular, or fibrovascular proliferation that develops gradually as the disease progresses, from the demarcation line into the vitreous above the retinal plane (Figure 4-15). It is due to proliferation of endothelial cells and spindle-shaped mesenchymal cells. The ridge extends beyond the retinal plane and may be accompanied by dilatation and tortuosity of the retinal vessels behind the equator, called **plus disease**. When plus disease exhibits changes greater than or equal to 5 contiguous or 8 cumulative clock-hours in zone 1 or 2, the condition is called **threshold disease**. Tufts of neovascularization posterior to the ridge, called **popcorn proliferation** may be seen.

Stage 3 is marked by a **ridge with extraretinal fibrovascular proliferation**. This stage is divided into *mild*, *moderate*, and *severe* phases. Fibrovascular proliferation in the vitreous, vascular shunts, segmental or contiguous neovascularization of the ridge, salmon-pink or red lesions, and increased tortuosity of the disc vessels occur. Occasionally, there may be small, isolated vascular malformations of neovascular tissue, called *preretinal globules*, posterior to the peripheral ridge. The macula and retinal vessels may be dragged toward the temporal side. Capillaries may extend from the inner retina to the vitreous cortex, which may become opaque and exhibit linear fibrous structures, usually located adjacent to a large pocket of liquefied vitreous.

Stage 4, retinal detachment, is divided into substages. In **stage IVA**, there is partial peripheral tractional nonrhegmatogenous retinal detachment that *does not involve the macula*, called *macula on*. In **stage IVB**, there is partial retinal detachment that *includes the macula*, called **macula off**. Retinal detachment may be effusive or tractional. It extends usually as a retinal fold from the disc toward the periphery. A neovascular tissue arises from the rear and grows into the vitreous toward *Weigert's ligament* on the posterior lens capsule.

Stage 5 features **total retinal detachment**, usually an exudative retinal detachment, which may result from vitreous traction. This detachment appears as an open or closed, funnel-shaped retina with massive vitreous hemorrhage and a solid retrolental membrane.

Spontaneous regression may occur in any stage. In an early phase, small neovessels may grow beyond the ridge and penetrate into the avascular retina, a condition called *prethreshold disease*. In a later phase, the ridge may be replaced by a vitreoretinal membrane, retina and macula may be dragged, vessels are straightened, and extensive pigmentary disruption may be present. An accentuated form of dragging in regressed ROP appears as a **falciform fold**. A highly malignant, fulminant, progressive type of ROP, in which the ridge formation and the vascular tortuosity may progress within a few days to a total rhegmatogenous retinal detachment, is called *rush disease*.

The **cicatricial phase** features *five grades*. In **grade 1, minor changes,** such as small areas of irregular retinal pigmentation, peripheral retinal patches, attenuated vessels, and myopia, occur. **Grade 2** features **localized fixed retinal detachment**, in which retinal vessels are pulled temporally and distorted, and tractional heterotopia of the macula, which is displaced temporally, and disc pallor are seen. In **grade 3**, there are **fixed retinal folds**, usually falciform, that extend to the temporal periphery, with vessels torn out of the nasal retina and incorporated into the folds. **Grade 4** is defined by an **incomplete retrolental mass** with fibrovascular membranes that extend toward the posterior pole of the lens, producing a progressively funnel-shaped retinal detachment that may partially cover the pupil. In **grade 5**, a **complete retrolental mass** is formed by a total retinal detachment; the mass is thickened and scarred. There is a vitreoretinopathy, which may produce dragging of the macula and temporal vessels toward the temporal periphery. Nystagmus, microphthalmia, high myopia, glaucoma, uveitis, cataract, corneal degeneration, or even phthisis bulbi may occur.

Symptoms

ROP may be asymptomatic. Symptoms that do occur can range from minimal visual disturbances to marked decreased vision to blindness.

Diagnosis

Fluorescein angiography reveals peripheral retinal vascularization and capillary nonperfusion.

Differential Diagnosis

The differential diagnosis should take into account such conditions as familial exudative vitreoretinopathy, incontinentia pigmenti (Bloch-Sulzberger syndrome), X-linked retinoschisis, leukokoria, congenital cataract, retinoblastoma, toxocariasis, persistent hyperplastic primary vitreous, pars planitis, Coats' disease, and vitreous hemorrhage.

Histopathology

The histopathology varies with the stage of the disease. In the early stages, there is a ridge—a thickening of the retina—at the junction between the vascularized and nonvascularized zones. Microvascular abnormalities, such as capillary tufts, collaterals, and capillarylike new vessels, develop and extend into the vitreous and fibroglial tissue. In the late stages, the vascular abnormalities persist, and the avascular retina organizes into a contracting scar. Young new vessels break through the internal limiting membrane, growing into the subvitreal space. Fibrovascular tissue (retinitis proliferans) is seen. Also seen is retinal detachment, which may be total and usually is rhegmatogenous with round or oval breaks, without operculum, located near the equator, although nonrhegmatogenous retinal detachment can occur. There is dragging or distortion of the macula, the optic nerve, and the posterior retinal vessels.

Treatment

ROP may regress, and no treatment is required. Cryotherapy of the anterior peripheral retina is recommended for active threshold stage 3 disease in zone 1 or for stage 2 with plus disease. For stage 3 disease, cryosurgical ablation of the entire peripheral avascular retina to the ridge of the neovascular tissue is appropriate. Diode laser photocoagulation is used for zone 1 ROP, applying spots to 360 degrees of the anterior avascular retina, placing the spots approximately one burn apart. Laser therapy is guided by indirect ophthalmoscopy. Scleral buckling and drainage of the subretinal liquid is used for nonrhegmatogenous retinal detachment in stage 4 or 5 disease. Lensectomy and vitreous membranectomy, accomplished by peeling off the preretinal membrane, may be performed, as may vitrectomy. Topical prednisolone acetate 1% is appropriate for some complications. Optimal administration of oxygen is necessary in the neonate. Vitamin E (tocopherol) therapy may be warranted.

Prethreshold Disease

Prethreshold disease is a form of ROP that may have any of the following characteristics: zone 1 ROP at any stage, less than *threshold dis-*

ease; zone 2 ROP at stage 3+, without *plus disease*; or zone 2 ROP at stage 3+, with fewer numbers of sectors at stage 3+ than are seen in *threshold disease.*

Threshold Disease

Threshold disease is a form of ROP that involves five contiguous clock-hour sectors (of 30 degrees each), or eight interrupted clock-hour sectors of stage 3 ROP in the presence of plus disease. It appears as a neovascularization usually located posterior to the equator, with progressive marked dilatation and tortuosity of the retinal vessels, called *plus disease*, and a ridge of extraretinal fibrovascular proliferation into the vitreous.

Plus Disease

Plus disease is a form of ROP that is characterized exclusively by a progressive dilatation and tortuosity of the retinal vessels. It appears as a neovascularization at the posterior pole, behind the equator, in which the vessels, particularly the arteries, are markedly dilated and tortuous. Plus disease is a pale stage of ROP stage 3. There is no iris engorgement, pupillary rigidity, vitreous haze, or retinal hemorrhage. Whenever plus disease is associated with any stage of ROP in zone 1, it is called *rush disease.*

Rush Disease

Rush disease is a fulminant, progressive form of ROP that may produce rhegmatogenous retinal detachment with breaks. It appears as a neovascularization with markedly dilated and tortuous vessels posterior to the equator (*plus disease*), located in zone 1. The vessels in rush disease may end in a flat, neovascular syncytial network.

Retinal Vasculitis

Retinal vasculitis is a diffuse vaso-occlusive retinal disease, either unilateral or bilateral, that primarily affects the veins but also can involve the arteries. It occurs frequently in men as an extension of an adjacent chorioretinitis. Retinal vasculitis occurs also in giant-cell arteritis, multiple sclerosis, systemic lupus erythematosus, polyarteritis nodosa, relapsing polychondritis, ankylosing spondylitis, Crohn's disease, pars planitis, acute retinal necrosis, necrotizing angiitis, tuberculosis, syphilis, cytomegalovirus retinopathy, other herpesvirus retinopathies, acquired immunodeficiency syndrome (AIDS), toxoplasmosis, sarcoidosis, dermatomycosis, Wegener's granulomatosis, Whipple's disease, Eales' disease, acute frosted retinal periphlebitis, Behçet's disease, masquerade syndrome, viral retinitis, diabetes, other collagen vascular diseases, infections, or idiopathic conditions.

Retinal vasculitis appears as retinal whitening, with creamy, sheathing exudates around the veins, which are dilated and tortuous, especially at the equator. Microaneurysms may be present. Arteries and capillaries may be markedly attenuated or occluded. A CRVO may also occur owing to thrombosis. Multiple superficial, small, flame-shaped hemorrhages may be scattered throughout the fundus. Areas of superficial retinal opacification, intraretinal edema, and cystoid macular edema may be seen. Cotton-wool spots may also be seen. Often, the optic disc is swollen. There may be cells in the vitreous and vitreous hemorrhage. Occasionally, areas of neovascularization of the retina or of the disc, retinal necrosis, and retinal detachment may also be seen. Sometimes, vitritis (marked by cells in a hazy vitreous) or an anterior uveitis is present. This retinal vasculitis may remit after varying periods.

Symptoms

Decreased vision is usually experienced by the patient.

Diagnosis

Fluorescein angiography may reveal segmental staining of the vessel walls, with irregular areas of hyperfluorescence, leakage of dye, cystoid macular edema, extensive peripheral capillary nonperfusion, and areas of neovascularization. Visual field examination may reveal a field defect.

Treatment

Corticosteroids consist of methylprednisolone, 40 mg every 2 weeks periocularly, or systemic prednisone, 60 mg/day PO. Laser photocoagulation is used for NVD and NVE. Systemic immunosuppressive drugs are used when vision is deteriorating: cyclosporin A (Sandimmune), 2.5–5.0 mg/kg/day PO; cyclophosphamide (Cytoxan), 1–2 mg/kg/day PO; chlorambucil (Leukeran), 0.1–0.2 mg/kg/day PO; or azathioprine (Imuran), 1.5–2.0 mg/kg/day PO.

Sickle Cell Retinopathy

Sickle cell retinopathy (also known as *sickle cell hemoglobin C disease, sickle cell thalassemia*, *sickle cell anemia*, and *sickle cell trait*) is a hereditary vascular retinopathy (Figure 4-16) in which the *normal hemoglobin* (HbA and HbA_2) has been replaced by an *abnormal sickle hemoglobin* (HbSS, HbSC, or HbS-Thal) that is markedly susceptible to changes in oxygenation. The condition occurs commonly in persons from the Mediterranean area and the West Indies and almost exclusively affects black patients.

Sickle cell retinopathy is due mainly to the sickling of the erythrocytes, in which the red cells become elongated into a sickle shape under the condition of reduced oxygen tension. It may also be caused by hemolysis and hemostasis, which may produce occlusion of the arteries, which in turn may cause retinal ischemia and consequent thrombosis by fibrovascular proliferation.

Clinical Forms

Sickle cell retinopathy appears in two clinical forms: nonproliferative and proliferative. **Nonproliferative sickle cell retinopathy** usually is seen as small peripheral arterial occlusions, hemorrhages, and iridescent deposits. Tiny red spots or lines of blocked small vessels, called the **disc sign of sickling,** may appear on the surface of the disc, a result of sickle-shaped deformity of the erythrocytes owing to deoxygenation. Hemorrhages that appear as red patches may be located distal to the point of the occlusion and be confined to the retina or may occur in the subhyaloid space, in a potential space between the internal limiting membrane and the nerve fiber layer, or in a space between the sensory retina and the RPE. These hemorrhages, called *salmon patches*, may appear as ovoid red spots of approximately 0.25–1.00 dd, which later turn pink, then orange, then white. They may resolve partially and may have a surrounding schisis cavity. Alternatively, as

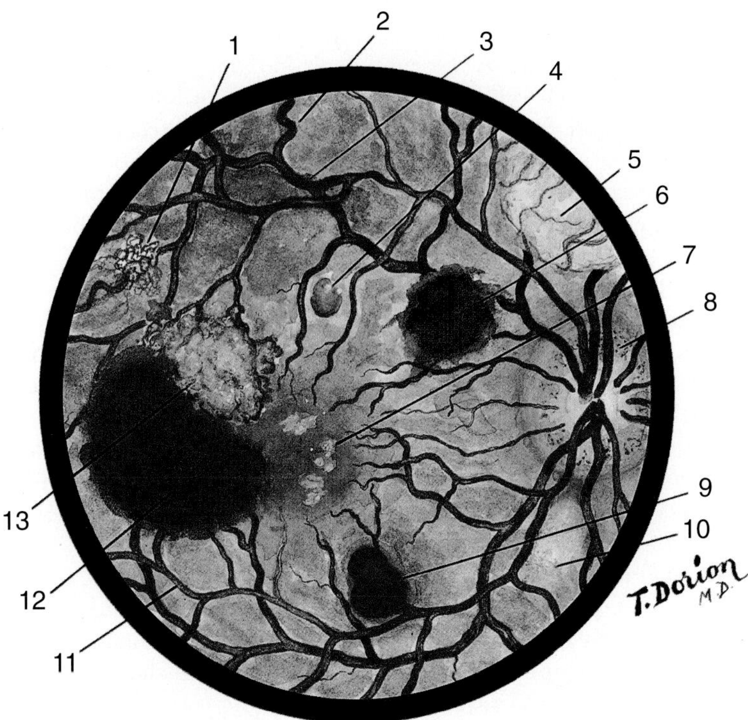

Figure 4-16. *Sickle cell retinopathy. (1) Peripheral neovascularization. (2) Vessel tortuosity at the periphery. (3) Arteriovenous anastomoses. (4) Iridescent spots. (5) Retinal detachment. (6) Black sunbursts. (7) Cotton-wool spots in the macula. (8) Disc sign of sickling. (9) Salmon patches. (10) Retinal whitening. (11) Silver-wire arteries. (12) Vitreous hemorrhage. (13) Sea fans.*

hemolysis occurs, they may disappear and leave at the periphery or in the macula fine, yellow, glistening refractile crystalline deposits of hemosiderin called **iridescent spots.**

In addition, there are areas of retinal whitening and vascular tortuosity at the periphery, due to AV shunting. Often seen are some black, circumscribed, ovoid lesions with stellate or spiculate borders, resembling chorioretinal scars. These lesions exhibit a perivascular accumulation of pigment, measure approximately 0.5–2.0 dd, and are located at the peripheral equatorial fundus. Called *black sunbursts*, they are produced by pigment migration due to dissection of a large intraretinal hemorrhage into a subretinal space. The lesions represent resolved subretinal hemorrhages with secondary RPE hyperplasia and hypertrophy. Cotton-wool spots may be present, mostly in the macula.

Proliferative sickle cell retinopathy is staged according to the **Goldberg classification. Stage 1**, *peripheral retinal artery occlusion*, is due to intravascular sickling, mostly between the equator and ora serrata. Arteries appear chalky as the *silver-wire reflex*. There is a retinal capillary nonperfusion. Background lesions such as salmon patches, iridescent spots, black sunbursts, and occluded vessels may be present.

Stage 2 is characterized by *peripheral AV anastomoses* that occur at the junction of perfused and nonperfused retina, mostly in the temporal quadrant. The anastomoses probably represent dilated preexisting capillaries rather than true neovascularization, and they shunt the blood from the occluded arteries to the veins.

Stage 3, *peripheral retinal neovascularization*, arises at the site of the arterial occlusion from the AV anastomoses, at the interface of the avascular and vascular retina, toward the ora serrata. Sometimes, isolated neovascular patches are seen that do not coalesce and appear as fine, naked, red, blending channels, more often located in the superotemporal region, resembling telangiectasis and microaneurysms; these resemble a coral formation and are called *sea fans*. Multiple arteries and veins may be incorporated in them. The sea fans may grow into the vitreous, may grow posteriorly to a detached vitreous cortex, or may undergo spontaneous regression and disappear completely.

Stage 4 features *vitreous hemorrhages*, which may be massive or minimal and which may arise mostly from bleeding sea fans.

Stage 5, *retinal detachment* (nonrhegmatogenous or rhegmatogenous), usually is due to vitreous retraction bands or fibrovascular proliferation. There may be small to moderate, ovoid or horseshoe-shaped tears or holes, located commonly in the equatorial or pre-equatorial areas. Sometimes, angioid streaks also are present.

Symptoms

Sickle cell retinopathy may be asymptomatic. Ocular symptoms, if they do occur, might include floaters, flashing lights, and reduced vision. Crises of severe abdominal pain or musculoskeletal discomfort are frequent.

Diagnosis

A CBC and fasting blood sugar test should be performed. A sickle cell preparation will likely be positive but can be negative in sickle cell trait or sickle cell hemoglobin C disease. Hemoglobin electrophoresis reveals the presence of homozygous hemoglobin S in the red cells. Chest roentgenograms are helpful. The angiotensin-converting enzyme level is increased. Fluorescein angiography may reveal almost total capillary closure at the periphery of the sea fans, AV anastomoses, preretinal neovascularization in the early phases, leakage of fluorescein in the late phases, and areas of hypofluorescence and hyperfluorescence corresponding to changes in the RPE.

Differential Diagnosis

Conditions that should be considered in the differential diagnosis are diabetes, sarcoidosis, retinal vein occlusion, retinal emboli, Eales' disease, ROP, chronic myelogenous leukemia, pars planitis, collagen vascular diseases, familial exudative vitreoretinopathy, and radiation retinopathy.

Histopathology

In **nonproliferative sickle cell retinopathy**, old resorbed hemorrhages (called *iridescent spots*) that contain proteinaceous material and hemosiderin-laden macrophages are present, deposited in acquired schisis cavities just beneath the internal limiting membrane. *Salmon patches* (hemorrhages in different stages of resorption) are located in the deep retinal and subretinal spaces. Areas of RPE hyperplasia, RPE hypertrophy, and perivascular pigment migration (*black sunbursts*) also are seen, as are areas of discontinuity in the internal limiting membrane through which the vessels extend into the vitreous (*sea fans*). AV communications arise at the junction of the perfused and nonperfused retina. Fibroglial tissue, numerous sickled erythrocytes, and few lymphocytes may be present near the sea fans.

In **proliferative sickle cell retinopathy**, stage 1, occlusions of major vessels occur, with fibrin thrombus that obstructs tertiary branches of the central retinal artery, which may be followed by AV loops, or venous beading. Stage 2 disease exhibits large AV anastomoses; stage 3, neovascularization and fibrous proliferation; stage 4, vitreous hemorrhages; and stage 5, fibrous proliferation that produces tractional retinal detachment.

Treatment

Treatment is not always helpful. Scatter, low-power (800-mW) argon or xenon laser photocoagulation with burns of 0.1 second in duration and 500 μm in size over a 360-degree circumference or by sectors may be used. Feeder-vessel photocoagulation also might be considered. Pars plana vitrectomy, cryotherapy, and segmental scleral buckling surgery are other treatment options.

Opticociliary Shunt

Opticociliary shunt is an abnormal connection between the choroidal and retinal circulation at the disc, in which the blood is shunted from a high-pressure area in the central retinal vein to a lower-pressure area in the choroidal circulation and exits the eye by the vortex veins. The shunt may be a congenital anomaly but more frequently is acquired secondary to a CRVO, sarcoidosis, arachnoid and optic nerve cyst, optic nerve coloboma, drusen, chronic atrophic papilledema, pseudotumor cerebri, or orbital tumors such as meningioma, melanoma, or juvenile pilocystic astrocytoma (glioma).

Opticociliary shunt appears as a pale, slightly swollen disc with blurred margins and collateral opticociliary veins deviated in the center of the disc, diverting the blood from an obstructed central retinal vein to the choroidal circulation. There may be some arterial attenuation.

Symptoms

Ocular symptoms include poor visual acuity and axial proptosis in optic nerve sheath meningioma.

Diagnosis

Visual field examination may reveal an altitudinal defect, grossly irreversible constriction, or, as in compressive orbital lesions and retrobulbar inflammations, central and cecocentral scotoma. Fluorescein angiography may reveal a shunt vessel diverting retinal venous blood around an obstructed optic nerve toward the choroid, but *no dye leakage* is seen. Gadolinium-enhanced fat-suppressed MRI may show an intraorbital optic nerve sheath meningioma.

Differential Diagnosis

Cavernous hemangioma and chronic open-angle glaucoma should be considered in the differential diagnosis.

Choroidal Detachment

Choroidal detachment (also known as *uveal effusion syndrome of Schepens and Brockhurst*, *uveal edema*, *ciliochoroidal effusion*, *uveal detachment*, and *uveal hydrops*) is a collection of fluid in a potential suprachoroidal space between the sclera externally and the choroid and ciliary body internally, which produces elevation of the choroid, RPE, and sensory retina. It occurs usually after trauma or intraoperatively or postoperatively, commonly 10–14 days after cataract surgery, and presents with a leaking, shallow anterior chamber and marked hypotony (often as low as 6 mm Hg). It also can occur after scleral buckling repair of a retinal detachment or may occur spontaneously bilaterally, in apparently healthy eyes, more commonly in men, in the absence of hypotony and without association with any general disorders. Choroidal detachment may occur in systemic diseases such as diabetes; in vascular diseases such as hypertension; in inflammatory diseases such as scleritis, Vogt-Koyanagi-Harada syndrome, and sympathetic ophthalmia; in nanophthalmos; or in carotid-cavernous fistula. It can occur spontaneously after perforation of a corneal ulcer, after rupture of a choroidal neovascular membrane in patients on anticoagulant therapy, in the presence of an intraocular neoplasm such as leukemia or metastatic carcinoma of the choroid, or in multiple myeloma.

Choroidal detachment might be caused by poor venous drainage, which may produce a fluid transudation into the suprachoroidal space. Alternatively, the cause may be a sudden hypotony and engorgement of the choroidal vessels, which are not able to retain the fluid. Other etiologies include increased pressure of the episcleral veins, which may disturb the circulatory homeostasis and the normal pressure relationship within the choroid and so produce transudation of the fluid in the suprachoroidal space, ultimately leading to choroidal detachment. A local stimulus, such as a limbal incision in cataract surgery or application of an excessive amount of thermal energy in panretinal argon laser photocoagulation, may produce a suprachoroidal fluid collection that results in choroidal detachment.

Clinical Types

Choroidal detachment may be hemorrhagic and transudative. **Hemorrhagic choroidal detachment** occurs after trauma or intraocular surgery and is the result of accidental rupture of a choroidal vessel that leaks into the suprachoroidal space. **Transudative choroidal detachment** occurs after retinal detachment surgery as a result of prolonged hypotony, after laser photocoagulation, or in scleritis, Vogt-Koyanagi-Harada syndrome, hypertension, nephritis, or myopia. It may resemble malignant melanoma.

There are three clinical types of choroidal detachment: *annular*, *globular,* and *flat*. **Annular choroidal detachment** appears as a gray ring with a smooth surface and well-defined borders, usually located at the peripheral retina, where the vessels and lamellae are lax and oriented tangentially. It involves the ciliary body as well as the peripheral choroid.

Globular choroidal detachments appear as large, solid, homogeneous, dark brown, hemispherical masses, with a smooth, immobile convex surface and well-defined borders (Figure 4-17). The detachments may be single or multiple (usually up to four). Globular choroidal detachments are located more frequently in the temporal quadrants, anteroinferior to the equator, and usually *do not involve the posterior pole*. They are not limited by the ora serrata, which can be seen without scleral depression, but are prevented from spreading by the vortex veins, which enter the sclera and create valleys, separating the hemispherical masses superiorly and inferiorly. Retinal vessels course over the choroidal detachment and appear normal. In the early

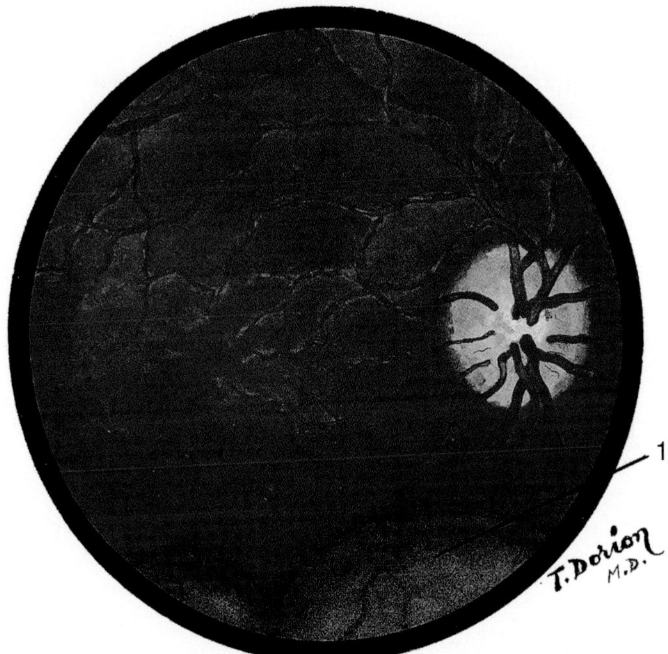

Figure 4-17. *Choroidal detachment. (1) Large bulbous elevations of peripheral fundus that come into contact with one another as "kissing" choroidal detachment.*

stages, there may be subretinal exudates. In severe cases, the mounds may fill the vitreous almost entirely, and the temporal and nasal masses may actually touch; this is called *kissing choroidal detachment.*

Flat choroidal detachment appears as a nonelevated, brown-gray mass, usually located at the posterior pole or in some isolated peripheral areas, where fluid exudation is limited by the density and relative shortness of the suprachoroidal lamellae.

Uveal effusion syndrome of Schepens and Brockhurst, or **uveal edema,** is a rare, bilateral, flat, peripheral choroidal effusion accompanied by a nonrhegmatogenous retinal detachment, with occasional retinal exudates and localized areas of RPE hypertrophy or hyperplasia. It is not associated with any surgery or trauma and occurs mainly in men.

Symptoms

Choroidal detachment may be asymptomatic, though decreased vision and severe pain are experienced by some patients.

Diagnosis

Fluorescein angiography reveals no leakage under the choroidal detachment. Gonioscopy, B-scan ultrasonography, and scleral transillumination of the globe may aid in the diagnosis. Chromic phosphate P_{32} might be used to differentiate from tumors.

Differential Diagnosis

Choroidal melanoma, choroidal hemangioma, and retinal detachment should be considered in the differential diagnosis.

Histopathology

The choroid is markedly thickened, with edema, intense diffuse and nodular lymphocytic and plasmatic infiltration, and foci of epithelioid cells exhibiting pigment phagocytosis but not necrosis, which may also be present in the pars plana. The inner choroidal layers demonstrate folds, oriented meridionally. The RPE also may show folds, hypertrophy, hyperplasia, and proliferation of nodular or linear proteinaceous material. The retinal outer plexiform layer and inner nuclear layer may house large macrophages, many of which contain pigment, whereas others are filled with a homogeneous proteinaceous material.

Treatment

The detachment may be merely observed, as it sometimes resolves within days. Treatment of the underlying cause, such as a cleft or wound leak (by patching, suturing, cyanoacrylate glue, or a bandage contact lens), is appropriate. Laser, cryotherapy, or diathermy may be used. Surgical drainage of the fluid by sclerotomy is a therapeutic option. Vitrectomy may be performed. Cycloplegics (atropine 1%, 1 drop three times a day) and corticosteroids (prednisolone acetate 1%, 1 drop topically four times a day, or systemically, 5 mg PO four times a day) can be administered.

High-Altitude Retinopathy

High-altitude retinopathy (also known as *acute mountain sickness*) is a vascular and hemorrhagic retinopathy that occurs in climbers (e.g., mountaineering, hiking, or skiing) after exposure for several weeks to high altitude, usually 10,000–25,000 ft. It may be associated with a high-altitude cerebral edema that rapidly improves on descent, a high pulmonary edema, corneal endothelial decompensation (which may require keratoplasty), or a cataract (which may occur as a result of reduced atmospheric absorption of ultraviolet light, thereby causing an increased ambient level and a higher dose of ultraviolet light to the lens).

High-altitude retinopathy is due to hypobaric hypoxia, in which the atmospheric pressure is decreased, producing a drop in the partial pressure of oxygen and an arterial oxygen saturation as low as 28 mm Hg (normal, 96 mm Hg). This state probably causes hypoxic vasodilatation, with a sudden rise in the intravascular pressure.

High-altitude retinopathy appears usually as a bilateral, extensive, macular and peripheral intraretinal hemorrhage and vitreous hemorrhage, varying only in degree of extent. Often, a solitary macular hemorrhage occurs alone. Outside the macular region, the hemorrhages usually are deep but may be superficial and flame-shaped. They may resolve spontaneously on return of the affected individual to a lower altitude. In time, a macular pigment dispersion may occur. Vessels may be engorged and tortuous, or an ischemic CRVO may be present. The optic disc may be hyperemic, or an early mild papilledema may be seen. Few exudates may be present throughout the posterior pole.

Symptoms

Ocular symptoms include bilateral decreased visual acuity, to finger counting, and blurred vision. Metamorphopsia and snow blindness (photophthalmia) also occur.

Diagnosis

Amsler grid distortion is a diagnostic indicator of high-altitude retinopathy. Fluorescein angiography may reveal widespread capillary nonperfusion, and electroretinography may show a permanent reduction in critical fusion frequency. Visual field examination may demonstrate a field defect. Dark adaptation may be abnormal. Retinal blood flow and retinal blood volume are increased, whereas mean retinal circulation time is decreased.

Treatment

Treatment consists of administering oxygen, diuretics (furosemide [Lasix], 40 mg/day PO; prednisone, 20 mg/day PO), and nonsteroidal anti-inflammatory drugs (etodolac [Lodine], 400 mg PO twice a day). Laser panretinal photocoagulation may be useful. Prophylactically, acetazolamide (Diamox), 500 mg PO for 48 hours before ascent, can be given to climbers to prevent cerebral edema. Sunglasses may be worn (e.g., UV light–absorption glasses) or, in an emergency, goggles made of cardboard with a thin slit will suffice.

Purtscher's Retinopathy

Purtscher's retinopathy (also called *traumatic retinal angiopathy* or *angiopathic retinopathy*) is a bilateral hemorrhagic retinopathy that usually occurs after chest-crushing or long-bone injuries (Figure 4-18). It probably is due to an abrupt rise in the intraluminal pressure of the orbital vessels resulting from a sudden and violent compression of the thorax which, through a fat embolus, may produce multiple arterial occlusions and acute capillary ischemia, possibly causing hemorrhage, edema, and exudation.

Purtscher's retinopathy appears, in the first 2 hours after the injury, as preretinal and intraretinal hemorrhages throughout the fundus, many of which surround the disc. Retinal edema, resembling cumulus clouds, may be present and may increase in size to more than 1 dd. Also many fluffy, yellow-white cotton-wool exudates may be seen at the posterior pole. Hemorrhages and exudates usually resolve completely in several weeks or months. A cherry-red spot may occur in the macula, caused by a fat embolus or a leukoembolus. Veins may appear dilated. The optic disc occasionally becomes atrophic.

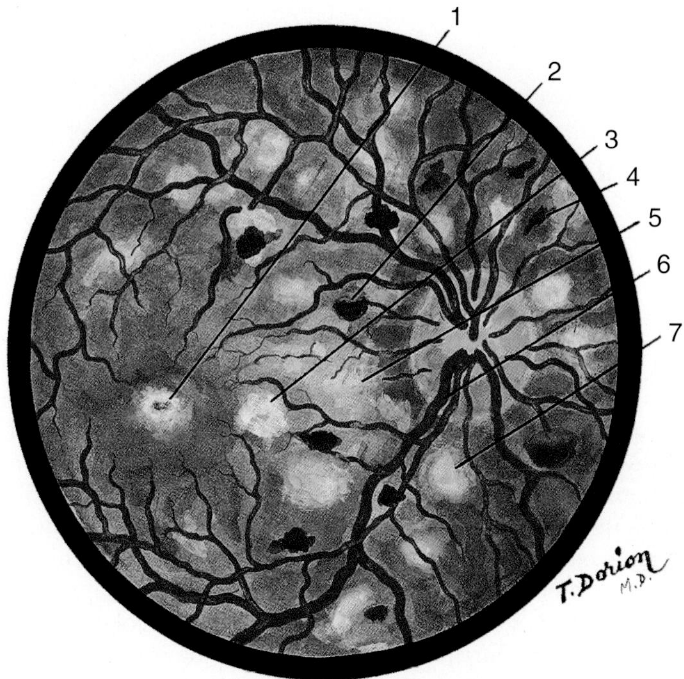

Figure 4-18. *Purtscher's retinopathy. (1) Cherry-red spot in the macula. (2) Preretinal hemorrhage. (3) Fluffy, cloudlike exudates. (4) Superficial hemorrhage. (5) Retinal edema. (6) Dilated veins. (7) Cotton-wool spots.*

Differential Diagnosis

Acute pancreatitis, collagen vascular disease, and globe perforation after a retrobulbar injection are considerations in the differential diagnosis.

Histopathology

Histologic evaluation confirms retinal infarctions in the nerve fiber layer of the retina. Blood pockets in the subhyaloid space or in the inner retinal layers also are present.

Treatment

No effective treatment has been identified.

Valsalva Retinopathy

Valsalva retinopathy is a hemorrhagic retinopathy occurring after heavy lifting, vomiting, coughing, or straining at stool. It may be associated with macroaneurysms or diabetic retinopathy.

Valsalva retinopathy is due to a rupture of the superficial retinal capillaries and a marked rise in the retinal venous pressure. It is caused by a **Valsalva's maneuver,** a rapid increase of the intrathoracic and intra-abdominal pressure during a forcible effort against a closed glottis.

The retinopathy appears as multiple retinal hemorrhages of various sizes (sometimes up to 1 or 2 dd) and various shapes (many of them dome shaped) or as preretinal hemorrhages with a horizontal fluid level, often partially hemolyzed and centered about the macula (Figure 4-19). Occasionally, massive fluffy clouding of retinal transudates may be present. Also, it may precipitate small areas of isolated, localized retinal edema. Hemorrhages resolve in a few days or weeks. Serous macular detachment may persist longer, but spontaneous reattachment usually occurs and leaves a normal fundus.

Symptoms

The predominant symptom of Valsalva retinopathy is a sudden decrease in the visual acuity after coughing, sneezing, heavy lifting, or straining at stool.

Diagnosis

Diagnosis via visual field testing may show a central scotoma. Fluorescein angiography reveals no leakage.

Histopathology

Histologic analysis reveals preretinal (subhyaloid) hemorrhages and intraretinal hemorrhages. Serous detachment of the internal limiting membrane is possible. Localized retinal edema may be present.

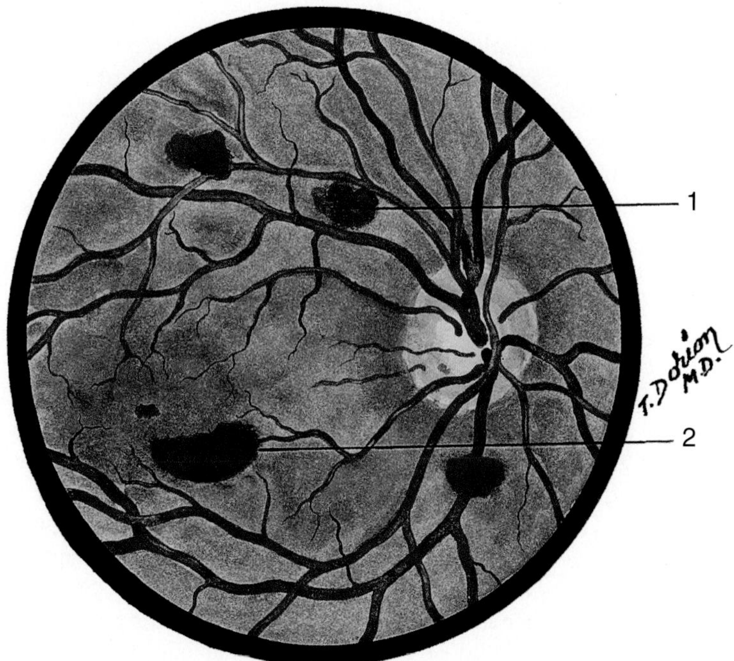

Figure 4-19. *Valsalva retinopathy. (1) Intraretinal hemorrhage. (2) Preretinal hemorrhage.*

Treatment

No treatment for Valsalva retinopathy is available, as the hemorrhage resolves spontaneously.

Shaken Baby Syndrome

Also termed *battered child syndrome*, *whiplash shaken infant syndrome*, and *child abuse retinopathy*, shaken baby syndrome is a hemorrhagic retinopathy that occurs after a violent shake of an infant; after a direct eye, head, or chest trauma; or after a nonaccidental trauma by intentional child abuse or a lack of reasonable care of a child by parents, babysitters, or other caretakers. Such cases usually exhibit a discrepancy and implausible history between the two parents in explanation of the child's injury and delay in seeking medical assistance.

The retinopathy is due to broken small retinal vessels that cause hemorrhages of all kinds—subretinal, intraretinal, preretinal, or vitreal—by repetitive acceleration and deceleration motions of the brain, which may produce tearing of the bridging dural vessels as a consequence of the shaking. At the same time, the vitreous forces may act in a perpendicular direction to the plane of the retina and may cause a separation of the internal limiting membrane, a retinal detachment, or a dialysis. These intraocular hemorrhages usually are secondary to an intracranial hemorrhage, such as a subarachnoid or subdural hemorrhage. They may also be due to a mechanical increase of the arterial and venous pressure or to a rise of the central venous pressure from thoracic compression or centrifugal forces.

The hemorrhages appear in various sizes and depth—from small, superficial splinter or flame-shaped hemorrhages to round, deep, dome-shaped, or geographic, lake-shaped extensive hemorrhages—or as hemorrhagic retinoschisis. Most of the time, the hemorrhages are white-centered (Roth's spots). Often, a large, sub–internal limiting membrane hemorrhage may occur at the macula. Also, vitreal hemorrhage may occur in isolation or associated with subdural, subarachnoid, or cerebral contusion. All these hemorrhages may clear in time, leaving residual scars (sometimes in the macula) or vitreal strands that may produce rhegmatogenous retinal detachment, tractional retinal tears, or ring-shaped retinal folds surrounding the macula (usually outside the retinal vascular arcades). The optic disc also may be affected. Initially, hemorrhages occur in the nerve sheath, followed by papilledema and optic atrophy associated with chorioretinal atrophy. Cotton-wool spots may be present.

Symptoms

Shaken baby syndrome symptoms include skin bruises, hyphema, chemical eye burns, and retinal detachment. Often, convulsions, coma, and other neurologic signs follow the trauma.

Treatment

Treatment should begin with consultations with a pediatrician, a neurologist, and other specialists for joint complex treatment. Administrative action might entail a change in the child's custody. In some cases, legal action may be mandated.

Herpes Zoster Retinitis

Herpes zoster retinitis is a vascular retinopathy that may affect the optic nerve. It is caused by *herpes zoster ophthalmicus*, a virus that results from the activation of a latent *varicella-zoster virus* (VZV), or *chickenpox VZV*, in the trigeminal ganglion. It spreads through the neurons of the ophthalmic nerve, the first division of the fifth cranial nerve. It occurs more commonly in elderly and debilitated persons, in AIDS patients, in acute retinal necrosis syndrome, and in neurologic disorders. It may be produced by direct viral invasion, by vasculitis, or by neuritis.

Herpes zoster retinitis appears as small, yellowish lesions located along the retinal vessels and usually in the outer retina. Initially, retinal vessels and the inner retina are spared. After a period (most commonly 3 weeks), these lesions enlarge as geographic areas of outer retinal necrosis. Variably sized and shaped intraretinal hemorrhages also may be present. The optic disc may become congested and acutely swollen, and an optic neuritis may develop. Occasionally, there is a hemorrhagic chorioretinitis with vitritis.

Symptoms

Symptoms include blurred vision. Visual acuity may be decreased markedly to light perception. Other symptoms include pain and redness, ulcerative skin lesions on eyelids, conjunctivitis, episcleritis, scleritis, keratitis, iridocyclitis, and glaucoma. Neurologic signs include cranial nerve palsies, encephalitis, contralateral hemiplegia, and postherpetic neuralgia.

Diagnosis

Diagnosis by visual field testing may reveal extensive constricted field defects.

Differential Diagnosis

Herpes simplex virus (HSV) should be considered in the differential diagnosis.

Histopathology

Histologic examination confirms a perivascular lymphocytic infiltration in the retina. Areas of retina are partially necrotic. Intraretinal hemorrhage and retinal vasculitis usually are present. The choroid may have inflammatory cells and the optic disc may be infiltrated by lymphocytes. The presence of a positive immunoperoxidase staining indicates herpes zoster.

Treatment

Herpes zoster retinitis may be treated by administration of acyclovir (Zovirax), 800 mg PO five times daily for 7 days, or 5–10 mg/kg IV every 8 hours for 7 days, plus prednisone, 60 mg PO for 3 days, tapered and followed by oral treatment. Also beneficial are famciclovir (Famvir), 500 mg PO three times a day for 1–2 weeks, and valacyclovir (Valtrex), 1,000 mg PO three times a day for 7 days. Foscarnet (Foscavir) may be given intravenously, 60 mg/kg 1-hour infusion. Corticosteroids are used in the treatment of all but immunocompromised patients and include prednisolone (Pred Forte) 1%, 1 drop four times a day. For treatment of glaucoma, beta-blockers may be administered (timolol [Timoptic] 0.5%, 1 drop twice a day, or Timoptic XE 0.25%, 1 drop once daily; betaxolol [Betoptic] 0.5%, 1 drop twice a day; levobunolol [Betagan] 0.5%, 1 drop twice a day; carteolol [Ocupress] 1%, 1 drop twice a day; epinephrine [Dipivefrin], 1 drop twice a day). Carbonic anhydrase inhibitors include acetazolamide (Diamox sequels), one 500-mg sustained-release capsule PO twice a day. Cycloplegics (e.g., atropine 1%, 1 drop three times a day) may be used, but *miotics are to be avoided.*

Acute Retinal Necrosis Syndrome

Also known as *Kirisawa's uveitis*, acute retinal necrosis syndrome (ARN) is a viral disease that occurs in healthy, immunocompetent persons of any age. The disorder often is bilateral, the second eye being involved after several weeks. It includes episcleritis, vitreous opacification, and a necrotizing retinitis.

The etiology of ARN may be unknown. Most commonly, it is caused by VZV or HSV type 1 and 2, or by *cytomegalovirus* (CMV), possibly by an immunocytopathologic process.

It appears in an early stage as small, opaque, multifocal, whitish yellow lesions scattered in the peripheral retina outside the temporal vascular arcades. In a later stage (in some 3 weeks), these lesions may spread rapidly, coalesce, and become opalescent and confluent in broad areas, in a circumferential progression up to 360 degrees. The posterior margin is irregular and scalloped, and a sharp transition occurs between the involved and the noninvolved retina. Full-thickness necrotizing retinitis, sometimes in a geographic pattern with posterior nummular infiltrates, may develop in a later stage. Initially, vessels are normal but, in time, a secondary retinal vasculitis may be present; often it is obliterative, with narrowed, whitened, and sheathed vessels accompanied by scattered hemorrhage along the vessel borders. Occasionally, white plaques—probably *immune reactants*—may be seen in the arteries.

For most of the time, the arterial circulation is compromised minimally. The inner retina and macula usually are spared. As the lesion progresses, the peripheral retina may become thinned, a pigmented epiretinal membrane is formed, and the vitreous may contract and become opacified, forming a *proliferative vitreoretinopathy with retinal folds, type* C. Exudative retinal detachment may occur. Possible retinal tears, located usually in the inferior posterior retina, may lead to a rhegmatogenous retinal detachment. Giant tears may appear along a demarcation area between normal and affected retina and may extend in perhaps 6 weeks to approximately three-fourths of the eye. An overlying marked vitritis, with abundant vitreous cells, usually is present. Optic disc edema is possible. The necrotizing retinitis regresses and may reveal an RPE stippling and atrophy (corresponding to the area of prior retinitis) and a fibroglial proliferative area, overlying a central scar.

Symptoms

Symptoms of ARN include blurred vision, with blindness within weeks if not treated; photophobia; unilateral or bilateral ocular or periorbital pain; increased IOP, and limbal flush. ARN may result in granulomatous keratic precipitates, relative afferent pupillary defect, and decreased color vision.

Diagnosis

Diagnosis on the basis of visual field testing may reveal a central scotoma. Serum titers for VZV, herpes simplex, toxoplasmosis, and CMV are indicated for diagnosis. Urine analysis should be performed for CMV, in addition to CT scan of the orbit. B-scan ultrasonography may reveal an enlarged optic nerve. Anterior chamber paracentesis may show antibodies of HSV-1. The following tests should be performed: CBC with differential cell count, FTA-ABS, RPR, ESR, and purified protein derivative of tuberculin (PPD) with anergy panel. Fluorescein angiography also should be performed.

Differential Diagnosis

Considerations in the differential diagnosis include Behçet's disease, sarcoidosis, toxoplasmosis, CMV retinopathy, ocular lymphoma (reticulum cell sarcoma), and pars planitis. Toxocariasis, ophthalmic artery occlusion, ocular ischemic syndrome, and commotio retinae (Berlin's edema) are other possible diagnoses.

Histopathology

Histologic evaluation confirms marked choroidal thickening, lymphocytic infiltration involving larger choroidal vessels, and intranuclear inclusions. In the cicatricial stage, an RPE proliferation and migration underlie a thinned peripheral necrotic retina. A nonpigmented epithelial membrane on the surface of the necrotic retina may be present. Immunoperoxidase staining for herpes zoster may be positive.

Treatment

Treatment for ARN includes administration of acyclovir (Zovirax), 800 mg PO five times daily for 7 days, then tapered for months; ganciclovir (Cytorene), 2.5 mg/kg IV every 8 hours for 10 days, or 500 mg PO every 4 hours; or foscarnet (Foscavir), 60 mg/kg IV every 8 hours for 4 weeks. Systemic corticosteroids include methylprednisolone, 250 mg IV four times a day for 3 days, followed by prednisone, 60 mg PO twice a day for 2 weeks. Aspirin, 650 mg PO per day for 2 months, may be used.

Retinal detachment can be treated by prophylactic application of a triple row of laser photocoagulation or pneumatically. Surgical intervention includes pars plana vitrectomy with silicone oil injection, scleral buckling, and optic nerve sheath decompression.

Topical cycloplegics include atropine 1%, 1 drop three times a day, and homatropine 1%, 1 drop three times a day. Beta-blockers used include timolol (Timoptic) 0.5%, 1 drop twice a day, betaxolol (Betoptic) 0.50%, 1 drop twice a day, and carteolol (Ocupress) 1%, 1 drop twice a day. Possible anticoagulants are heparin, 1,500 U/hour IV, under control of prothrombin time, partial thromboplastin time, bleeding time, blood urea nitrogen, and platelet count, and then warfarin (Coumadin), 2.5–7.5 mg PO per day for 2 weeks.

Wyburn-Mason Syndrome

Also known by such other names as *racemose hemangioma, congenital AV anastomosis*, *Bonnet-deChaume-Blanc syndrome*, and *cirsoid aneurysm*, Wyburn-Mason syndrome is a familial, nonhereditary, unilateral, nonprogressive or slowly growing congenital communication between the afferent and efferent retinal vessels. It is an AV shunt in which the blood flows directly from the involved vein, without any intervening capillaries (Figure 4-20). Usually, it is associated with similar malformations of the ipsilateral midbrain, the basofrontal region, or the posterior fossa; of the orbit, or the pulsatile vascular nevi of the face, which is the distribution of the trigeminal nerve (cranial nerve V).

The syndrome probably is due to a failure in the differentiation of the anterior plexus of the cerebrovascular primordium in the embryo. It appears as markedly dilated and tortuous normal or malformed vessels that project forward from the retina, involving a small area of one quadrant, or from the entire fundus. It results in a complete loss of the normal vascular pattern and abnormal A/V ratio (normal, 2:3). Rarely, the dilated and tortuous vessels may regress and then recur.

The syndrome may appear as a single peripheral AV anastomosis, sometimes with a hairpin loop that connects the AV segment, or as a complex system that may obscure all retinal details (like filling the fundus with a **bag of worms**). At the disc, it may appear as a knot of retinal tissue. There may be macular hemorrhages or vitreous hemorrhages, exudates, CRVO, retinal edema, or sclerosis.

Symptoms

Decreased visual acuity usually is the predominant symptom of Wyburn-Mason syndrome.

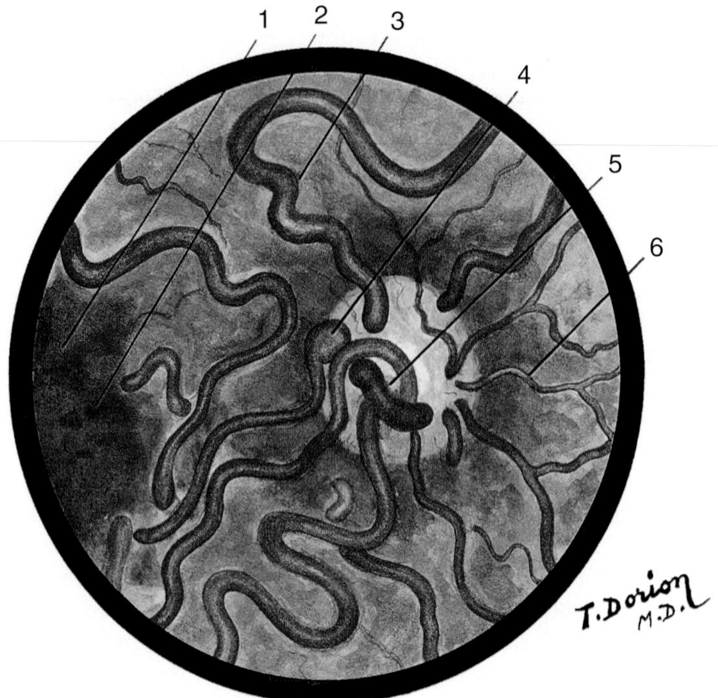

Figure 4-20. *Wyburn-Mason syndrome. (1) Vitreous hemorrhage. (2) Macular hemorrhage. (3) Malformed, markedly dilated vessels, with complete loss of normal vascular pattern. (4) Arteriovenous anastomosis. (5) Knot of retinal tissue at disc. (6) Normal retinal vessels.*

Diagnosis

Visual field analysis may show hemianopic field defects. Fluorescein angiography reveals dilated veins and significant capillary closure of the adjacent retina but *no leakage*. MRI of the brain may show intracranial vascular malformations. Electroencephalography is used to confirm the diagnosis.

Differential Diagnosis

The leading consideration in the differential diagnosis is retinal capillary hemangioma.

Histopathology

Histologic evaluation shows cirsoid, racemose, serpentine, plexiform, or cavernous hemangiomas of the retina and of the optic nerve. There may be abnormalities or complete absence of the capillary bed between the arteries and the veins.

Treatment

Treatment of Wyburn-Mason syndrome is not necessary.

Giant-Cell Arteritis

Giant-cell arteritis (GCA; also termed *temporal arteritis* or *cranial arteritis*) is an idiopathic vascular retinopathy, an inflammatory obliterative arteritis (Figure 4-21). It involves extradural branches of the external carotid artery, such as the temporal artery or the ophthalmic artery, the medium and large muscular arteries of the head, and the proximal part of the vertebral artery, and occurs more frequently in white women older than 60. It may be associated with polymyalgia rheumatica.

GCA is triggered by damage of the extraocular vessels and not by direct involvement of the retinal vasculature. When the posterior ciliary arteries supplying the optic nerve are involved, an ischemic optic neuropathy may develop. It appears as an arteriosclerotic fundus, with marked narrowing of the retinal vessels and sometimes with CRAO or BRAO, venous stasis retinopathy, intraretinal hemorrhages, or (less frequently) cotton-wool spots. The disc occasionally may be swollen slightly, with blurred margins and a mild papilledema. Conversely, it may be pale or completely infarcted with striate peripapillary hemorrhages or an AION or optic malacia. Sometimes, the disc may have a flat atrophic excavation, with sharply delineated margins. Often, GCA may precipitate a **pseudo–Foster-Kennedy syndrome**, with an ischemic papillitis in one eye and optic atrophy in the other. Occasionally, the posterior pole may be unaffected, the area of occlusion being retrobulbar.

Symptoms

Symptoms include excruciating pain over the temporal artery, headache, and morning neck stiffness. It may produce tenderness in the

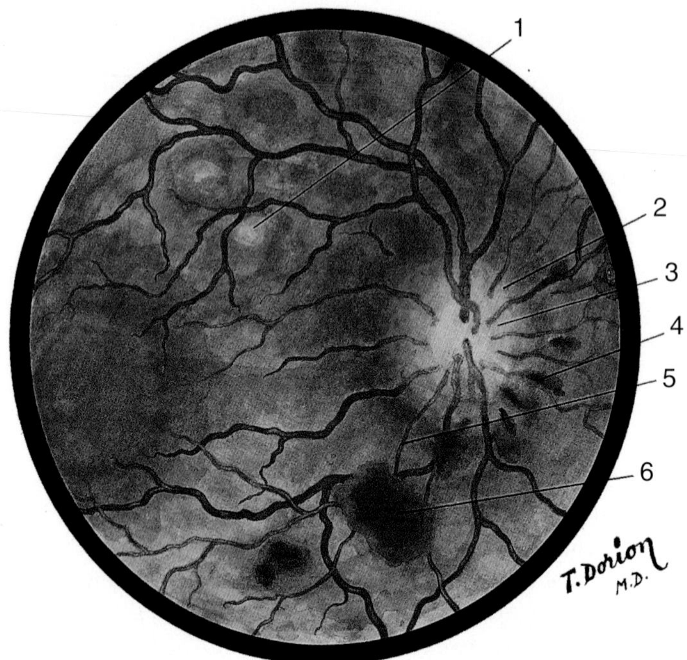

Figure 4-21. *Giant-cell arteritis. (1) Cotton-wool spots. (2) Slightly swollen disc, with blurred margins. (3) Disc pallor. (4) Striate peripapillary hemorrhages. (5) Marked narrowing of retinal vessels. (6) Intraretinal hemorrhages.*

forehead and temporal scalp areas when the hair is combed. The temporal artery is visible as a firm strand and is tortuous, nodular, and pulseless. Jaw claudication may result in pain in chewing. Other symptoms are sudden vision loss, amaurosis fugax, scotomas, and markedly rapid decrease in visual acuity in 3–12 weeks. Cortical blindness may ensue. GCA is known to trigger nausea, fever, anorexia, weight loss, malaise, myalgia, brain stem stroke, ophthalmoplegia, diplopia with sixth and third nerve palsy, tonic pupil, and angina.

Diagnosis

Diagnostic signs are a Westergren ESR elevated above 100 mm/hour (normal, 35–40 mm/hour) and an elevated fibrinogen level in plasma (normal,

200–400 mg/dl). A CBC may show a normocytic hypochromic anemia. The white blood cell count may be increased. Serum alkaline phosphatase is increased. Protein electrophoresis reveals a marked elevated *serum alpha$_2$-globulin* and *beta-globulin.* The level of C-reactive protein is raised, and the liver enzyme level may be elevated. Doppler ultrasonography is used to detect the side of artery obliteration. Temporal biopsy may reveal extensive giant-cell and mononuclear cell infiltration in the vessel wall.

Orbital biopsy may be performed. Relative afferent pupillary defect or *Marcus-Gunn pupil* consists of a constriction of both pupils when the light is directed at the normal eye and a dilatation of both pupils when the light then is rapidly transferred to the affected eye. Visual field testing may reveal an altitudinal field defect. Fluorescein angiography may show slightly delayed filling of the optic disc and peripapillary circulation with leakage. Ocular plethysmography is a further diagnostic test for the presence of GCA.

Differential Diagnosis

Considerations in the differential diagnosis include polyarteritis nodosa, nonarteritic ischemic neuropathy, papillitis, CRVO, CRAO, and optic nerve tumor.

Histopathology

Histologic analysis confirms a granulomatous vasculitis of the temporal artery. It is accompanied by thrombosis, intimal hyperplasia, and infiltration by multinucleated giant cells, plasma cells, and lymphocytes. Further characterizing signs include disruption and reduplication of the elastic lamina, then the infiltration of cells spreads into the media and adventitia, occluding the lumen. When involved, the disc may exhibit gliosis, glitter cells, fat-laden histiocytes, or total atrophy. The macula may display a marked atrophy of the ganglion cell layer and the nerve fiber layer.

Treatment

Treatment calls for *immediate bilateral excision and biopsy of a portion of temporal artery.* Also viable are a biopsy of the facial artery or of the superficial posterior occipital artery. Hospitalization is indicated.

Systemic corticosteroids should be administered, starting with prednisolone, 100 mg/day or 1 mg/kg/day PO, IM, or IV, tapering to a maintenance dose of 20 mg/day (or less) for at least 6 months. An alternate regimen is methylprednisolone, 250 mg IV every 6 hours in 12 doses (in the hospital), before switching to oral prednisone, 60 mg/day.

Antiulcer medication should be given, such as an H_2 blocker (e.g., ranitidine [Zantac], 150 mg PO twice a day). Iron, folic acid, and vitamin B_{12} are beneficial for treatment of anemia. Consultation with an internist is essential.

Suggested Reading

Balles MW, Puliafito CA, D'Amico DJ, et al. Semiconductor diode laser photocoagulation in retinal vascular disease. Ophthalmology 1990;97:1553–1555.

Blake J. General Injuries. In A Sorsby (ed), Modern Ophthalmology, vol 2 (2nd ed). Philadelphia: Lippincott, 1972;617–634.

Brown GC. Retinal arterial obstruction. Focal Points 1994;3:3–11.

Butler FK, Harris DJ Jr, Reynolds RD. Altitude retinopathy on Mount Everest. Ophthalmology 1992;99:739–746.

Capone A Jr, Wallace RT, Meredith TA. Symptomatic choroidal neovascularization in blacks. Arch Ophthalmol 1994;112:1091–1097.

Collins ML, Nelson LB, Parlato CJ. Ophthalmic and Systemic Manifestations of Child Abuse. In W Tasman, EA Jaeger, MM Parks, et al. (eds), Duane's Clinical Ophthalmology, vol 5. Philadelphia: Lippincott–Raven, 1996;44:1–10.

Dukker JS, Fischer DH. Acute Retinal Necrosis. In W Tasman, EA Jaeger, MM Parks, et al. (eds), Duane's Clinical Ophthalmology, vol 3. Philadelphia: Lippincott–Raven, 1996;28:1–6.

Fogle JA, Green WR. Ciliochoroidal Effusion. In W Tasman, EA Jaeger, MM Parks, et al. (eds), Duane's Clinical Ophthalmology, vol 4. Philadelphia: Lippincott–Raven, 1996;63:1–6.

Gafliano DA, Jampol LM, Rabb MF. Sickle-Cell Disease. In W Tasman, EA Jaeger, MM Parks, et al. (eds), Duane's Clinical Ophthalmology, vol 3. Philadelphia: Lippincott–Raven, 1996;17:1–33.

Gass JD, Blodi BA. Idiopathic juxtafoveolar retinal telangiectasis. Ophthalmology 1993;100:1536–1539.

Greven CM, Weaver RG, Owen J, Slusher MM. Protein S deficiency and bilateral branch retinal occlusion. Ophthalmology 1991;98:33–34.

Hunter PA. Infections of the Outer Eye. In DJ Spalton, RA Hitchings, PA Hunter (eds), Atlas of Clinical Ophthalmology (2nd ed). London: Wolfe, 1994;4.22.

Jaeger E. Venous Obstructive Disease of the Retina. In W Tasman, EA Jaeger, MM Parks, et al. (eds), Duane's Clinical Ophthalmology, vol 3. Philadelphia: Lippincott–Raven, 1996;15:1–21.

Katz B, Hoyt F. Intrapapillary and peripapillary hemorrhage in young patients with incomplete posterior vitreous detachment. Ophthalmology 1995;102:349–354.

Lewis H, Schachat AP, Haimann MH, et al. Choroidal neovascularization after laser photocoagulation. Ophthalmology 1990;97:503–511.

Lieb WE, Flaharty PM, Sergott RC, et al. Color Doppler imaging provides accurate assessment of orbital blood flow in occlusive carotid artery disease. Ophthalmology 1991;98:548–552.

Loose IA, Schroeder RD. Retinopathy and distant extraocular trauma. In W Tasman, EA Jaeger, MM Parks, et al. (eds), Duane's Clinical Ophthalmology, vol 3. Philadelphia: Lippincott–Raven, 1996;32:1–4.

Mames RN, Snady-McCoy L, Guy J. Central retinal and posterior ciliary artery occlusion after particle embolization of the external carotid artery system. Ophthalmology 1991;98:527–531.

McAlister IL, Constable IJ. Laser-induced chorioretinal venous anastomosis for treatment of nonischemic central retinal vein occlusion. Arch Ophthalmol 1995;113:456–468.

McNamara JA. Treatment of Advanced Stages of Prematurity (ROP). In W Tasman, EA Jaeger, MM Parks, et al. (eds), Duane's Clinical Ophthalmology, vol 6. Philadelphia: Lippincott–Raven, 1996;108:1–10.

McNamara JA, Moreno R, Tasman W. Retinopathy of Prematurity. In W Tasman, EA Jaeger, MM Parks, et al. (eds), Duane's Clinical Ophthalmology, vol 3. Philadelphia: Lippincott–Raven, 1996;20:1–11.

McNamara JA, Tasman W, Brown G, Federman JL. Laser photocoagulation for stage 3+ retinopathy of prematurity. Ophthalmology 1991;5:576–580.

Palena PV, Ausburger JJ. Phakomatoses. In W Tasman, EA Jaeger, MM Parks, et al. (eds), Duane's Clinical Ophthalmology, vol 3. Philadelphia: Lippincott–Raven, 1996;34:1–10.

Palmer EA. Current management of retinopathy of prematurity. Focal Points 1993;3:2–12.

Palmer EA. Retinopathy of prematurity. Focal Points 1982;12:1–11.

Palmer EA, Flynn JJ, Hardy RJ, et al. The cryotherapy for retinopathy of prematurity cooperative group. Ophthalmology 1992;99:329.

Patz, A. Retrolental Fibroplasia (Retinopathy of Prematurity). In A Sorsby (ed), Modern Ophthalmology, vol 2 (2nd ed). Philadelphia: Lippincott, 1972;3–10.

Rosenbaum JT. Practical diagnostic evaluation of uveitis. Focal Points 1993;6:1–11.

Schatz H, Fong ACO, McDonald R, et al. Cilioretinal artery occlusion in young adults with central retinal vein occlusion. Ophthalmology 1991;98:594–601.

Sebeg J. Vitreous Pathology. In W Tasman, EA Jaeger, MM Parks, et al. (eds), Duane's Clinical Ophthalmology, vol 3. Philadelphia: Lippincott–Raven, 1996;39:5–21.

Sorsby A. Genetically Determined Anomalies. In A Sorsby (ed), Modern Ophthalmology, vol 2 (2nd ed). Philadelphia: Lippincott, 1972;43–85.

Troost BT, Glaser JS. Aneurysms, arteriovenous communications, and related malformations. In W Tasman, EA Jaeger, MM Parks, et al. (eds), Duane's Clinical Ophthalmology, vol 2. Philadelphia: Lippincott–Raven, 1996;17:16–22.

Wyhinny GJ, Jackson JL, Jampol LM, Caro NC. Subretinal neovascularization following multiple evanescent white-dot syndrome. Arch Ophthalmol 1990;108:1384–1385.

Zion VM. Phakomatoses. In W Tasman, EA Jaeger, MM Parks, et al. (eds), Duane's Clinical Ophthalmology, vol 5. Philadelphia: Lippincott–Raven, 1996;36:1–13.

5

Inflammatory Retinopathy

Pars Planitis

Pars planitis is also called *intermediate uveitis*, *peripheral uveitis*, *basal uveovitritis*, *chronic cyclitis*, and *vitritis*. Of unknown etiology, it is a moderate inflammation of the anterior vitreous and peripheral retina and usually is bilateral. It follows an indolent course, with remissions and exacerbations or even spontaneous resolution, sometimes after 20 years or more. Pars planitis occurs more commonly in otherwise healthy children and in young adults and more frequently in the winter. The anterior segment may not be affected or may show only minimal to mild inflammation. Pars planitis may occur in multiple sclerosis, Whipple's disease, ocular lymphoma (reticulum sarcoma), Lyme disease, and sarcoidosis and may be associated with the haplotype HLA-DR2, DQW1.

Pars planitis may be produced by an inflammatory process, a degenerative cystic formation, or a fibrous proliferation with neovascularization. A deficiency of cell-mediated immunity against the *retinal S-antigen*, an immunologic reaction to vitreous cells, or an allergy to its own retina may be the cause.

Pars planitis appears as a white membrane or as fluffy yellowish cottonball exudates located in the deep vitreous and over the pars plana and the inferior retina. The early stage evinces discontinuous yellowish gray exudates or clumps called *snowballs* or *snowbanking*, which appear abruptly just anterior to the ora serrata over the inferior pars plana. In a later stage, as the process continues, these exudates may coalesce into a massive plaque of smooth, gelatinous, white-gray membrane covering the ora serrata. Vitreal opacities, organization, hemorrhage, or even scars may develop, usually at the vitreous base. At the peripheral retina, degenerative cysts, areas of neovascularization, or sometimes exudative retinal detachment may appear. The disc may appear mildly hyperemic, showing neovascularization, peripapillary edema, or papilledema. Vessels may appear tortuous, dilated, or segmented (with sheathing as a retinal periphlebitis) or may exhibit small, pale, gelatinous exudates along the vascular walls. There may be retinal artery attenuation, neovascularization at the peripheral retina, retinal vasculitis, occlusion of the terminal retinal venous branches, and phlebitis. Foveal reflex usually is absent. Cystoid macular edema, with patchy dispersion of pigment, may also be present. Pars planitis may precipitate vitreous hemorrhages, proliferating retinal astrocytes, or collapsed vitreous. Intraocular pressure may be increased as a secondary glaucoma, and there may be posterior vitreous detachment.

Symptoms

Pars planitis may be asymptomatic. It also may result in asthenopia, blurred vision, floaters, pain, redness, photophobia, decreased vision, and cataract.

Diagnosis

Diagnosis is obtained by indirect ophthalmoscopy with scleral depression. Slit-lamp examination with a Goldmann three-mirror lens is used to confirm diagnosis. Fluorescein angiography may reveal staining and diffuse leakage from retinal vessels and capillaries in all quadrants, in the optic nerve head, and in the macula. Diagnostic tests should include chest roentgenograms and serum lysozyme titers. Angiotensin-converting enzyme level is increased. Additional tests include fluorescent treponemal antibody absorption test, immunofluorescent antibody test, enzyme-linked immunosorbent assay, antinuclear antigen, HLA-B27 antigen test, and polymerase chain reaction (PCR).

Differential Diagnosis

The differential diagnosis should include toxoplasmosis, toxocariasis, filariasis, multiple sclerosis, amyloidosis, inflammatory bowel disease,

Lyme disease, cataract, retinal detachment, juvenile chronic arthritis, ankylosing spondylitis, and ocular lymphoma (reticulum sarcoma).

Histopathology

Histologic examination reveals a chronic nongranulomatous inflammation of the vitreous base, with fibrocytes and scattered mononuclear cells adjacent to a hyperplastic nonpigmented pars plana epithelium. Also, T-lymphocyte cuffing may be seen. The disc is swollen, with perivascular infiltrates. There is edema and pigment disorganization at the macula. The retina may be detached, with a separation between retinal pigment epithelium (RPE) and sensory retina. The internal limiting membrane may be wrinkled. The vitreous contains snowballs composed of collapsed condensed vitreous, blood vessels, scattered lymphocytes, spindle-shaped cells, glial cell proliferation, neovascularization from the retina, new collagen, and hyperplastic nonpigmented pars plana epithelium.

Treatment

No treatment is required for pars planitis. For cystoid macular edema, corticosteroids may be administered. They may take the form of *periocular* depot injections or posterior sub–Tenon's capsule injections, up to six doses of methylprednisolone (Depo-Medrol), 80 mg/ml 1 ml, or triamcinolone, 40 mg/ml 0.5 ml every 2 weeks, repeated for at least 4 months. *Systemic* therapy may take the form of prednisone, 60 mg/day PO for 4 weeks. High-dose pulse IV methylprednisolone in a single dose can be administered. *Topical* agents include prednisolone 1% (Pred forte) 1 drop PO four times a day. Acetazolamide (Diamox sequels), one 500-mg time-released capsule PO daily, can also be used.

Retinal cryopexy also is beneficial, using a single freeze-thaw cycle per application to the areas of snowbanking or neovascularization within the vitreous base. Immunomodulating agents, such as cyclophosphamide or cyclosporine, 5 mg/kg/day, selectively depress the proliferation of activated T-lymphocytes. Treatment can also include antimetabolites, such as methotrexate, 15 mg PO daily for a 5-day course. Surgical options include vitrectomy and cataract extraction by phacoemulsification, isolated or combined with pars plana vitrectomy, *but intraocular lens implantation in the posterior chamber should be performed only in an eye that has remained quiescent for 6–12 months before surgery.*

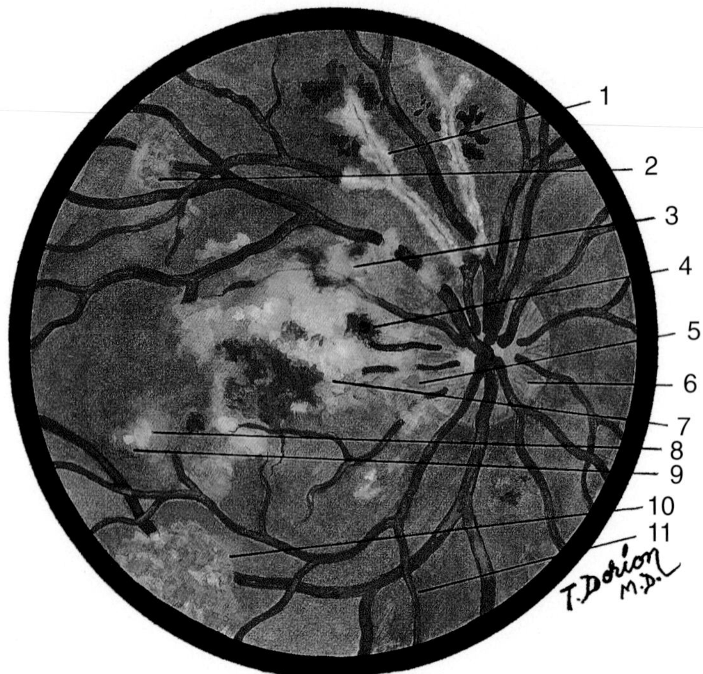

Figure 5-1. *Cytomegalovirus (CMV) retinitis. (1) Frosted-branch angiitis. (2) Brushfire retinitis. (3) Retinal creamy infiltrates. (4) Blotchy hemorrhage. (5) Juxtapapillary lesion. (6) Optic neuritis. (7) Pizza-pie lesion. (8) Healed lesion. (9) Satellite lesion. (10) Granular retinal infiltrate with retinal pigment epithelium atrophy. (11) Arterial attenuation.*

Cytomegalovirus Retinitis

Cytomegalovirus (CMV) retinitis is either congenital or acquired and can emerge as unilateral or bilateral chorioretinitis (Figure 5-1), which occurs more frequently in immunocompromised men, such as patients with acquired immunodeficiency syndrome (AIDS). It may be associated with prematurity, cerebral calcifications, chorioretinitis, splenomegaly, purpura, hemolytic anemia, interstitial pneumonitis, microphthalmos, cataract, optic atrophy, and optic disc malformations.

CMV retinitis is caused by an opportunistic neurotropic virus, CMV, that contains DNA. The **congenital** form is due to a transplacental infection and usually appears as a *central retinitis*. The **acquired** form occurs often after a kidney transplant, in diabetes, from an infected maternal cervix during delivery, or by nasal droplet infection, sexual transmission, or blood transfusion and appears as a *peripheral retinitis*.

The two clinical types of lesions in CMV retinitis are **active** (a rapidly progressive, necrotic lesion with hemorrhage and usually located at the posterior pole) and **indolent** (a slowly progressive, infiltrative lesion usually located at the peripheral retina).

In its early stage, CMV retinitis appears as scattered opaque, white-gray, granular patches of round or oval dots located deep in the retina. These dots have irregular, sharply demarcated and ragged edges, are variably sized, and usually are noncontiguous. As the disease progresses, the patches become multiple, multifocal, dry, yellow-white, and densely opaque and are located perivascularly in irregular sheathing. They may coalesce and extend in the periphery or at the posterior pole or at both locations, including the peripapillary area. Perivenous creamy infiltrates, retinal necrosis, and (rarely) cotton-wool spots may be present. Blotchy hemorrhages, retinal vasculitis, or arterial attenuation also may be seen. Sometimes, there is a whitening of the vessels (called *frosted-branch angiitis*) with both active and inactive lesions. A thin glial membrane and slate retinal scars may appear in time. The macula may contain multiple focal lesions, which may resolve to a pigmented macular scar. Often, the disorder may result in a juxtaposition of whitish granular necrosis and red retinal hemorrhage (called *pizza-pie*, or *cheese-and-ketchup*, or *tomato-ketchup*) lesion. Occasionally, areas of retinal edema or nonrhegmatogenous retinal detachment may occur, or rhegmatogenous retinal detachment with breaks may be found, located in the area of atrophic healed lesions. Sometimes, there are focal granular infiltrates, which enlarge along a line and leave the destroyed retina and the atrophic RPE behind with some bleeding at the edges; this condition is called *brushfire retinitis*. As the old lesions heal, new lesions called *satellite lesions* appear at their margins. The optic disc may be congested as an optic neuritis with juxtapapillary retinitis. The vitreous generally is quiet but, occasionally, proliferative vitreoretinopathy with fixed retinal folds may be present. Choroid, pars plana, and ora serrata usually are spared.

Symptoms

Patients with CMV retinitis may complain of mild floaters. The disorder may trigger decreased visual acuity, possibly as poor as no light perception.

Diagnosis

The disorder may be diagnosed as relative afferent pupillary defect. Virus may be isolated from urine, throat swab, tears, or liver biopsy. An indirect fluorescent antibody test may be positive. Complement fixation antibody titers may be positive (>1:64), and the T-lymphocyte count will be low (<50/µl). CD4 count will be less than 50 cells/mm.

Differential Diagnosis

Considerations in the differential diagnosis should include toxoplasmosis, rubella, syphilis, and herpes simplex infection.

Histopathology

Histologic analysis should reveal a coagulative necrotizing retinitis, with scant lymphocytes, neutrophilic infiltration, and large cytomegalic cells with tiny, multiple *basophilic intracytoplasmic* **inclusion bodies** and large *eosinophilic intranuclear inclusions* (called *virions*). Subendothelial hemorrhage, pigment dispersion, retinal fibrosis, and atrophy also are present. Destruction of the axons in the nerve fiber layer may be found. The macula may evince a hyperplastic scar, and calcium deposits may be seen in the retinal layers.

Treatment

Treatment includes such antiviral antimetabolites (virostatics) as ganciclovir (Cytovene) given initially as 2.5 mg/kg/day IV for 10 days, followed by a maintenance dose of 5 mg/kg/day IV for 5 days weekly; or as 500 mg PO every 4 hours or 1,000 mg PO three times a day; or by intravitreal injections; or by a sustained slow-release implant. An alternative agent may be used, such as foscarnet (Foscavir), 60 mg/kg IV every 8 hours, followed by a maintenance dose of 90–120 mg/kg every 24 hours, depending on renal toxicity. Combination ganciclovir-foscarnet therapy is viable, *given sequentially, not simultaneously, because the drugs are physically incompatible.* Vidarabine (Vira-A) may be administered. Interferon inducers (Poly I:C) may decrease viruria. Surgical options include pars plana vitrectomy with silicone oil injection for reti-

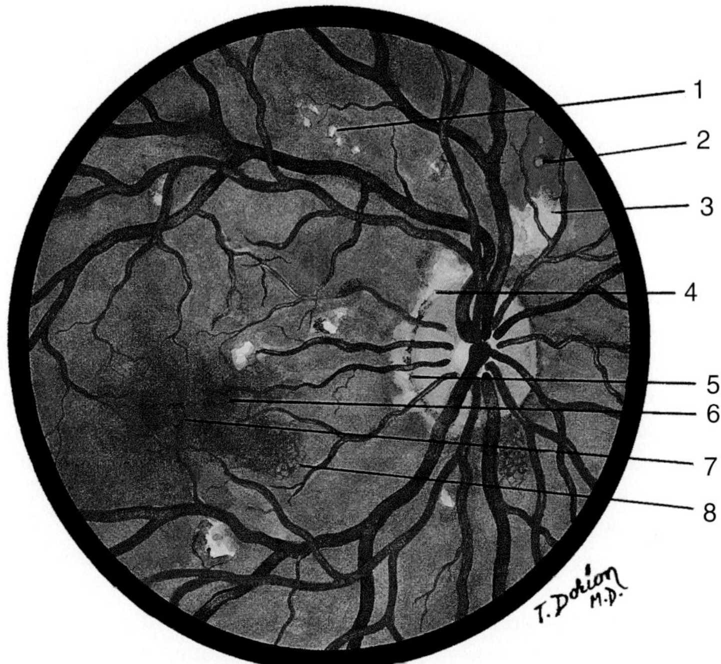

Figure 5-2. *Histoplasmosis. (1) Typical histospots. (2) Atypical histospots. (3) Scarring. (4) Peripapillary chorioretinal atrophy. (5) Pigmented line at the disc margin. (6) Subretinal hemorrhage. (7) Retinal pigment epithelium detachment. (8) Chorioretinal neovascularization.*

nal detachment. Treatment may be directed to reducing the immunocompromising drugs for cancer chemotherapy or after kidney transplant.

Histoplasmosis

Also termed *presumed ocular histoplasmosis syndrome*, histoplasmosis is an infectious disease (Figure 5-2) caused by a soil fungus, *Histoplasma capsulatum*, endemic in the Ohio-Mississippi Valley (and occasionally in Europe), or by exposure to chickens, pigeons, and parakeets or to bird droppings. There may be a relationship between the systemic infection and the ocular disease.

Three types of histoplasmosis ocular lesions are identified: *chorioretinopathy*, *solitary granuloma*, and *diffuse endophthalmitis.*

Clinical Types

Histoplasmosis chorioretinopathy is formed by a triad of histospots, peripapillary chorioretinal atrophy, and subretinal hemorrhage. **Histospots** appear as small, punctate, round or oval peripheral chorioretinal atrophic lesions with pigment located centrally or eccentrically; they may even be nonpigmented, of some one-eighth to one-fourth disc diameter in size. Histospots may be typical or atypical. *Typical histospots* appear as sharply circumscribed, punched-out lesions with a uniformly flat or excavated bottom. *Atypical histospots* appear as creamy-yellow lesions with indistinct margins and with a slightly elevated (rather than excavated) bottom.

Peripapillary chorioretinal atrophy appears as a white-yellow or green-yellow zone that usually *reveals a pigment line at the disc margin*, as opposed to the **crescent** in some normal eyes, wherein *the pigment is located at the outer border of the scar.*

Subretinal hemorrhage appears as an extremely dark gray or purple-red dusky hemorrhage arising from chorioretinal neovascularization. It may extend onto the macula.

Occasionally, a *disciform maculopathy* may occur, appearing as a circumscribed, slightly elevated white-yellow or gray area, as choroidal infiltration, or as a serous retinal detachment. The macula may appear mottled, with or without marginal hemorrhages, exudative maculopathy, or subretinal choroidal neovascularization. It may be a dark, greenish or blackish ring of RPE detachment. The vitreous is clear.

Solitary granuloma, a second type of histoplasmosis, appears as a unique grayish-yellow tumor that varies in size and elevation, with relatively well-defined margins, usually located in the midperiphery.

Diffuse endophthalmitis is the third type of histoplasmosis, is very rare, and has none of the foregoing lesions. It appears as a focal or disseminated retinitis, mostly at the periphery and associated with vitritis, and as iridocyclitis.

Symptoms

No symptoms accompany the onset of histoplasmosis, unless the macula is involved.

Diagnosis

Fluorescein angiography may demonstrate leakage. The complement fixation test is negative. Chest roentgenograms may show calcifications. Both the histoplasmin skin test and the HLA-B27 test may be positive.

Differential Diagnosis

Considerations in the differential diagnosis are other granulomatous diseases, such as tuberculosis, sarcoidosis, coccidioidomycosis, and cryptococcosis. Other possible diagnoses are high myopia, age-related macular degeneration, multifocal choroiditis, and drusen.

Histopathology

Histologic appraisal shows aggregation of lymphocytes surrounding focal zones of downgrowth of retinal cells, presumed to be *astrocytes*, into the choroid (Figure 5-3). There are lipid deposits, histiocytes, and breaks and cracks in Bruch's membrane. Scattered RPE melanin granules and RPE detachment or proliferation may be present. Chorioretinal atrophy with gliotic scarring occurs. Usually, photoreceptors and the choriocapillaris are destroyed in areas of punched-out lesions. Additionally, retinal detachment, fibrovascular organization, and hyalinization may be present. Occasionally, *Histoplasma* fungus may be seen in a lymphocytic perivascular infiltrate.

Treatment

Antifungal treatment with amphotericin B (Fungizone) is not efficient. Antihistamine intradermal desensitization with histoplasmin is beneficial. Acute maculopathy calls for systemic prednisone, 50–150 mg PO in the morning, or prednisolone acetate, 40 mg via retrobulbar injection every week in one or two doses.

Xenon or argon laser photocoagulation can be used for subretinal choroidal neovascular membranes that appear 200 μm or more outside the foveal avascular zone of the macula, or for juxtafoveolar membranes that appear within 200 μm of the center of the foveal avascular zone. Surgical excision of subfoveal choroidal neovascular membranes

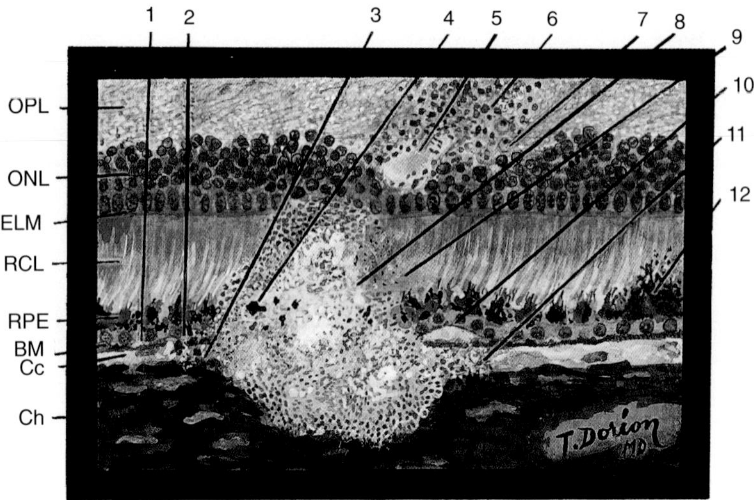

Figure 5-3. *Histopathologic findings in histoplasmosis. (1) Lipid deposits on Bruch's membrane. (2) Breaks and cracks in Bruch's membrane. (3) Focal lymphocytic aggregation surrounding an area of downgrowth of retinal cells, presumed to be astrocytes. (4) Melanin granules. (5) Vessel. (6) Perivascular lymphohistiocytic infiltrate. (7) Nest of* Histoplasma capsulatum. *(8) Chorioretinal atrophy with punched-out lesions and gliotic scars. (9) Destroyed rod and cone layer. (10) RPE detachment. (11) Destroyed choriocapillaris. (12) RPE proliferation. (OPL, outer plexiform layer; ONL, outer nuclear layer; ELM, external limiting membrane; RCL, rod and cone layer [photoreceptors]; RPE, retinal pigment epithelium; BM, Bruch's membrane; Cc, choriocapillaris; Ch, choroid.)*

is an alternative. Patients should avoid aspirin, coughing, Valsalva's maneuver, or nonpressurized ascent above 800 feet.

Sympathetic Ophthalmia

Sympathetic ophthalmia is a uveitis of unknown origin that occurs in both eyes. It appears anytime between perhaps 9 days to more than 40 years after an ocular perforating wound or an intraocular operation usually in one eye only (Figure 5-4).

Sympathetic ophthalmia probably is triggered by an infection due to a virus or bacteria or by a cell-mediated autoimmune mechanism of hyper-

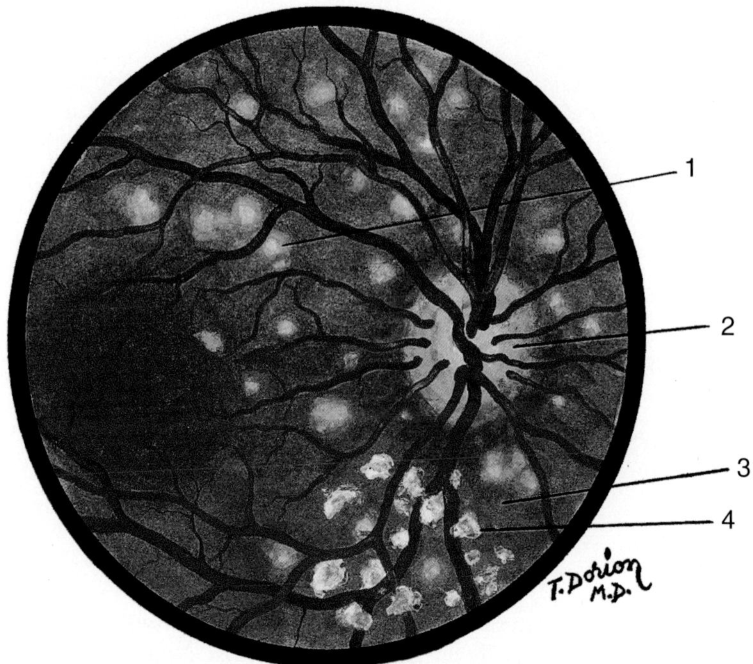

Figure 5-4. *Sympathetic ophthalmia (1) Dalen-Fuchs nodules. (2) Pale, swollen disc. (3) Hazy vitreous. (4) Atrophic choroidal scars.*

sensitivity to the uveal pigment (called *sympathizing reaction*) in which the injury of one eye programs the body against the uveal tissue of both eyes.

The appearance of sympathetic ophthalmia is that of several small, slightly elevated, yellow-white or creamy, fluffy spots (**Dalen-Fuchs nodules**). They are located at the posterior pole and the peripheral retina and may coalesce. Gliosis and choroidal scars may be present. The optic disc may be pale and swollen, and the vitreous may be hazy and may contain vitreous cells.

Symptoms

Sympathetic ophthalmia symptoms include photophobia, pain, and redness. Blurred vision may ensue in the noninjured eye, *the sympathizing eye.*

Diagnosis

A history of trauma or surgery is common in sympathetic ophthalmia. Scar of the wound of entry in the injured eye (*the exciting eye*), mutton-fat keratic precipitates, and cells and flare in the anterior chamber in both eyes may be seen. Complete blood cell count (CBC) should be performed, as should a fluorescent treponemal antibody absorption test and angiotensin-converting enzyme titers. Chest roentgenograms, fluorescein angiography, and B-scan ultrasonography are recommended.

Differential Diagnosis

Differential diagnosis should consider the Vogt-Koyanagi-Harada syndrome, phacoanaphylactic endophthalmitis, sarcoidosis, and syphilis.

Histopathology

Histologic analysis reveals **nonnecrotizing granulomatous uveitis**. The choroid usually is markedly thickened and infiltrated. *Nodular infiltration* is represented by Dalen-Fuchs nodules, which are composed mainly of epithelioid cells and giant cells and are located between RPE and Bruch's membrane. *Diffuse infiltration* consists of T-lymphocytes that are interspersed with mononucleated epithelioid cells and multinucleated giant cells, which sometimes may contain melanin granules. Usually, the disorder is located at the posterior choroid, in randomly organized granulomas, and is perivascular. The vitreous may exhibit cells. Optic nerve atrophy also may be present, and the retina and choroid usually are spared.

Treatment

Treatment is enucleation of the severely injured, sightless eye within 9 days after trauma. Topical, periocular, and systemic corticosteroids should be administered if the inflammation has appeared in the second eye, *the sympathizing eye*. Topical cycloplegics include scopolamine (Isopto-Hyoscine) 0.25%, 1 drop three times per day, and atropine 1%, 1 drop three times per day. Systemic immunosuppressive agents, such as methotrexate, 15 mg PO daily for a 5-day course are administered.

Herpes Simplex Retinopathy

Herpes simplex retinopathy is a bilateral infectious retinochoroiditis. It is congenital or acquired at the time of delivery by exposure in the birth canal and is caused by *herpes simplex virus* (HSV) *type 1*. It may be associated with keratitis, encephalitis, or hepatitis and may occur in newborns and adults.

In the *newborn*, HSV appears as large, yellow-white patches located (sometimes fulminatingly) at the equatorial retina and capable of coalescing into a massive, diffuse white area. The disorder evinces numerous intraretinal exudates of various sizes and shapes, retinal edema, or necrotizing retinitis. Retinal arteries are dilated markedly, and retinal vasculitis and retinal neovascularization often are present. Choroidal hemorrhages may be seen. The vitreous may reveal diffuse opacities and an extensive vitritis, and the optic disc may be atrophic. Sometimes, a disseminated intraocular coagulopathy may develop. The disease may be lethal.

In *adults*, HSV appears as numerous fluffy white areas scattered throughout the fundus. Flame-shaped intraretinal hemorrhage may be present. Retinal vessels are engorged markedly and are sheathed. Areas of retinal neovascularization also may be seen. Diffuse granular pigmentation (and sometimes widespread areas of retinal necrosis) and overlying vitreous involvement may be present. Retinal detachment and posterior vitreous detachment occasionally may occur. After healing, the retina remains thinned and reduced to a glial scar tissue. RPE is hyperpigmented. HSV may affect immunosuppressed patients with AIDS, and it may be systemic.

Symptoms

HSV may be asymptomatic, or patients may present with unilateral red eye, photophobia, decreased vision, tearing, eyelid rash, or keratitis.

Diagnosis

Blood culture for virus should be performed. Other diagnostic tests include enzyme-linked immunosorbent assay, PCR assay of the aqueous, and serology for HSV antibodies.

Differential Diagnosis

Considerations for the differential diagnosis should include toxoplasmosis, rubella, CMV, and syphilis.

Histopathology

Histologic evaluation reveals a full-thickness necrotizing retinitis. It also shows an extensive retinal hemorrhagic necrosis, especially in the inner layers, with infiltration of polymorphonuclear leukocytes, plasma cells, and lymphocytes. Photoreceptors usually are spared. Vascular inflammation is minimal, with swollen endothelial cells that may obstruct the lumen. There may be a focal necrosis of the RPE. The choroid may demonstrate infiltration of plasma cells, polymorphonuclear cells, and intranuclear inclusions in choroidal cells.

Treatment

Treatment can be effected with acyclovir, 30 mg/kg PO in three divided doses or 200 mg PO five times daily for 10 days. Additional agents include vidarabine (Vira-A), 15 mg/kg/day IV for 10 days, and foscarnet (Foscavir), 60 mg/kg IV every 8 hours for 10 days.

Progressive Outer Retinal Necrosis

Progressive outer retinal necrosis (*PORN syndrome*) is an extremely rapidly progressive, acute, peripheral necrotic retinopathy. Usually, it occurs in AIDS patients as a variant of necrotizing herpetic retinopathy, with poor prognosis leading to blindness. It may be caused by *varicella-zoster virus*, and the disorder may recur.

It appears as multiple, discrete, white-yellow, opaque foci or patches. These lack granular borders, are located deep in the outer retina, and initially spare the inner retina. The patches range in size from less than 50 μm to 1,000 μm and usually are located at the periphery (with or without macular involvement), at the posterior pole, or at the optic disc. They may coalesce in larger areas of full-thickness necrosis and form a whitish outer retinal sheen. The necrosis may extend very quickly 360 degrees around the globe, through which the retinal vessels clearly are visible. Small perivascular hemorrhages may accompany the disorder and, occasionally, retinal detachment may occur. Often, there is perivascular sheathing in the necrotic area or adjacent to it. In time, these lesions resolve, leaving a lucency around the veins. Visible are large, white, atrophic plaques in which early removal of necrotic debris and a retinal edema adjacent to the vessels results in the appearance of **cracked mud**. A mild optic neuritis and minimal vitritis may be present.

Symptoms

Initially, bilateral blurred vision may emerge as a symptom. Additional symptoms include severe, irreversible rapid visual loss, possibly to no light perception in 1 month if not treated aggressively. Unilateral or bilateral ocular pain also may result.

Diagnosis

Diagnosis is derived from culture or PCR identification of varicella-zoster virus. Low CD4 lymphocyte counts (<50 cells/mm) are characteristic.

Histopathology

Histologic analysis provides evidence of a complete atrophy of sensory retinal layers. The RPE is disorganized and shows pigmentary changes. Retinal vessels are sclerotic in the necrotic area. Plaques of retinal scarring are present, and preretinal fibrosis overlying the posterior pole also is seen.

Treatment

Treatment consists of antiviral therapy. Agents include acyclovir, 800 mg PO five times daily for 10 days, or 10 mg/kg IV every 8 hours; foscarnet (Foscavir), 60 mg/kg IV every 8 hours for 4 weeks; ganciclovir (Cytovene), 500 mg PO every 4 hours, or 2.5 mg/kg IV for 10 days (or ganciclovir intraocular device); or vidarabine (Vira-A), 15 mg/kg/day IV for 10 days. Combined antiviral therapy is beneficial. Other interventions include laser photocoagulation and repair of retinal detachment by silicone oil tamponade.

Brushfire Retinitis

Brushfire retinitis is a slowly progressive, necrotizing retinitis that occurs in CMV retinitis. It appears mostly in immunocompromised persons, such as AIDS patients. It probably is caused by a direct cell-to-cell transfer of the infected virions of the DNA virus (CMV).

Brushfire retinitis appears as a yellow granular area of focal infiltrates (usually with no hemorrhage) and as an advancing active edge in the peripheral retina, mostly anterior to the equator. It enlarges slowly along a line, leaving behind areas of RPE atrophy and destroyed, burned-out retina.

Symptoms

The major symptom of brushfire retinitis is decreased visual acuity, which may be irreversible.

Diagnosis

Visual field examination may reveal a progressive vision loss, usually temporally.

Treatment

Treatment is similar to that of CMV retinitis, including administration of ganciclovir and foscarnet.

Candidiasis

Candidiasis is an insidious, indolent chorioretinitis. It is mostly bilateral and slowly progressive and is caused by the fungus *Candida albicans* (Figure 5-5). It occurs frequently in patients receiving chemotherapy, immunosuppressive cytotoxic drugs, steroids, parenteral hyperalimen-

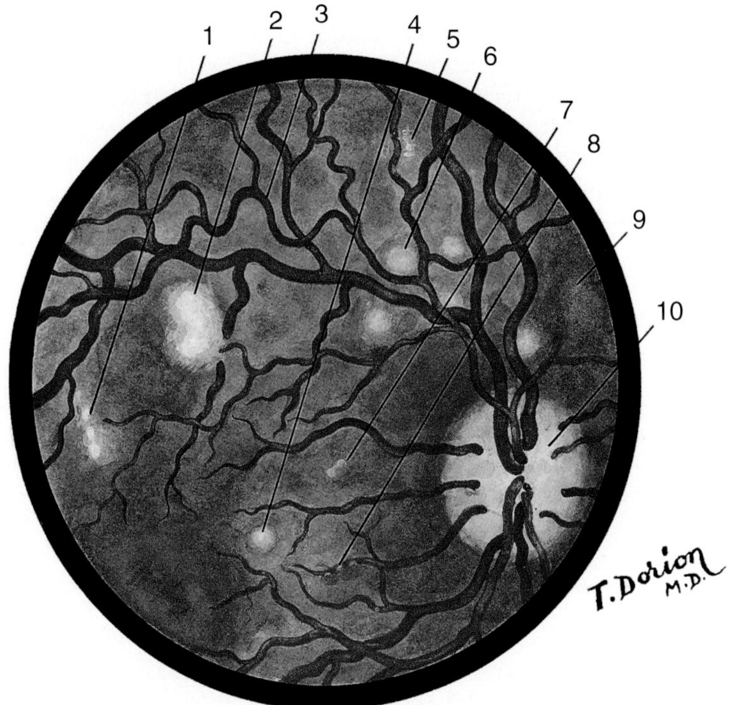

Figure 5-5. *Candidiasis. (1) String of pearls. (2) Snowball in the vitreous. (3) Tortuosity of the vessels. (4) Headlight in the fog. (5) Perivascular infiltrate. (6) Cotton-wool spots. (7) Isolated nerve fiber layer infarct. (8) Perivascular plaques (or Kyrieleis arteriolitis). (9) Hazy vitreous. (10) Pallor of the disc.*

tation, or hemodialysis. Additionally, candidiasis can occur after abdominal surgery and prolonged antibiotics; with indwelling catheters, irradiation, intravenous drug abuse, diabetes, and esophageal ulcers; and in debilitating diseases, malnutrition, malignancies, and immunocompromised persons with AIDS.

Candidiasis probably is due to the direct effect of the fungus on the retina, choroid, and optic nerve. The fungal infection usually enters the eye through the chorioretinal circulation and may affect also the heart valves, the female genital tract, and the central nervous system.

Initially, candidiasis may appear as small, round to oval, irregular, homogeneous, yellow-white retinal lesions. These lesions, resembling cotton-wool spots, have fluffy margins and small adjacent retinal exudates and are scattered over the fundus. The lesions may appear deep into the retina and may enter the vitreous. Also visible are perivenous infiltrates and periarterial sheathing or plaques, called **Kyrieleis arteriolitis.** These infiltrates may spread to involve the optic nerve, which may become pale. Sometimes, Roth's spots, focal areas of superficial arteritis, tortuosity, perivasculitis, papillitis, and endophthalmitis, may occur. Rarely, isolated nerve fiber layer infarcts may be seen. The vitreous may demonstrate diffuse cellularity and haze (or vitreous microabscesses) as **snowball** opacities that may be linked together as a **string of pearls** or as vitreous infiltrate, called *headlight in the fog.*

Symptoms

The predominant symptom of candidiasis is decreased visual acuity. Floaters and sometimes bilateral pain also accompany the disorder.

Diagnosis

Diagnosis of *C. albicans* is obtained from culture of blood, urine, or intravenous site or by vitreous biopsy. A CBC should be performed, and blood urea nitrogen (BUN) and creatinine levels should be assessed. Liver function tests should be run. Echocardiography should be used to rule out valvular involvement.

Histopathology

A granulomatous choroiditis and a necrotic retinitis are demonstrated on histologic evaluation. There may be retinal nerve fiber infarctions. Budding blastopores and pseudohyphae may be present. Fungus usually is located in the choriocapillaris but may be present also through Bruch's membrane.

Treatment

Candidiasis is treated with amphotericin B, 5–10 mg/day IV, while the BUN level is monitored (normal, 8–25 mg/dl); this level may increase by as much as 40 mg/dl (in which case the drug should be discontinued). Alternatively, amphotericin B, 5 μg intravitreally, may be given. Other agents are flucytosine, 150 mg/kg PO daily, divided in three doses for 3 weeks; fluconazole (Diflucan), 150 mg/day PO in a single dose; or ketoconazole, 200–400 mg/day PO. Cycloplegics include atropine 1% three times daily.

Other interventions include pars plana vitrectomy. Systemic corticosteroids may be administered after 48 hours of antifungal therapy. Antibiotics, such as rifampin (Rifadin), 20 mg/kg PO every 12 hours, are also used.

Cryptococcosis

Cryptococcosis is also termed *torulosis* or *European blastomycosis*. It is a bilateral chorioretinitis caused by the fungus *Cryptococcus neoformans*, also called *Torula histolytica*. It occurs in disseminated pulmonary diseases, meningitis, immunocompromised patients (e.g., those with AIDS), tuberculosis, and syphilis. It affects kidney transplantation patients under immunosuppressive therapy and occurs after corticosteroid or broad-spectrum antibiotic therapy or after exposure to pigeons.

Cryptococcosis appears as multiple, small, yellow or gray-white retinal and subretinal exudates with irregular fluffy borders. The exudates often are elevated 2–3 mm and are scattered over the fundus. The disorder may be accompanied also by retinal angiectasis, marked arterial attenuation, and perivascular infiltrates. *C. neoformans* fungus may be seen within the retina. The optic disc usually is pale and sometimes is severely swollen, with surface hemorrhage that in time may become atrophic. A later stage may demonstrate a subretinal exudative fluid, serous retinal detachment, and endophthalmitis.

Symptoms

Symptoms of cryptococcosis include blurred vision and eventual decreased visual acuity to hand movement or no light perception. Light flashes and floaters are noticeable. Pain, redness, hypopyon, and rubeosis iridis can result. Large keratic precipitates (mutton-fat precipitates) appear. Ophthalmoplegia also may occur.

Diagnosis

Diagnostic workup would include blood culture on Sabouraud's dextrose agar medium. Urinalysis and cerebrospinal fluid analysis should be performed. On biopsy, fungus identification can be obtained by mucicarmine stain or India ink preparation, which demonstrate the fungus's characteristic mucopolysaccharide capsule. Fluorescein angiography may reveal hypofluorescence in the early phase and, in the late phase, staining and dye leaking. B-scan ultrasonography may show a medium internal reflectivity, moderate acoustic hollowness, and no choroidal excavation.

Histopathology

Histologic analysis shows focal or diffuse granulomatous necrotizing lesions located in the choroid and retina. *C. neoformans* may be present as a budding organism with a thick gelatinous capsule and giant cells in a granulomatous retinal lesion or within the optic nerve sheath. There also may be intraretinal hemorrhage, uveitis, retinal detachment, optic atrophy, or endophthalmitis.

Treatment

Treatment is effected by antifungal therapy with amphotericin B (Fungizone), 0.075–0.300% 1 drop every hour topically, then tapered; or 1 mg every 48 hours subconjunctivally for two doses; or 1 mg in 500 ml 0.5% dextrose in water IV over 4 hours for 4–12 weeks while monitoring the BUN level (with a pretreatment with hydrocortisone, 25 mg IV, and a narcotic to minimize the adverse effects); or 5 μg intravitreally. Other treatment options include fluconazole (Diflucan), 200 mg PO for 12 weeks; flucytosine (5-FC; Ancobon), 10 mg/ml 1 drop every hour topically, then tapered, or 100–150 mg/kg/day PO every 6 hours in four divided doses; or itraconazole (Sporanox), 200 mg PO twice a day for 6 months, or 1%, 1 drop every hour topically, then tapered.

Aspergillosis

Aspergillosis is a retinochoroiditis and vitritis caused by the fungus *Aspergillus fumigatus*. This bacterium produces a systemic disease—an opportunistic infection—that occurs from contact with infected soil or manure and sometimes in intravenous drug abusers, in patients on corticosteroids and undergoing immunosuppressive therapy after kidney transplantation, in CMV retinitis patients, in debilitated patients with leukemia and other hematologic disorders, and in conjunction with Goodpasture's syndrome, alcoholism, bronchopneumonitis, prematurity, chronic sinus disease, and polyps. The disorder may occur also in healthy persons living in hot, humid climates and may be lethal.

Aspergillosis is due to an infectious destructive effect of the hyphae of that fungus on the retina, choroid, and vitreous. It appears as small white lesions that may have a hemorrhagic center and is disseminated into the retina. The lesions may progress to microabscesses that may be found also in the choroid. The hyphae of the fungus might produce retinal necrosis and exudative retinal detachment. Intraretinal hemorrhages may occur. During the extension of the infection, the vitreous becomes involved, and an endophthalmitis may develop. In this late stage, the fundus may appear as a **pseudohypopyon**. Cells usually are present in the vitreous.

Symptoms

Symptoms include blurred vision, ocular pain, redness, eyelid swelling, chemosis, iritis, keratic precipitates, hypopyon, rubeosis iridis, and proptosis.

Diagnosis

Diagnosis is confirmed by marked eosinophilia in the peripheral blood (up to 80%; normal, 1–3%) and an elevated serum IgE level. Positive skin test corroborates the diagnosis.

Histopathology

Necrosis in the retina is revealed on histologic evaluation. There is marked perivasculitis and abscesses in the choroid. Septate, branching hyphae are possible in the subretinal space and in the choroid, retina, and vitreous. Multiple polymorphonuclear leukocytes may be present in the vitreous and beneath the internal limiting membrane. The optic nerve may be necrotic, with macrophages phagocytosing disintegrating myelin.

Treatment

Antifungal therapy consists of amphotericin B (Fungizone), 1.0–1.5 mg/kg IV every 4 hours for 3 months, or 5 μg intravitreally; flucytosine (5-FC; Ancobon), 100–150 mg/kg/day in four divided doses; itraconazole (Sporanox), 200 mg PO twice a day; ketoconazole (Nizoral), 200–800 mg/day in a single dose for weeks or months; or rifampin (Rifadin), 300 mg PO twice a day. Pars plana vitrectomy and drainage of abscess also are viable interventions.

Brucellosis

Also called *Malta fever* or *Bang's fever*, brucellosis is a nodular choroiditis with optic neuritis and, rarely, a severe endophthalmic panuveitis. The disorder usually occurs as a systemic, acute, or (more often) insidious infection after direct contact with infected hoofed farm animals, such as goats, sheep, cattle, and swine. It appears in slaughterhouse workers from contact with infected meat, in farmers and veterinarians after contact with placentae of infected animals, or after ingestion of unpasteurized milk or cheese.

Brucellosis is caused by a direct inflammatory effect of a gram-negative bacillus: *Brucella melitensis* (in goats), *B. suis* (in hogs), or *B. abortus* (in cattle). The bacterium may enter through abraded skin, through mucous membranes, or through the respiratory tract.

The disorder appears as single or multiple tiny choroidal nodules that are yellow-white, are slightly elevated, and are surrounded by a moderate retinal exudation or a circumscribed area of subretinal edema. Often, the optic disc is moderately congested and swollen, with blurred margins, having the appearance of an optic neuritis or a mild papilledema. A few small retinal hemorrhages may be scattered at the posterior pole. These are self-limited and resolve leaving pigmented scars.

Symptoms

Among the many symptoms are decreased vision, nodular iritis, nummular keratitis, dacryocystitis, fever, chills, night swelling, headache, abdominal pain, constipation, arthralgia, weakness, weight loss that may persist for years, anorexia, cervical and axillary lymphadenopathy, hepatosplenomegaly, and depression. Abscesses in the bones, spleen, or brain may occur.

Diagnosis

The agglutination test is positive when it reveals fourfold elevated titer (usually >1:100). IgG antibodies are observed in the acute phase. Blood culture may be positive in the early stage of the disease. A CBC may show an absolute or relative lymphocytosis and serum glutamic pyruvic transaminase may be elevated.

Differential Diagnosis

The differential diagnosis should consider influenza, tularemia, Q fever, enteric fever, Hodgkin's disease, tuberculosis, malaria, and psychoneurosis.

Histopathology

Histologic analysis reveals a granulomatous or nongranulomatous uveitis, with intensive nodular lymphoid cell infiltration into the choroid. There is a swelling of the optic nerve fibers, and there may be subretinal edema.

Treatment

Treatment includes tetracycline, 2 g/day PO for 3 weeks; streptomycin, 0.5 g IM every 12 hours; ampicillin, 100 mg PO every 8 hours; and trimethoprim-sulfamethoxazole (Bactrim DS), PO twice a day for 2 weeks. Topical corticoids are beneficial, as is prednisolone acetate 1% (Pred forte), 1 drop four times a day. Bed rest and adequate nutrition are necessary.

Suggested Reading

Anand R, Font RL, Fish RH, Nightingale SD. Pathology of cytomegalovirus retinitis treated with sustained release intravitreal ganciclovir. Ophthalmology 1993;100:1032–1039.

Brod RD, Clarkson JG, Flynn HW, Green WR. Endogenous Fungal Endophthalmitis. In W Tasman, EA Jaeger, MM Parks, et al. (eds), Duane's Clinical Ophthalmology, vol 3. Philadelphia: Lippincott–Raven, 1996;11:1–27.

Culberston WW. Viral retinitis. Focal Points 1988;12:1–12.

Donahue SP, Greven CM, Zuravleff JJ, et al. Intraocular candidiasis in patients with candidemia. Ophthalmology 1994;101:1302–1309.

Engstrom RE Jr. The progressive outer retinal necrosis syndrome. Ophthalmology 1994;101:1488–1492.

Gilles CL, Bloom JN. Uveitis in Childhood. In W Tasman, EA Jaeger, MM Parks, et al. (eds), Duane's Clinical Ophthalmology, vol 4. Philadelphia: Lippincott–Raven, 1996;56:4–6.

Godfrey WA. Acute Anterior Uveitis. In W Tasman, EA Jaeger, MM Parks, et al. (eds), Duane's Clinical Ophthalmology, vol 4. Philadelphia: Lippincott–Raven, 1996;40:7–8.

Hooper PL. Pars planitis. Focal Points 1993;12:2–11.

Macular Photocoagulation Study Group. Five year follow-up of fellow eyes of individuals with ocular histoplasmosis and unilateral extrafoveal or juxtafoveal choroidal neovascularization. Arch Ophthalmol 1996;114:677–688.

McDonald HR, Bustos SD, Sipperley JO. Vitrectomy for epithelial membrane with candida chorioretinitis. Ophthalmology 1990;4:466–469.

Patel SS, Rutyen AR, Marx JL, et al. Cytomegalovirus papillitis in patients with acquired immune deficiency syndrome. Ophthalmology 1996;103:1476–1482.

Specht CS, Mitchell KT, Bauman AE, Gupta M. Ocular histoplasmosis with retinitis in a patient with acquired immune deficiency syndrome. Ophthalmology 1991;98:1356–1360.

Woods AC. Brucellosis. In A Sorsby (ed), Modern Ophthalmology, vol 2 (2nd ed). Philadelphia: Lippincott, 1972;145–150.

6

Degenerative Retinopathy

Age-Related Macular Degeneration

Age-related macular degeneration (ARMD), also known as *senile macular degeneration*, is a degenerative lesion of the macula that occurs bilaterally but *not necessarily simultaneously*, sometimes developing over several years. It is of multiple etiologies and occurs more commonly in sclerotic, elderly patients. It may be caused by an abnormal cellular metabolism of the retinal pigment epithelium (RPE) or of the photoreceptors, which may produce an RPE proliferation, accumulation of fibrotic neovascular tissue, thickening and splitting of Bruch's membrane, choroidal neovascularization, RPE detachment, and scar formation. *There is no evidence of any inflammatory process.* ARMD may have a genetic basis. Environment may be important, as the phenotype in Japan is different from that in Western Europe or North America.

There are usually two clinical types, dry and wet. **Dry** (or **atrophic, nonexudative**, or **nonvascular**) **macular degeneration** (Figure 6-1) appears as a pale macula, with patchy irregular, sharply demarcated areas of mottled pigmentation, scattered clumpings, and depigmentation. There may be drusen, which appear as small, discrete, round, slightly elevated, hard, yellow spots or sometimes as large, nodular, laminar or cuticular lesions with ill-defined borders. Foveal reflex is absent. There may be various punched-out areas of RPE atrophy or choroidal atrophy with a total choroidal loss that is irregular, called **geographic** or **areolar macular atrophy**. Occasionally, small intraretinal cysts filled with an edematous fluid are seen, which may lead to a

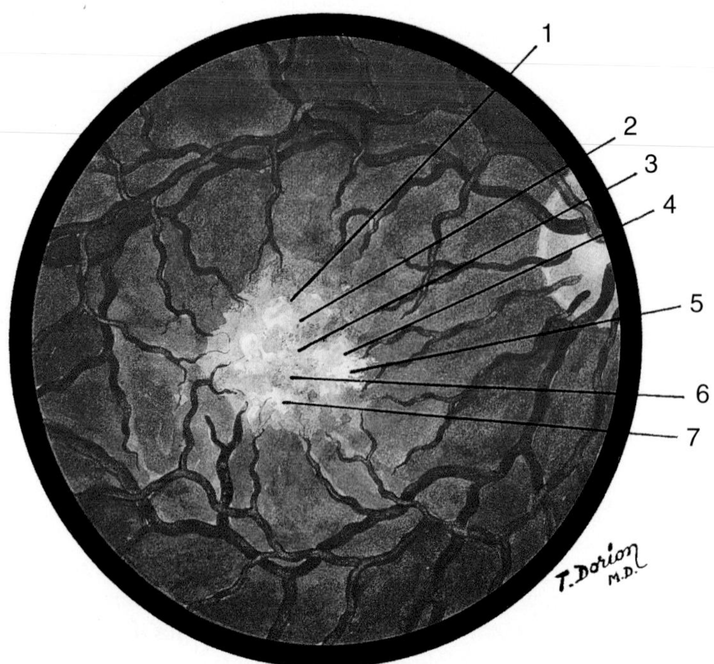

Figure 6-1. *Dry, atrophic, age-related macular degeneration. (1) Geographic, areolar macular atrophy. (2) Mottled pigmentation and depigmentation. (3) Choroidal sclerosis. (4) Drusen. (5) Choroidal atrophy. (6) Cystoid macular degeneration. (7) Scarring.*

macular hole formation, usually in the inner wall of a macrocyst; this is called **cystoid macular degeneration.** Retinal vessels are barely visible as a gray membrane. Choroidal vessels are sclerosed and the blood supply is reduced, giving the appearance of a **central choroidal sclerosis.** Sometimes the lesions in the macula appear oval in shape and transversally oriented, have minimal pigment, and are asymmetric in the two eyes; this condition is called **Haab's macula.**

In **wet** (or **exudative, neovascular, disciform,** or **Kuhnt-Junius**) **macular degeneration,** the macula appears glassy with an irregular surface and is elevated with subretinal fluid accumulation, which may lead to a serous or hemorrhagic macular detachment. Foveal reflex is absent. Retinal vessels often anastomose on the macular surface. Choroidal vessels may invade the retina. Subretinal hemorrhage may be present, and

sub-RPE neovascularization can occur. The sub-RPE neovascularization is usually of two types: *classic*, with demarcated boundaries, or *occult*, in which the margins are not as well defined. There may be retinal detachment or RPE detachment, both appearing as round, sharply demarcated blisters, with smooth dome-shaped contour, with or without RPE tears. **Circinate macular retinopathy** also may occur. At a later stage, a gray-white disciform scar, called **macular pseudotumor** and measuring approximately 3.5 mm in diameter and 0.5 mm in thickness, may develop.

Symptoms

ARMD may be asymptomatic. Alternatively, visual acuity may be lost, or lines and edges may be visually distorted.

Diagnosis

Visual field examination may show a central or paracentral scotoma. Amsler grid testing is useful. Fluorescein angiography may reveal, in the early phase, an elevation of the RPE with uniform pooling of dye and a smooth contour; in the middle phase, pinpoints of speckled hyperfluorescence with fluorescein leakage are seen; in the late phase, the pooling of the dye may obscure the boundaries of the choroidal neovascularization, and there is staining of fibrous tissue. Indocyanine green angiography may reveal an occult form of neovascularization.

Differential Diagnosis

Drusen, histoplasmosis, myopia, choroidal rupture, angioid streaks, choroidal tumor, and laser scars should be considered in the differential diagnosis.

Histopathology

In **dry, atrophic ARMD**, the retina is thinned at the macula, with pigmentary disturbances such as hypopigmentation of the RPE, RPE atrophy, RPE detachment or tears and, in some areas, RPE hypertrophy

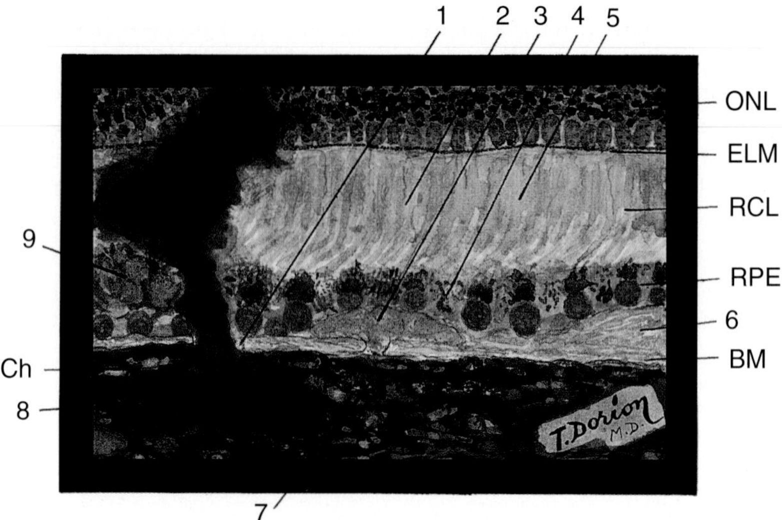

Figure 6-2. *Histopathologic findings in wet, Kuhnt-Junius, age-related macular degeneration. (1) Defects in Bruch's membrane (BM), with subretinal leakage. (2) Degenerated cone processes. (3) Placoid, disciform, sub-RPE degeneration. (4) Abnormal RPE cells. (5) Absence of the cone processes. (6) Sub-RPE fibrovascular tissue. (7) Choroidal neovascularization. (8) Choroidal hemorrhage extending through defects in BM into retina and into vitreous. (9) Adenomatous RPE hyperplasia. (ONL, outer nuclear layer; ELM, external limiting membrane; RCL, rod and cone layer [photoreceptors]; RPE, retinal pigment epithelium; Ch, choroid.)*

or hyperplasia. Bruch's membrane is thickened on its inner face, where a reticulum of parallel membranes and altered collagen fibers, embedded with basal laminar deposits of *calcium* and *lipofuscin*, may be present. Microcystoid spaces in the outer plexiform layer of Henle may be present, as may macrocysts as retinoschisis.

Wet, disciform ARMD (Figure 6-2) presents histologically as RPE proliferation that may grow in a flat pattern, as placoid sub-RPE degeneration, or as adenomatous RPE hyperplasia. Cone processes usually are degenerated or completely absent. There is a choroidal neovascularization, with sub-RPE and subretinal leakage through defects in Bruch's membrane. Accumulation of abnormal fibrotic neovascular tissue and RPE cells may be seen. A disciform scar composed of a thin sub-RPE fibrous and fibrovascular tissue often is present. Occasionally, a hemorrhage may extend into the choroid and break through the retina into the vitreous.

Treatment

Prophylactic treatment of bilateral soft drusen is appropriate. Photodynamic therapy by injection of Verteporfin, a photosensitizing dye and liposomal benzoporphyrin derivate monoacid A (BPD-MA), may be helpful. This drug is selectively absorbed and retained within the choroidal neovascularized tissue but not in normal retinal or choroidal vasculature. Injection must be repeated every 3 months, followed by irradiation and nonthermal laser light, as an exciting source of the neovascularized tissue, which will liberate oxidative energy, thereby causing thrombus formation and indirect obliteration of the new vessels.

Laser photocoagulation, using minimal-intensity burns, is used for an extrafoveolar choroidal neovascular membrane occurring 200–2,500 μm from the center of the foveolar avascular zone. External-beam irradiation with 1,000 cGy to the macula, for subretinal neovascularization, is a treatment that is not yet well established.

Surgical excision to remove the subfoveolar choroidal neovascular membrane may be beneficial, but it also removes the RPE, which will lead to atrophy of the choriocapillaris and subsequent photoreceptor degeneration. An option is surgical macular translocation, by a C-strapped retinotomy in the temporal retina, and subsequent upward and downward movement of the retina, placing the macula in a location with normal RPE. Then laser is applied around the edges of the flap, and silicone oil is injected to maintain a retinal reattachment. Neuronal cell and RPE cell transplantation may be used.

Pharmacologic therapy may be done with interferon. Treatment with an antibody to *vascular endothelial growth factor* and antagonists to integrins may avoid laser-induced retinal damage. Low-vision magnifying glasses, vitamin supplementation, zinc, and antioxidants might be helpful.

Choroideremia

Choroideremia (also known as *progressive chorioretinal degeneration* and *progressive tapetochoroidal dystrophy*) is a bilateral, congenital,

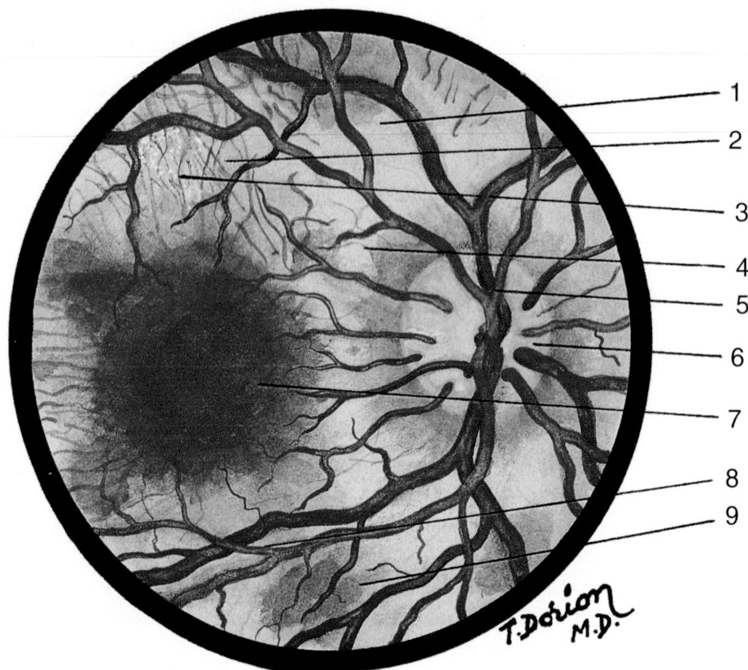

Figure 6-3. *Choroideremia. (1) Extensive chorioretinal atrophy. (2) Bare white sclera. (3) Choroidal vessels traversing sclera. (4) Sclerosed choroidal vessels. (5) Normal retinal vessels. (6) Pale disc. (7) Island of normal macula. (8) Arterial attenuation. (9) Island of normal choroid.*

hereditary, X-linked recessive, progressive chorioretinal atrophy (Figure 6-3). It occurs mostly in male individuals of 4–30 years; hence, men cannot pass the gene to their sons, but all their daughters will be carriers. In women, choroideremia is benign, asymptomatic, and nonprogressive. It is not associated with any other anomaly.

Choroideremia is caused by a degenerative process, the primary defect probably being in the RPE. It appears as large patches of depigmented choroidal atrophy with well-defined margins, located initially at the equator but then expanding toward the periphery and centrally yet sparing the macula. In the midperiphery, occasionally one sees a combination of mottled pigmentation and depigmentation or irregular, minute, square chunks of pigment granules and pale areas up to 0.5 dd in size, called a **salt-and-pepper lesion**.

Sometimes, a macular pigment aggregation forms a dark ball. Choroidal vessels either are sclerosed and exposed or are absent. Retinal vessels usually are normal, but the arteries may be narrowed and slightly thinner than in the normal retina or, in the late stage, retinal artery attenuation may be present. As the degeneration progresses, the bare white sclera, traversed by a few choroidal vessels and pigment clumping, may be seen. Small islands of retina and choroid may remain in the macula and in the periphery.

The optic disc is normal and flat, although rarely a ringlike halo of RPE loss, similar to that in myopia, is seen. At a later stage of disease, the disc may become pale and atrophic.

Symptoms

Night blindness is present from childhood and progresses to blindness over a long period, with complete loss of vision in approximately 35 years.

Diagnosis

Electroretinography (ERG) is abnormal, showing an absence of rod **scotopic activity** (noncolor vision) and a progressive diminution of **photopic activity** (color vision). Visual field examination may reveal progressive constriction of the peripheral vision. Color vision is mostly normal. Fluorescein angiography may show an extensive choroidal atrophy, with visualization of choroidal vasculature and areas of hypofluorescence.

Differential Diagnosis

Conditions that must be considered in the differential diagnosis include retinitis pigmentosa, gyrate atrophy, albinism, and thioridazine (Mellaril) retinopathy.

Histopathology

On histologic examination, there is marked choroidal atrophy that in some areas is total. Extensive retinal degeneration, especially in the outer retinal layers, is apparent. Atrophy of the choriocapillaris and RPE throughout the entire fundus except the macula may be present. Retinal vessels are normal, although occasionally there is arterial attenuation. Choroidal vessels are sclerosed or absent. The optic disc is initially normal, but optic atrophy may develop in advanced stages.

Treatment

No treatment is helpful. The patient might wear dark glasses for comfort. Genetic counseling is appropriate.

Retinitis Pigmentosa

Retinitis pigmentosa, also known as *pigmentary degeneration of the retina* and *dystrophia retinae pigmentosa,* is a *tapetoretinal degeneration*, a bilateral, hereditary, autosomal recessive, dominant, or X-linked disease that occurs symmetrically and is slowly progressive (Figure 6-4). Rarely, it may be unilateral, sectorial, even hypopigmented, in which case it is called **retinitis pigmentosa sine pigmento**. Retinitis pigmentosa may be associated with open-angle glaucoma, posterior subcapsular cataract, disc drusen, pars planitis, myopia, keratoconus, polydactyly, Laurence-Moon-Bardet-Biedl syndrome, Usher's syndrome, Hallgren's syndrome, Refsum's syndrome, Bassen-Kornzweig syndrome, or Kearns-Sayre syndrome. It probably is caused by abnormal genes at various loci within the human genome, often including the *X*, *3*, *6*, and *8 chromosomes*.

Retinitis pigmentosa appears as jet-black or brown pigment flecks, usually crowded paravascularly, resembling **bone spicules**. These are located in the equatorial region and spread toward the midperiphery and pericentrally, occupying more commonly one quadrant of each fundus. *The macula generally is spared, except in X-linked retinitis pigmentosa*, which is the worst form. In this form, there is macular atrophy, cystoid macular edema (CME), cellophane maculopathy, or partial-thickness macular holes. In classic retinitis pigmentosa, there may be blotchy hypopigmentation along the vascular arcades. Retinal vessels are barely visible. Arteries are diffusely narrowed and threadlike, with thickened walls. Choroid vessels may appear prominent, sclerosed, and obliterated. There also may be exudative vasculopathy, such as telangiectasia, serous retinal detachment, or lipid deposits at the periphery. The optic disc usually is pale and waxy yellow owing to edema or retinal ischemia, or it may exhibit drusen.

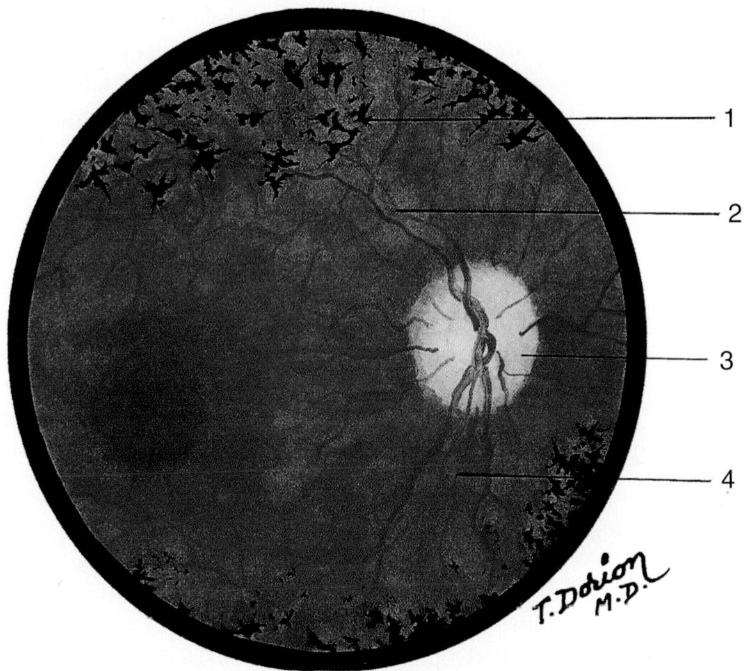

Figure 6-4. *Retinitis pigmentosa. (1) Bone spicule pigmentation at the equator and midperiphery. (2) Retinal vessels, barely visible. (3) Waxy, pale disc. (4) Arterial attenuation.*

Symptoms

Night blindness is present from early youth, and loss of peripheral vision occurs early as well. Then, gradually, visual field constriction to **gun-barrel vision** develops.

Diagnosis

Visual field examination reveals constriction of the visual field with a partial ring scotoma in the midperiphery that corresponds to the equatorial pigmentation and eventually may progress to the entire field, the central visual field being last to be lost. ERG amplitude is reduced or extinguished.

On electro-oculography (EOG), a light rise is completely absent, and only baseline fluctuations are seen. Dark adaptation reveals a curve that is flatter than normal, with only a minor rise, and the *Kohlrausch's kink* is absent. Fluorescein angiography may show a mottled hyperfluorescence at the posterior pole and in the pre-equatorial region.

Differential Diagnosis

Among the conditions that should be considered in the differential diagnosis are pseudoretinitis pigmentosa, phenothiazine toxicity, rubella, syphilis, Refsum's syndrome, toxemia of pregnancy, Vogt-Koyanagi-Harada syndrome, Kearns-Sayre syndrome, and Bassen-Kornzweig syndrome. Congenital stationary night blindness, gyrate atrophy, choroideremia, and vitamin A deficiency are other considerations.

Histopathology

Histologic evaluation reveals progressive disappearance of the photoreceptors, even atrophy, especially of the rods. There is a perivascular degeneration and a hypertrophic proliferation of the RPE. Hyperplasia and a migration of filament-filled macrophages into the retina is seen. Atrophic maculopathy also may be present.

Treatment

No treatment has been found to be effective. Subconjunctival placental extract is controversial. Light deprivation can afford comfort; this is effected by the wearing of protective, dark eyeglasses or opaque contact lenses. Cataract extraction with implantation of an intraocular lens (IOL) in the posterior chamber might be tried. Acetazolamide (Diamox), one 250-mg tablet PO four times per day, may be administered for CME. Vitamin A, 15,000 IU/day, is given. Low-vision aids and genetic counseling should be offered.

Retinitis Pigmentosa Inversa

Retinitis pigmentosa inversa, also known as *central* and *pericentral retinitis pigmentosa*, is a hereditary, autosomal recessive dystrophy in which pigmentary changes similar to those of retinitis pigmentosa occur

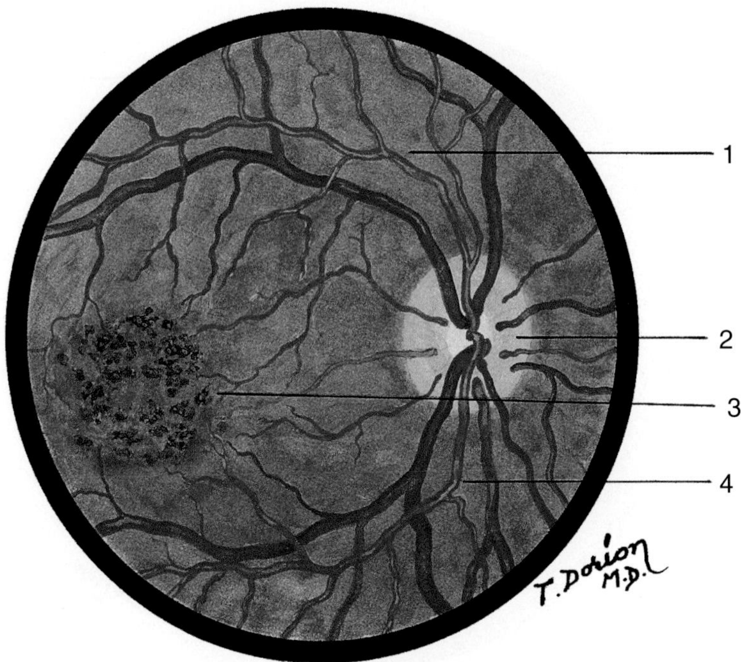

Figure 6-5. *Retinitis pigmentosa inversa. (1) Normal peripheral retina. (2) Normal optic disc. (3) Mottled macular pigmentation. (4) Normal retinal vessels.*

only in the macula and central retina (Figure 6-5). It is usually associated with cone dystrophy.

Retinitis pigmentosa inversa appears as bone-spicule pigmentation, or trabeculi, or black dots, like a fine mottled pigmentation, *scattered within the macula but without any peripheral pigment accumulation. Retinal vessels, peripheral retina, and optic disc are all normal*, in contradistinction to classic retinitis pigmentosa.

Histopathologically, there is degeneration and disorganization of the RPE in the macula and in central and pericentral retina.

Pseudoretinitis Pigmentosa

Pseudoretinitis pigmentosa, also known as *exogenous pigmentary degeneration*, is a unilateral or bilateral degenerative disorder in which

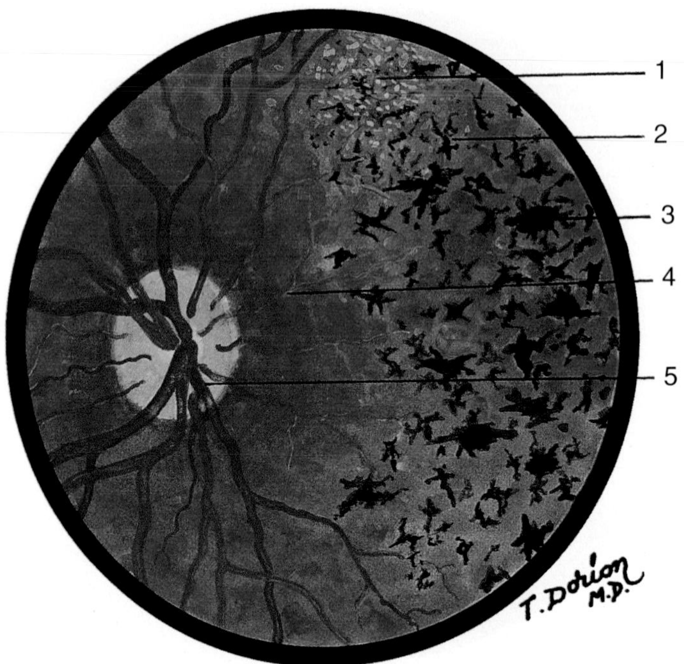

Figure 6-6. *Pseudoretinitis pigmentosa. (1) Salt-and-pepper lesion. (2) Bone-spicule pigmentation. (3) Pigment aggregates. (4) Atrophic retinal vessels in the nasal retina. (5) Normal retinal vessels at the disc.*

the fundus appearance mimics that of retinitis pigmentosa (Figure 6-6). It occurs after trauma, especially a concussive ocular injury that occurs early in life, or after face-mask anesthesia. It also develops in syphilis, rubella, pigmented paravenous choroidal atrophy, chorioretinitis, eclampsia, encephalitis, vaccination or influenza, Vogt-Koyanagi-Harada syndrome, Curschmann-Steinert disease, Kearns-Sayre syndrome, Usher's syndrome, drug intoxication (e.g., with thioridazine [Mellaril], chlorpromazine, chloroquine, a phenothiazine derivative called *NP 207*, sodium iodate), or after a previous retinal detachment.

Pseudoretinitis pigmentosa probably is due to a direct effect of inflammation, to toxic effects of drugs or, as in facemask anesthesia, to an ophthalmic artery occlusion by pressure on the eye that transmits compression of the vessel.

In *trauma*, pseudoretinitis pigmentosa appears as an accumulation of pigment at the posterior pole, as bone spicules, large aggregates, or multiple, small pigmented dots interspersed with fine depigmented areas, called a **salt-and-pepper lesion.** Vessels of the nasal retina may be atrophic but, in the macula and disc, vessels usually are normal. There may be gliosis. In *choroiditis*, the condition appears as a generalized retinal degeneration.

Diagnosis

In the diagnosis, ERG is extinguished.

Histopathology

In pseudoretinitis pigmentosa, a selective loss of the rod and cone layer (photoreceptors) is seen on histologic workup. There is also pigment migration into the retina. There may be a generalized RPE degeneration, with phagocytic cells containing granules that stain positively with periodic acid–Schiff (PAS) stain. The outer retinal layers are more often affected.

Lattice Degeneration

Lattice degeneration, also known as *palisade degeneration*, is a hereditary, congenital, usually bilateral and symmetric, peripheral vitreoretinal degeneration (Figure 6-7). It may be associated with Ehlers-Danlos syndrome, Marfan's syndrome, and Stickler's syndrome. Lattice degeneration may be caused by an abnormal formation of the retinal internal limiting membrane or by cystic degeneration.

The condition appears as a network of arborizing, crisscrossing white lines that represent sclerotic vessels with sharply delineated margins, located side by side as palisades, in rows, more commonly in the 11- to 1-o'clock and 5- to 7-o'clock sectors, at the peripheral retina. Occasionally, there may be an obliterative fibrosis of the blood vessels, called *lattice-wicker*. Reddish and blackish pigment clumps or yellow dots and patches are seen. Twenty or more polymorphic, elongated, excavated troughs surrounded by a narrow rim are disposed in two to four rows, intersecting with one another and usually concentric. They lie parallel to the ora serrata anterior to the equator, are concentrated

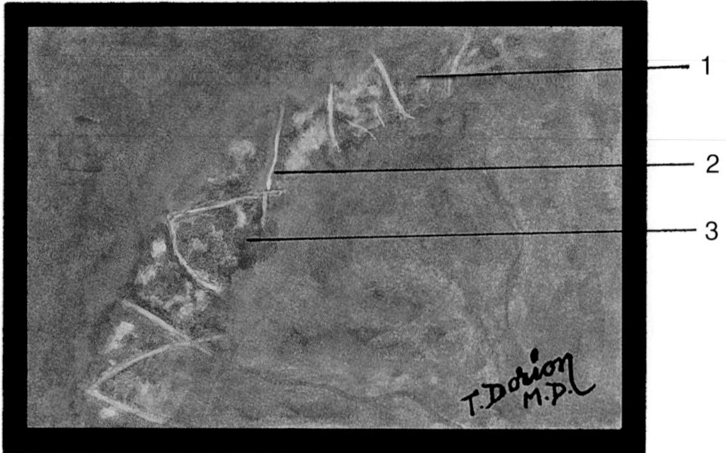

Figure 6-7. *Lattice degeneration. (1) Peripheral vitreoretinal degeneration. (2) Sclerotic vessels. (3) Pockets of liquefied vitreous.*

mostly toward the vertical meridian, and *always are at the vitreoretinal interface*. They may occupy less than 30 degrees or up to 270 degrees of the eye. Occasionally, they are located more posteriorly, along the major retinal vascular arcades, and are called *perivascular lattice degeneration*. At other times, they are located more anteriorly, within the vitreous base, and are called *vitreous base elevation*.

In some areas of the retina, these glistening white spots give a **snail-track** appearance. Rarely, punched-out areas of retinal thinning and vitreous pockets of fluid are evident. The vitreous fibrils usually are condensed and firmly adherent, which can cause subsequent shrinkage of the vitreous, vitreous detachment, retinal holes, or horseshoe-shaped tractional tears measuring approximately 0.066–0.100 dd, which may produce a retinal detachment.

Histopathology

On histologic evaluation, the retina is thinned. There is discontinuity of the retinal internal limiting membrane and atrophy and gliosis of the inner retinal layers (Figure 6-8). Full-thickness retinal holes may appear within the area of lattice. Retinal vessels are thickened, sclerosed, or

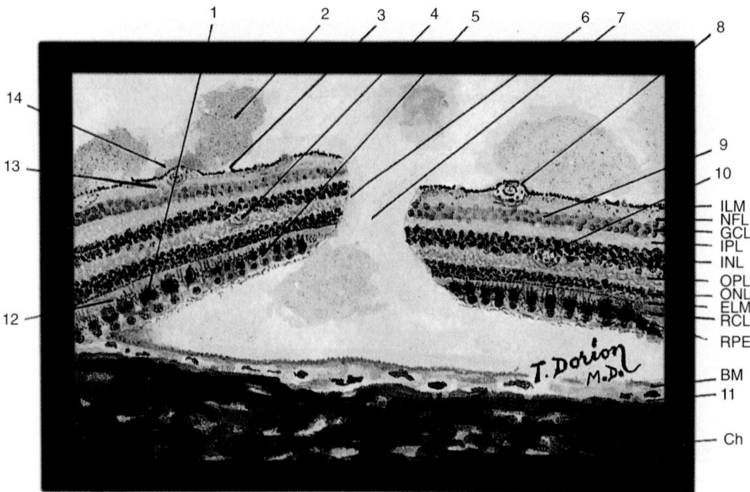

Figure 6-8. *Histopathologic findings in lattice degeneration. (1) Hypertrophic or hyperplastic retinal pigment epithelium (RPE) beneath the lesion. (2) Pockets of liquefied vitreous, with strong vitreous adhesions at its margins. (3) Discontinuity of the internal limiting membrane (ILM). (4) Hyalinized vessels. (5) Normal RPE beneath the lesion. (6) Thinned retina. (7) Full-thickness retinal hole. (8) Thick-walled blood vessel. (9) Atrophy of the inner retinal layers. (10) Sclerosed blood vessel, with perivascular pigment. (11) Choriocapillaris, intact. (12) Loss of photoreceptors. (13) Glial proliferation in the inner retinal layers. (14) Condensation of the vitreous at the sites of the lesion. (NFL, nerve fiber layer; GCL, ganglion cell layer; IPL, inner plexiform layer; INL, inner nuclear layer; OPL, outer plexiform layer; ONL, outer nuclear layer; ELM, external limiting membrane; RCL, rod and cone layer [photoreceptors]; BM, Bruch's membrane; Ch, choroid.)*

hyalinized. The RPE usually is normal beneath the lesions, but it may also be hypertrophic or hyperplastic. Pockets of liquefied vitreous may be seen, with strong vitreous adhesions at its margins.

Treatment

Cryothermy or photocoagulation may be used as prophylactic therapy in case of retinal detachment in the fellow eye, if the lattice degen-

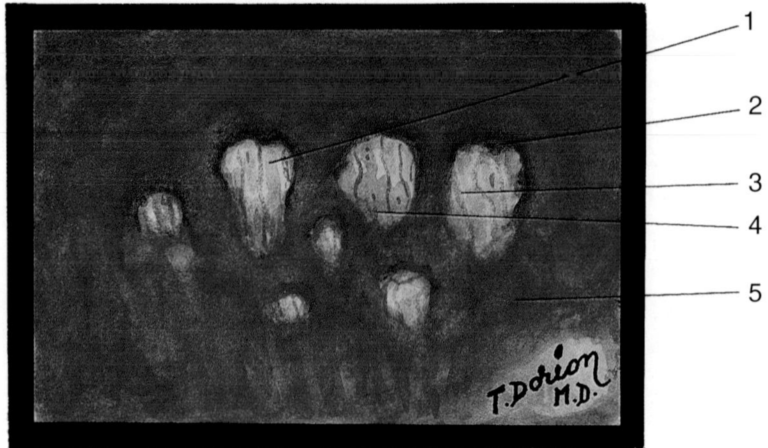

Figure 6-9. *Paving-stone degeneration. (1) Retinal thinning and retinal pigment epithelium loss. (2) Rim of retinal pigment epithelium hypertrophy. (3) Prominent visible choroidal vessels. (4) Linear pigmentation. (5) Normal retina.*

eration is extensive in high myopia, or if there is a family history of retinal detachment.

Paving-Stone Degeneration

Paving-stone degeneration, also known as *cobblestone degeneration*, *peripheral chorioretinal atrophy*, and *equatorial choroiditis*, is an atrophy (often bilateral) of the outer retinal layer (Figure 6-9) of the peripheral retina. It has no clinical significance. *It is not a predisposing factor in retinal detachment*; in fact, paving-stone degeneration may actually limit the retinal detachment's spread.

Paving-stone degeneration may be due to an insufficiency or occlusion of the choroidal vessels, which may cause focal postischemic atrophy of the RPE and the outer retinal layer of sensory retina. Alternatively, it may be due to obliteration of the choriocapillaris that supplies that portion of the retina.

Paving-stone degeneration appears as nonelevated, discrete, round or oval, pale, yellow-white or sometimes reddish and depigmented, sharply demarcated single patches, or clusters of small patches, measuring approximately 0.1–1.5 mm (1 dd) or more. These patches display a partial rim of dark pigmentation and may be likened to **pseudobreaks**. They are located usually between the ora serrata and the equator anteriorly and inferiorly, at 5- to 7-o'clock, in rows parallel to the ora serrata. There are prominent, visible choroidal vessels at the base of the lesion. In addition, spaces of normal retina appear between the patches, which may coalesce to form larger patches. A circumferential band with convex scalloped margins or incomplete septa or linear pigmentation also is seen.

Histopathology

A circumscribed ischemic area is noted in a thinned retina, with loss of RPE and outer retinal layers, including the photoreceptors, external limiting membrane, outer nuclear layer, and outer plexiform layer. The RPE ends abruptly at the area of degeneration. There may be pigment migration. The remaining inner retinal layers, which are normal, adhere to Bruch's membrane, which usually is intact, and to the RPE at the edge of the lesion. The choriocapillaris is absent or partially obliterated. There may be a hypertrophy or hyperplasia of the RPE at the margin of the lesions. The vitreous is normal.

Treatment

Treatment is not necessary.

Best's Vitelliform Dystrophy

Best's vitelliform dystrophy (known also as *vitelliform foveal dystrophy, vitelliruptive macular degeneration, exudative central detachment of retina, macular pseudocysts,* and *exudative foveal dystrophy*) is a bilateral, symmetric, progressive, autosomal dominant, degenerative lesion of unknown cause that occurs commonly in the macula of hypermetropic patients. It is due to an accumulation of *lipofuscin* granules in the RPE cells, which produces dysfunction of the RPE.

Clinical Stages

Best's vitelliform dystrophy occurs in four evolutionary stages. In **stage 1**, the *previtelliform* stage, the fundus appears normal, but the ERG is abnormal. Alternatively, there may be discrete foveal pigment mottling and depigmentation within the macula.

In **stage 2**, the *vitelliform*, *egg-yolk*, or *poached-egg* stage, one sees a single, round, homogeneous, cystlike, well-demarcated, submacular, opaque lesion with a shiny surface. This lesion appears as an accumulation of yellow material, and retinal vessels may course over it.

Stage 3 may be divided into four substages, *A–D*. **Stage 3A**, *scrambled egg* or *fried egg*, appears as a polymorphic, degenerated lesion owing to the destruction of the cyst, which may exhibit subretinal neovascularization, pigmentary dispersion, hemorrhage, and drusen or may appear as a bright orange deposit, resembling the yolk of a sunnyside-up fried egg. The lesion measures up to 1–2 dd.

Stage 3B, *pseudohypopyon* (Figure 6-10), appears as a round lesion, often with stellate margins. The lesion consists of an irregular material organized in layers as a result of its rupture in the subretinal space and its subsequent partial absorption, partial reformation, and liquefaction, with a horizontal fluid level.

Stage 3C reveals a discrete accumulation of a yellowish vitelliform material, usually in the center of the macula. **Stage 3D** is similar to stage 3C, but choriocapillaris atrophy may be seen.

Stage 4, or *macular star*, appears as whitish, triangular, irregular atrophic patches that occasionally may progress to a full-thickness macular hole.

Symptoms

Visual acuity may be decreased, but some patients experience no symptoms.

Diagnosis

ERG usually is normal. Dark adaptation may be mildly disturbed. EOG appears decreased, with an abnormal light-peak to dark-through ratio

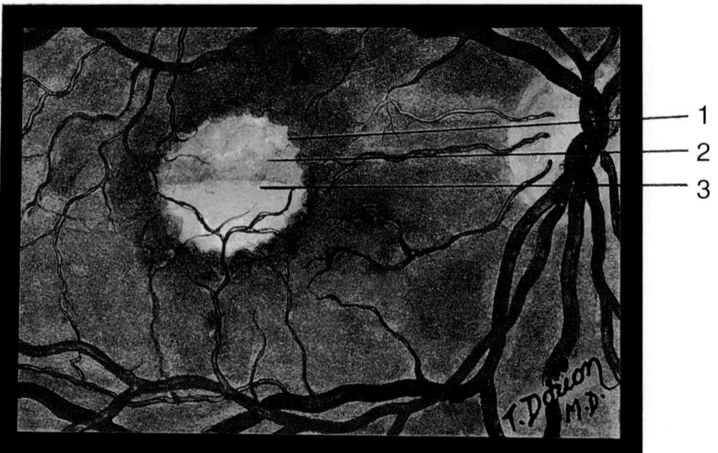

Figure 6-10. *Best's vitelliform dystrophy, stage 3B: pseudohypopyon. (1) Stellate margins. (2) Layered material. (3) Horizontal fluid level.*

of 1.20–1.59 that is consistent with altered RPE function (normal: >2). (The light-peak to dark-through EOG ratio is the ratio between the voltage amplitudes of slow oscillations generated by constant eye movement in a patient who was preadapted to room light level [35–70 lux] for 15 minutes, and the amplitudes obtained for another 15 minutes in a dark room.) Fluorescein angiography may show a window defect, a blockage of transmission owing to lipofuscin deposits, but no leakage.

Differential Diagnosis

In the differential diagnosis, preretinal hemorrhage in a resolving stage should be considered.

Histopathology

On histologic evaluation, a defect is seen at the level of the RPE, which is disorganized and atrophic and in which pigment cells are enlarged and engorged, with secondary lysosomes and an excessive amount of *lipofuscin* granules. There may be lipofuscin in the macrophages, in the subretinal space, or free within the choroid. Choroidal neovascularization may be present. In a late stage, a hypertrophic, glial, or vascularized fibrous scar tissue usually is present. Giant drusen in the RPE contain vessels.

Treatment

No effective treatment exists. Low-vision aids are recommended. Laser photocoagulation for choroidal neovascularization is appropriate. Genetic counseling should be offered.

Angioid Streaks

Angioid streaks are asymmetric, almost exclusively bilateral, pigmented, stationary or slowly progressive stripes resembling blood vessels (Figure 6-11) and occur more commonly in middle-aged men. They usually are associated with Groenblad-Strandberg syndrome (pseudoxanthoma elasticum), Paget's disease (osteitis deformans), Ehlers-Danlos syndrome, sickle cell anemia, thalassemia, thrombocytopenic purpura, senile elastosis, acromegaly, familial hyperphosphatemia, or lead poisoning.

Angioid streaks are caused by linear ruptures in Bruch's membrane, due to defects or pathologic alterations of the membrane by an unknown mechanism. A possible pull of the extraocular muscles may create forces against a fixed point of the optic disc.

The streaks appear as reddish to dark brown or slate-gray bands of irregular contour, width, and configuration but usually are curvilinear and wider than the blood vessels. They are bordered by a gray-white proliferation of fibrous tissue. Extending like a star outward from the peripapillary area of the disc, the streaks stretch toward the equator, forming a network of jagged branches that mimic the retinal vessels. Generally, they are radially oriented, but they also can be concentric to the optic disc. The streaks may resemble **lacquer cracks**.

Angioid streaks are located beneath the retina, deeper than the retinal vessels but above the choroidal vessels, throughout the posterior pole, traversing the macula without affecting vision. They *do not extend to the optic disc*. Sometimes, they may appear as broad, pale areas with fine, darker margins around the disc in a starfish pattern. They may be associated with small atrophic areas resembling **histospots** or may display subretinal crystalline deposits. Retinal vessels course

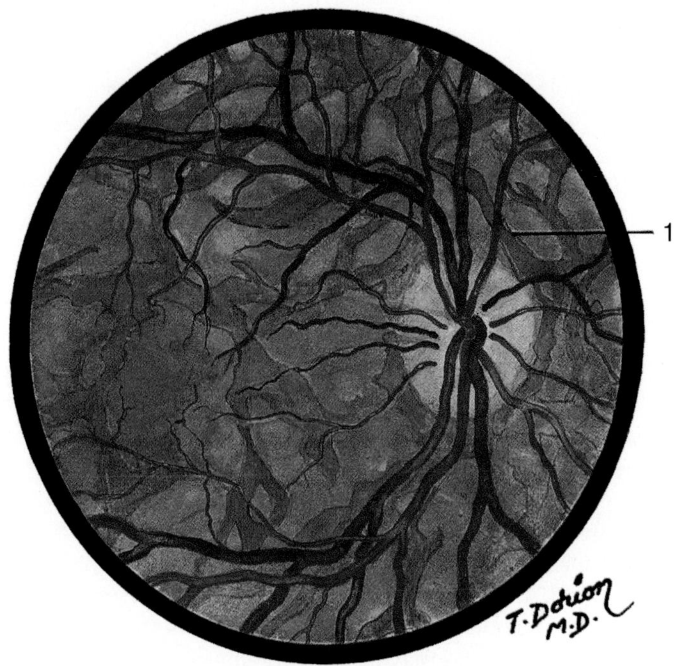

Figure 6-11. *Angioid streaks. (1) Ruptures in Bruch's membrane, resembling blood vessels.*

normally over the angioid streaks. There may be macular hemorrhages (spontaneous or traumatic) or neovascular membranes, frequently at the papillomacular bundle area. Occasionally, the streaks are associated with pigmentary anomalies, such as dull, yellowish, mottled dots (described as *moth-eaten*) or small, round, yellowish, larger spots (called *salmon patches*), or stippling pigmentation, diffuse or localized, usually throughout the macula, that resembles the cutaneous changes in pseudoxanthoma elasticum (called *peau d'orange*).

Symptoms

Usually angioid streaks are asymptomatic. Symptoms that might occur include loss of central vision if there is direct macular involvement or macular subretinal neovascularization.

Diagnosis

Fluorescein angiography may reveal early hyperfluorescence and late staining of the angioid streaks. Indocyanine green videoangiography also may reveal the streaks. Alkaline phosphatase levels, urinalysis for calcium, hemoglobin electrophoresis, and sickle cell preparation are other diagnostic tests that should be performed.

Histopathology

Bruch's membrane appears thickened and calcified and is interrupted by breaks in the fibroelastic layer or by cracklike dehiscences. Fibrovascular tissue, if present, may proliferate through these breaks into the subretinal space, extending beneath the RPE. The RPE may be normal, partially degenerated, or hypertrophic, elevated by the growth of the fibrovascular tissue. The choriocapillaris may be replaced by connective tissue. Occasionally, neovascularization may develop through the breaks in Bruch's membrane, and this may produce a serous or a hemorrhagic extravasation that later can result in a disciform macular scar. Some secondary changes may also be present in the photoreceptors.

Treatment

Laser photocoagulation for neovascularization that does not involve the macula may be helpful. Treatment of the underlying disease is appropriate.

Retinoschisis

Retinoschisis (also known as *X-linked juvenile retinoschisis*, *congenital hereditary retinoschisis*, *congenital vascular veils*, *primary retinal splitting*, *inherited retinal detachment*, and *anterior dialysis of the young*) is a progressive, bilateral, congenital or acquired splitting of the retina. It may be macular or peripheral, primary or secondary, infantile or senile. When it occurs in young adults, the condition is called *presenile retinoschisis*. It is not associated with any systemic disorders.

Retinoschisis is due to a degenerative process in which fluid of **hyaluronic acid** may accumulate in the outer plexiform layer to form a large intraretinal cyst, to a destructive process of the connective tissue with compensatory glial proliferation, to a defect in the Müller cells, to chorioretinitis as a result of poor circulation, or to trauma.

Retinoschisis appears as a cavity or a splitting of the retina in which there is an intraretinal loss of at least 1.5 mm in length (or approximately 1 dd). The retinoschisis has two walls or leaves: The *inner wall* is thin and immobile, whereas the *outer wall* is thicker and marked by large breaks and holes, similar to a honeycomb. Both walls may collapse to produce a *rhegmatogenous retinal detachment.* Vessels may be sheathed, with white opacities that are the footplates of Müller cell columns and are called *snow flecks*. Retinoschisis may resolve spontaneously.

Various Forms

Primary retinoschisis occurs as a developmental anomaly in nonmyopic men, with cyst formation. In the early stage, it appears as a mild cystoid degeneration or as a flat tubular retinal detachment, located usually inferotemporally at the periphery. In a later stage, it appears as a fixed, smooth, convex elevation that is sharply delineated and transparent, with delicate, vascularized, fenestrated membranes, or **vascular veils**, located at the ora serrata; the latter may be mistaken for retinal tears.

Secondary retinoschisis occurs after choroiditis, retinal detachment, choroidal tumor, retinopathy of prematurity, Coats' disease, angiomatosis retinae, diabetes, parasitoses, or aplastic anemia.

Congenital retinoschisis occurs as an X-linked recessive disorder in which the retinal splitting is in the nerve fiber layer. It appears as a stellate, spoked-wheel, or bicycle wheel–like macular edema that does not show any leakage on fluorescein angiography. Retinal vessels may float in the vitreous, giving the appearance of *vascular veils*.

Acquired retinoschisis usually is located at the periphery, near the ora serrata, in the inferotemporal fundus.

Infantile or **juvenile retinoschisis** probably is congenital, an X-linked disorder that occurs only in male individuals, who are hypermetropic; the disorder is apparent at birth. It appears as multiple stellate disinsertions with sharp edges, like a cartwheel with radiating spokes and a hub that corresponds to the foveola. Glistening silver-gray spots scattered throughout the retina, latticelike degeneration, syneresis, chorioretinal scars, and vitreous detachment are seen. Vessels have irregular contours and are dendritic and telangiectatic, with occluded segments. Microaneurysms also may be present.

Senile or **adult retinoschisis** occurs after 40 years of age as a peripheral degenerative disorder that spares the macula. Located mostly in the inferotemporal retina, it is associated with hypermetropia. Adult retinoschisis appears in two clinical forms—*typical* and *reticular*—which may occur together.

Typical degenerative retinoschisis appears as a round or oval, smooth, fusiform, dome-shaped elevation with an optical empty cavity. The elevated inner wall of the retinoschisis is dome-shaped and superficially smooth, reveals small breaks, tiny yellow-white *snow flecks*, or *frosting*, and contains retinal vessels. Its outer wall is irregular, composed only of the internal limiting membrane and the nerve fiber layer. The outer wall of the retinoschisis looks like *beaten metal*, with single or multiple large holes of varying sizes and rolling over of the edges, which gives the appearance of *fish eggs* or *frog eggs*. The retinal vessels turn white on scleral depression, a phenomenon known as *white with pressure*. There is often a surrounding peripheral cystoid degeneration and a rhegmatogenous retinal detachment. In typical degenerative retinoschisis, the split is in the nerve fiber layer.

Reticular degenerative retinoschisis appears as a bullous retinal elevation with prominent reticular cystoid degeneration of the nerve fiber layer. The retinoschisis inner wall is thin, with extremely attenuated vessels that usually are sclerotic or occluded and course in an arborization pattern. Its outer wall is irregular, pitted, or pocked, with excavation in a *honeycomb* appearance. The outer wall is characterized by single or multiple holes with dendritic figures and rolled posterior edges. As in typical degenerative retinoschisis, the retinal vessels turn white with scleral depression.

Macular retinoschisis has a characteristic spoked-wheel appearance, sometimes with a macular heteropsia.

Peripheral retinoschisis usually involves large and small breaks in a lacelike pattern. Retinal vessels are irregular and thinned. There also is glial proliferation in a wormlike figure, which may extend beneath the inner retinal layers.

Symptoms

Retinoschisis may be asymptomatic. Those who experience symptoms may report decreased vision, loss of the peripheral visual field, amblyopia (in children), and strabismus.

Diagnosis

Visual field testing may show an absolute scotoma. Fluorescein angiography reveals no leakage or staining of the macular cysts. Fundus contact lens examination is useful.

Differential Diagnosis

Goldmann-Favre syndrome and rhegmatogenous retinal detachment should be considered in the differential diagnosis.

Histopathology

Splitting of the retina at the outer plexiform layer and in the adjacent nuclear layers as well as in the nerve fiber layer is evident histopathologically. The split retina has two walls: The outer wall is thicker and serrated and has holes with rolled margins This wall is composed of the inner nuclear layer, outer plexiform layer, outer nuclear layer, external limiting membrane, and rod and cone (photoreceptor) layer. The inner wall is thinner and has irregular, attenuated, or telangiectatic breaks between the vessels. The RPE has a granular salt-and-pepper appearance and, occasionally, has proliferated. The macula exhibits radiated plications that are bilateral and symmetric, formed by fine folds of the internal limiting membrane. There is a band of typical cystoid degeneration within the nerve fiber layer, which always separates the retinoschisis from the ora serrata.

Treatment

Repair of retinal detachment may be effected by light photocoagulation, diathermy, cryotherapy, or scleral buckling. Amblyopia can be treated by patching. Genetic counseling should be offered.

Cone-Rod Dystrophy

Cone-rod dystrophy (*progressive cone-rod degeneration*) is a bilateral, autosomal dominant or recessive, and occasionally sporadic degenerative disorder characterized by a slowly progressive deterioration of the cones and rods (photoreceptors). Onset is usually between the ages of 4 and 8 years or in teens and young adults of approximately 30 years. Two distinct processes—*cone dystrophy* and *rod dystrophy*—can occur, although cone dystrophy is less common than rod dystrophy. Cone-rod dystrophy may be associated with systemic diseases such as aryl sulfatase deficiency, mucolipidosis type IV, and Batten's disease.

Cone-rod dystrophy appears initially as a normal macula or discrete, mild to moderate perifoveolar pigmentations and absent foveal reflex. The condition may progress to macular hyperpigmentation or to a diffuse, central amorphous pigmentary atrophy or, rarely, to widespread areas of chorioretinal atrophy. The dystrophy commonly is located in the inferior retina.

In a later stage, the appearance is of clumps, retinal flecks, or pigmented bone-spicule areas resembling retinitis pigmentosa. There may be bilateral and symmetric oval areas of macular atrophy that give rise to a metallic appearance called *beaten-bronze atrophy*. In an advanced stage, there is a geographic atrophy of the macula. Often, there are areas of hyperpigmented foveolar mottling surrounded by concentric rings of atrophic hypopigmentation, and hyperpigmentation, similar to those in chloroquine retinopathy; this is called *bull's-eye maculopathy*. The optic disc may be normal, or there may be a slightly temporal pallor. Retinal vessels are moderately attenuated.

Symptoms

Nystagmus occurs in infants with cone-rod dystrophy. Decreased visual acuity to counting fingers occurs. Other symptoms include photophobia, abnormal color vision (sometimes total achromatopsia), defective vision during the day in bright light (**hemeralopia**), and night blindness (**nyctalopia**).

Diagnosis

An ERG may reveal a severe loss of cone function (or even absent cone function), such as a flat tracing in response to a 30-cycles/second stimulus, reduced flicker response, and reduced single-flash photopic response, but only a moderate loss of rod function. The EOG may be subnormal.

Fluorescein angiography may reveal, in the early phase, an increased transmission of choroidal fluorescence as windows defects, without leakage of dye or fluorescein staining. In a later phase, there may be widespread RPE hypertrophy and hypotrophy in the macula, with an annular pattern of hyperfluorescence that corresponds clinically with *bull's-eye macula.*

Visual field testing shows a paramacular ring scotoma, grossly constricted fields, and pseudoaltitudinal defects. Dark-adaptation curves are monophasic in late-stage dystrophy, with slightly elevated rod thresholds. The Farnsworth-Munsell 100-hue test for color vision is useful.

Differential Diagnosis

ARMD, Stargardt's disease, chloroquine toxicity, rod monochromatism, retinitis pigmentosa inversa, retinitis pigmentosa sine pigmento, central areolar choroidal dystrophy, and congenital optic atrophy should all figure in the differential diagnosis. Malingering and hysteria also should be considered.

Histopathology

Histologic assessment reveals that cones and rods are absent from the macula and from the paramacular region. The RPE may be degenerated or absent, and the outer retinal layers may be atrophied.

Treatment

Treatment is not effective. Low-vision aids and gray-tinted eyeglasses might be suggested to improve vision and reduce photophobia. Miotics, such as pilocarpine 0.5–1.0%, four times a day during the day, also help to achieve these goals.

Fundus Albipunctatus

Fundus albipunctatus, also known as *albipunctatus dystrophy*, is an autosomal recessive dystrophy of unknown etiology that is usually bilateral and that occurs in two forms: *stationary* and *progressive.* It probably is due to a chronic deficiency of vitamin A.

Fundus albipunctatus appears as multiple, discrete, small, punctate, white-yellow deep dots or flecks (Figure 6-12). The dots or flecks are

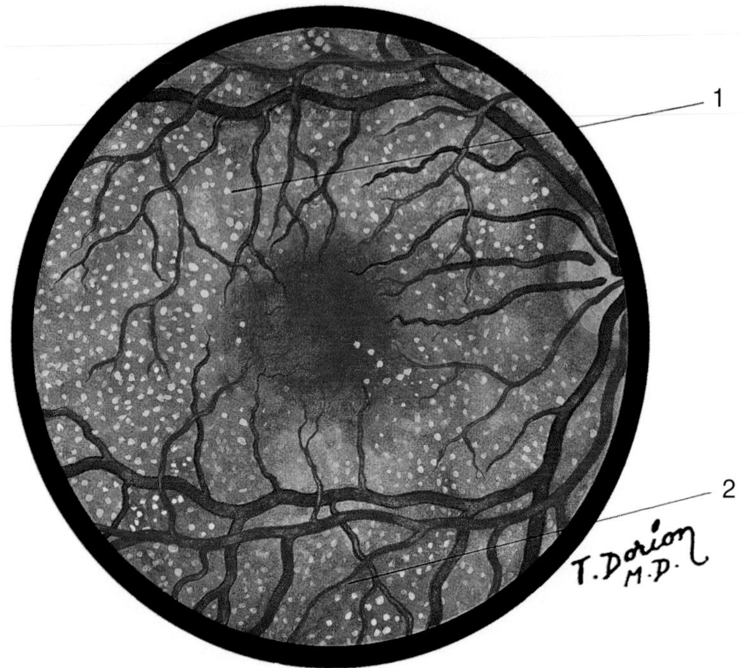

Figure 6-12. *Fundus albipunctatus. (1) Numerous deposits at the retinal pigment epithelium level and choriocapillaris. (2) Arterial attenuation.*

slightly irregular but commonly are of uniform size and are located at the midperiphery, with maximum density at the equator. Occasionally, they are oriented radially around the macula or crowded on the retina as *moth-eaten* lesions. When progressive, they may become more numerous or, conversely, their number may decrease or they may even disappear. Arteries often are attenuated. The optic disc may be normal or pale and atrophic.

Histopathologically, amorphous deposits are located deep in the retina, at the level of the RPE and choriocapillaris.

High Myopia

High myopia, also called *malignant myopia*, is a progressive chorioretinopathy that occurs frequently when the refractive error exceeds 6 D (Figure 6-13). High myopia is caused by a degenerative process.

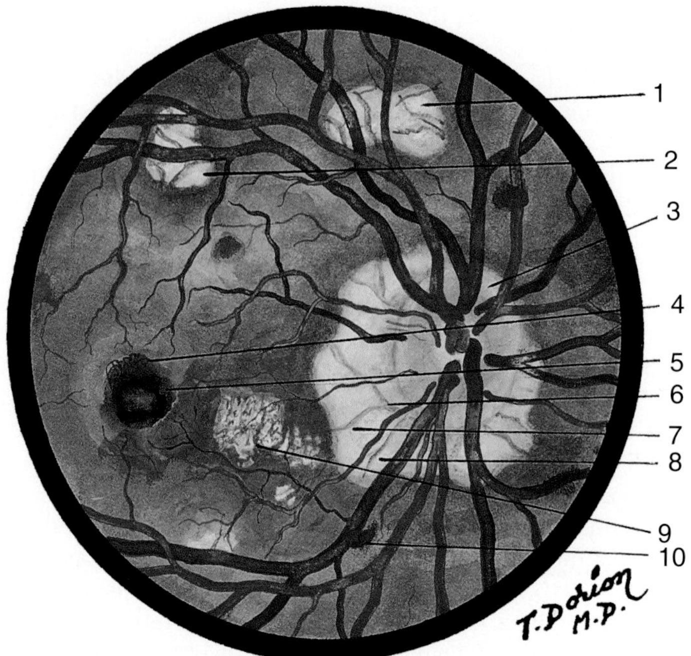

Figure 6-13. *High myopia. (1) Choroidal degeneration. (2) Punched-out choroidal atrophy. (3) Ovoid disc. (4) Choroidal neovascularization. (5) Fuchs' spot. (6) Thinned choroidal vessels. (7) Crescent. (8) Exposed sclera. (9) Lacquer cracks. (10) Subretinal hemorrhage.*

The optic disc usually appears ovoid with a longer vertical than horizontal axis. It sometimes is oblique or tilted and is yellow-pink. Nasal edges of the disc may be normal or may be overlapped by choroidal tissue; rarely, there is choroidal atrophy. In young persons, the nasal retina and the choroid are pilled, producing a light reflex called the **Weiss-Otto reflex**. Occasionally, the retina is pulled over the edges of the optic disc, producing supertraction of the nasal vessels and a distorted course. The temporal edges of the disc appear flattened, with a pale, depigmented area of choroidal atrophy: This area exhibits irregular margins and usually measures approximately one-third disc diameter up to several disc diameters. The area of choroidal atrophy may be circumpapillar, in which case it is called *crescent*.

At the temporal side, the choroid does not reach the disc margins, exposing a bare sclera over which thinned, sclerosed, or stretched choroidal vessels cross. The sclera also may bulge and become ectatic, lined by a thin atrophic choroid and producing an eversion of the disc and lamina cribrosa called *staphyloma*.

Central retinal vessels may be exposed posterior to their bifurcation on the disc or may be obliterated. Several small, spindle-shaped or flat hemorrhages from the choroidal vessels may be scattered throughout the fundus, more often in the macula or near the disc.

The macula may demonstrate choroidal neovascularization. Alternatively, a deep, black, round or elliptic macular lesion that is sharply circumscribed and has irregular margins may be seen; such a lesion, called **Fuchs' spot**, displays few *hemosiderin* deposits and occurs in an area of previous choroidal neovascularization or after recurrent deep hemorrhage. That lesion may be covered by fibrosis, which may change color from gray to red or yellow.

The retina may remain normal for several years until the degenerative process develops. Then peripheral retinal degeneration with multiple small cysts, called **Blessig-Ivanoff cysts**, might occur. Some lesions, such as **tension lines** (white lines that are located mostly at the posterior pole), may develop many years after myopia has ceased to progress.

The choroid usually is stretched and thinned. It may exhibit areas of round or irregular, yellow-white depigmentation or a punched-out, pigmented ring of choroidal atrophy. Also seen are occasional small breaks in Bruch's membrane, which appear as branching, irregular, yellow-white lines, more commonly in a horizontal or a stellate pattern, with connective tissue growing through these ruptures, which are called *lacquer cracks*. Areas of chorioretinal degeneration, usually of four types, may be present: *white without pressure*, *pigmentary degeneration*, *paving-stone degeneration*, and *lattice degeneration*.

The vitreous usually is fluid.

Symptoms

Visual acuity is decreased, especially at distance.

Diagnosis

Myopia may be diagnosed by performance of manifest and cycloplegic refraction and intraocular pressure measurement. Slit-lamp examination with a Hruby or contact lens also should be conducted. Fluorescein angiography and visual field testing are useful.

Differential Diagnosis

Tilted disc, ARMD, gyrate atrophy, and histoplasmosis are included in the differential diagnosis.

Histopathology

On histologic examination, the retina may appear thinned, more commonly near the disc, with some degree of degeneration of the outer layers. The RPE may be depigmented owing to a gradual degeneration of the melanocytes and consequent loss of pigment, or it may be absent in the atrophic area of the temporal crescent. The RPE may be normal or might exhibit proliferation at the disc margins. *The RPE and Bruch's membrane do not extend to the temporal margin of the disc.*

Bruch's membrane may have tears through which vessels may grow inward from the choroid. Nasally, the RPE may overlap the disc. The RPE at the macula, at the site of Fuchs' spot, may display proliferation or hyperplasia. The choroid usually is atrophic and thinned, with loss of stroma. Choroidal vessels are less numerous than normal, stretched, and sclerosed, and the intervascular spaces are larger. Occasionally, there may be choroidal vessel occlusion.

Treatment

Visual acuity can be corrected with minus concave lenses. Keratomileusis, radial keratotomy, scleral shortening or reinforcement, laser photocoagulation, or cryotherapy might be used for shortening the axial length of the eye, thus improving vision. Complications should be treated appropriately.

North Carolina Macular Dystrophy

North Carolina macular dystrophy is a familial, autosomal dominant macular dystrophy that is slowly progressive. This dystrophy and *hereditary macular degeneration and aminoaciduria*, *Lefler-Wadsworth-Sidbury foveal dystrophy*, *dominant progressive foveolar dystrophy*, and *central*

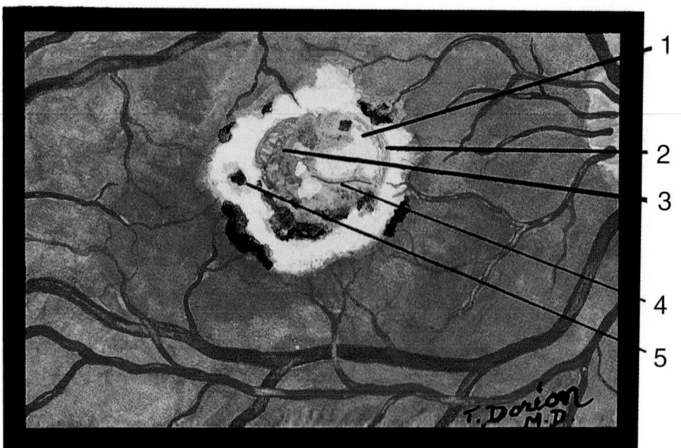

Figure 6-14. *North Carolina macular dystrophy, grade 3. (1) Total retinal pigment epithelium and choroidal atrophy. (2) Staphyloma-like lesion. (3) Choroidal neovascularization. (4) Large choroidal vessel. (5) Subretinal hemorrhage.*

areolar pigment epithelial dystrophy (CAPED) are clinical entities that represent forms of **regional choroidal dystrophy**. All are very similar.

North Carolina macular dystrophy appears, in the early stage, as a mild, nonspecific macular granular pigmentation. Later, often after years, a central areolar, circular or oval depigmented area of RPE atrophy that is sharply demarcated may develop. The choroid is visible, and larger choroidal vessels may appear yellow-white. Drusen are seen in the macula, which has a disciform shape, as a coloboma or staphyloma, with an outpouching atrophic area. Occasionally, subretinal hemorrhage and choroidal neovascularization also are present.

North Carolina macular dystrophy is considered to occur in three grades or stages: **grade 1**, in which the lesions are drusen and there is macular granular dispersion; **grade 2**, in which the drusen become confluent, and pigment clumping and early RPE atrophy are present; and **grade 3**, in which there is total atrophy of the RPE and of the choriocapillaris in the macula (Figure 6-14).

Histopathologically, RPE atrophy and choriocapillaris atrophy are seen in the macula. Pigmentary dispersion and RPE derangement also are seen. Fine or confluent drusen appear in the choroid and retina. Occasionally, subretinal hemorrhage may be seen. Also, choroidal neovascularization may be present.

Retinitis Proliferans

Retinitis proliferans is a retinal lesion consisting of fibrosis and neovascularization and extending into the vitreous, which occurs after hemorrhage in diabetes, Eales' disease, trauma, and other metabolic, toxic, or inflammatory diseases. It may be caused by retinal hypoxia, hemorrhage, or neovascularization, with proliferation of fibrous glial connective tissue that may destroy the internal limiting membrane.

Retinitis proliferans appears as bands of fibrous tissue and opaque white membranes between the retina and vitreous. There is massive preretinal fibroglial neovascularization, located more often at the posterior pole, at the disc, or along the temporal vascular arcades.

Vitreous hemorrhage usually is present. Parallel pipe-stem sheathing of retinal vessels may also be present. At a late stage of disease, the fibrous tissue becomes thicker and may produce a macular distortion, traction retinal detachment, or a posterior vitreous detachment.

Symptoms

Loss of visual acuity is the prominent symptom.

Histopathology

On histologic examination, thick, preretinal, large fibrovascular bands are seen on the posterior surface of a detached vitreous. Vitreous hemorrhages are present. The internal limiting membrane usually is destroyed. Retinal detachment may also be present.

Treatment

Laser photocoagulation or vitrectomy can be beneficial.

Peripheral Cystoid Degeneration

Peripheral cystoid degeneration is a band of intraretinal cystoid spaces within the sensory retina, approximately of equal dimensions in any direction, located initially in the temporal retina, usually at 0.5 dd from the ora serrata. This band slowly may spread posteriorly behind the equator or may affect the macula. The spaces have thin inner and outer walls, which may become thinner as the degeneration progresses. Often, dentate processes also are present. Each cyst may have a neck that connects it to the band of spaces smaller than the greatest diameter of the cyst. If it does not have a neck, it is called a *microcyst* when the diameter is less than 0.5 mm or *retinoschisis* if the diameter exceeds 1.5 mm (1 dd) and the retina is split into two layers.

Peripheral cystoid degeneration may be caused by the traction and movement of the ora serrata during accommodation.

Clinical Forms

Peripheral cystoid degeneration appears in two clinical forms: *typical* and *reticular*. **Typical peripheral cystoid degeneration** (**Blessig-Ivanoff cysts**) appears as bilateral, translucent, dark reddish dots that may coalesce to form myriad tiny, interlacing tunnels. The dots are located in the superotemporal retina and have rounded domes corresponding to the cysts and stippled depressions corresponding to the pillars. The affected retina is up to three times thicker than normal. Strands and grayish opacities resembling snowflakes may appear in the vitreous.

Reticular cystoid degeneration appears mostly as single or multiple bilateral, prominent linear or reticular structures, irregular in angle, with a fine, stippled surface, posterior to and continuous with a typical cystoid degeneration. This reticulum corresponds to the retinal vessels and is demarcated posteriorly by the vessels. The interseptal pillars may break and, by this mechanism, may form a reticular degenerative retinoschisis called **bullous retinoschisis**.

Histopathology

In **typical cystoid degeneration**, intraretinal spaces and channels are seen, located primarily in the Henle's fiber layer, which is the outer zone of the retinal outer plexiform layer between the compressed bundles of the photoreceptor axons and Müller glial cells. These spaces and channels may extend to the inner and outer nuclear layer and from the internal to the external limiting membrane. They may contain *hyaluronic acid*. Septa may occur between these spaces, composed of glial-axonal tissue rich in *cytochrome oxidase*. Degeneration of the cone outer segment may occasionally be present. The spaces may coalesce, forming macrocysts or retinoschisis. Often, Müller cell microvilli and fragments of the photoreceptor inner segment may be seen external or internal to the limiting membranes. The superficial capillary plexus usually courses through the cystoid cavities. The RPE commonly is preserved. In **reticular cystoid degeneration**, small cystoid spaces located in the nerve fiber layer may extend from the internal limiting membrane to the outer plexiform layer. As in typical cystoid degeneration, these spaces contain *hyaluronic acid*, which may represent a degenerative neural tissue. There is degeneration of the nerve fiber layer.

Incontinentia Pigmenti

Incontinentia pigmenti, also known as *Bloch-Sulzberger syndrome* or *Franceschetti-Jadassohn syndrome*, is a rare, congenital, X-linked trait or autosomal-dominant abnormality, a mesodermal and ectodermal dysplasia with ocular involvement (e.g., retinal detachment and vascular retinopathy) as well as systemic abnormalities, skin lesions, alopecia, delayed dentition and malformed teeth, nails, and bones, and central nervous system disorders (e.g., mental retardation, seizures, spastic paralysis, congenital heart disease, pheochromocytoma). Incontinentia pigmenti occurs mostly in white female infants (97%) at birth or shortly thereafter. It is lethal in boys, resulting in spontaneous abortion. Its cause is unknown.

Incontinentia pigmenti can appear as one of two clinical types: *Naegeli* and *Bloch-Sulzberger.* The **Naegeli type** is not congenital, occurs in both genders, is characterized by onset at approximately 2 years of age, and is associated with a reticular cutaneous pigmentation, without other abnormalities. The **Bloch-Sulzberger type** is congenital, occurs almost exclusively in girls, and is associated with systemic disorders and ocular defects.

Incontinentia pigmenti appears as a total retinal detachment, seen as a retrolental unilateral white mass with neovascularization and fibrous proliferation, which may simulate a pseudoglioma. Small, patchy, mottled or diffuse areas of pigmentation, occasionally with sub-RPE clumping and depigmentation, may be present throughout the fundus. Retinal vessels may appear dilated and tortuous. Abnormal arteriovenous anastomoses may be present. There may be a preretinal fibrous tissue at the equator and no retinal supply behind that area. Intraretinal hemorrhages of varying shapes and sizes may be present at the junction of vascularized and nonvascularized retina. Occasionally, a peripheral retinal necrosis is seen. Hypoplasia of the macula, with severe retinal dragging, may also be seen. The optic disc may be atrophic.

Symptoms

Symptoms include esotropia, leukokoria, cataract, blue sclera, microphthalmos, nystagmus, and conjunctival pigmentation.

Diagnosis

Recurrent vesiculobullous and verrucous skin lesions that may resolve spontaneously, leaving irregular patches or whorls of hyperpigmentation, are diagnostic. Fluorescein angiography may reveal a peripheral capillary nonperfusion, with a transition zone between perfused and nonperfused retina.

Differential Diagnosis

Pseudoglioma and retinopathy of prematurity should be considered in the differential diagnosis.

Histopathology

Histopathologically, there is a total exudative retinal detachment. Retinal dysplasia with rosettes and fibrous tissue may be present, as may obliterative endarteritis. In addition, primary RPE abnormalities, with nodular pigment proliferation and deposits of *lipofuscin*, are seen. There may be areas of exudative chorioretinitis. Intraretinal hemorrhages and, rarely, retinal necrosis may occur.

Treatment

No specific treatment is available, although laser photocoagulation might be beneficial.

Doyne's Honeycomb Choroiditis

Doyne's honeycomb choroiditis (also known as *malattia leventinese*, *dominant drusen of Bruch's membrane*, *Holthouse-Batten superficial choroiditis*, *Hutchinson-Tay central guttate choroiditis*, *familial drusen*, *crystalline retinal degeneration*, *iridescent crystals of the macula*, and *hyaline dystrophy*) is a bilateral, symmetric, progressive, autosomal dominant–pattern central retinal dystrophy. The disorder occurs in young persons of 20–30 years of age. It may be an early manifestation of ARMD.

Doyne's honeycomb choroiditis appears as a honeycomb pattern of multiple, deep, yellow, variably sized lesions; usually, they are large and scattered throughout the posterior fundus. At a later stage, some drusen become calcified, with a crystalline appearance, whereas some other drusen may disappear and leave behind small geographic areas of RPE atrophy. There is a pigment proliferation that appears as fine lines—macular, paramacular, or peripapillary—at the nasal edge of the disc. Occasionally, choroidal neovascularization may develop.

Symptoms

Doyne's honeycomb choroiditis may be asymptomatic in its early stage. Decreased visual acuity is a predominant symptom.

Diagnosis

Visual field tests are normal, as is color vision testing. ERG also is normal, but EOG may be subnormal, especially in advanced stages. Dark adaptation is normal. Fluorescein angiography may reveal multiple, sharply defined fluorescent spots—some of them confluent—and RPE transmission defects but no dye leakage.

Differential Diagnosis

Considerations in the differential diagnosis include ARMD, fundus flavimaculatus, retinitis punctata albescens, and Best's vitelliform dystrophy.

Histopathology

Histologic analysis demonstrates focal collections of eosinophilic homogeneous material of *cerebrosides* and *sialic acid*, located between the RPE and Bruch's membrane (often only at the macular region). The RPE may reveal a varying degree of thinning and depigmentation.

Treatment

No treatment is available for Doyne's honeycomb choroiditis.

Tapetochoroidal Degeneration

Tapetochoroidal degeneration (previously called *tapetum*, which in Greek means "rug") is a hereditary degeneration of the choroid and RPE. The disorder probably is due to atrophy of the choriocapillaris, which reduces the blood supply to overlying RPE and the outer retina; to a defect in lipid transportation; to a defect in the rod membrane and faulty or absent visual pigments; or to neovascularization beneath the RPE or between RPE and sensory retina, which may produce a degeneration of the retina.

Tapetochoroidal degeneration appears as a granular, diffuse depigmentation. It displays a circumferential band, usually extending from the ora serrata to the equator. Its anterior border is irregular, owing to the patchy pigmentation within the vitreous base. Its posterior border usually is smooth and well defined.

The tapetochoroidal degenerative diseases are retinitis pigmentosa, Laurence-Moon-Bardet-Biedl syndrome, Refsum's syndrome, Bassen-Kornzweig syndrome, Spielmayer-Vogt-Mayou syndrome, progressive external ophthalmoplegia, Usher's syndrome, choroideremia, gyrate atrophy, Stickler's syndrome, Bietti's crystalline retinopathy, and Leber's congenital amaurosis.

Histologic analysis shows degeneration of the RPE, with loss of pigment granules in the RPE cells. There is a thickening of Bruch's membrane. The choriocapillaris is atrophic and thinned. The disorder triggers a loss of photoreceptors.

Leber's Congenital Amaurosis

Leber's congenital amaurosis (also known as *hereditary retinal aplasia*, *heredoretinopathia congenitalis*, and *dysgenesis neuroepithelialis reti-*

nae) is a congenital, bilateral, generalized tapetochorioretinal degeneration or a group of such disorders. The condition usually is autosomal recessive but also may be dominant. It occurs at or shortly after birth or in early childhood and is more common in boys.

Leber's congenital amaurosis often is associated with cataract, nystagmus, hypermetropia, deafness, cardiomyopathy, polycystic kidney disease, osteopetrosis, and other skeletal anomalies. It probably is due to failure of sensory retina development and to choroid and pigmentary degeneration.

The disorder appears as a pigmentary stippling, with yellow flecks located outside the vascular arcades, or as retinitis pigmentosa–like bone spicules or subretinal clumps located at the periphery. The fundus background sometimes may appear normal, as *blonde fundus*, or as a nummular pigmentary pattern, such as *salt-and-pepper*, *marbleization*, or *mosaicism*. Less frequently, it may appear as choroideremia, gyrate atrophy, fundus albipunctatus, or albinismlike lesions. The optic disc may be pale and slightly swollen. Retinal arteries may be narrowed. The macula may lose the foveolar reflex and may exhibit an increased granularity, mottled hyperpigmentation and hypopigmentation, colobomas, localized RPE defects, a full-thickness hole, RPE geographic atrophy, snail-trail brilliance, or rarely, bull's-eye maculopathy. There may be chorioretinal atrophy.

Symptoms

Severe vision loss from 20/80 to no light perception occurs. There is pendular or searching nystagmus. Pupillary constriction to light is absent. Pigmentary retinopathy, photophobia, sunken eyeballs, cataract, keratoconus, and keratoglobus all may occur. Some patients may suffer sensory hearing loss, mental retardation, epilepsy, growth arrest, and hepatomegaly.

Diagnosis

The ERG waves usually are markedly reduced or extinguished and flat, showing no response to light stimuli. Hyperthreoninemia and hyperthreoninuria are indicative of Leber's congenital amaurosis.

Differential Diagnosis

In the differential diagnosis, cortical blindness should be considered.

Histopathology

On histologic evaluation, the outer retinal layers display degeneration, particularly of the photoreceptors, which may be missing and replaced by amorphous material. In the retinal outer nuclear layer, the nuclei may be oval and abnormal and, in the inner nuclear layer, abnormal structures also may be seen. The RPE may be degenerated and atrophic and lack the basal folds. Retinal and choroidal vessels usually are sclerotic. There may be retinal and choroidal atrophy and gliosis.

Treatment

No known treatment exists.

Retinal Tufts

Also called *granular patches*, *globular masses*, *granular tissues*, and *rosettes*, retinal tufts are peripheral vitreoretinal abnormalities consisting of internal projections of the retina. They usually are stationary and commonly are designated as three clinical types: *cystic*, *noncystic*, and *zonular traction*.

Clinical Types

A **cystic retinal tuft** is a congenital, localized, unilateral, single or multiple, gray-white, nodular internal projection of the retina. It demonstrates a dull, irregular surface that extends from a vitreous attachment at the apex of the tuft to a base that is more than 0.1 mm in diameter. *It is larger than the noncystic tuft.* Its appearance is chalky white and displays scant pigmentation. The lesion is elevated, usually surrounded by cystic degeneration and secondary retinal detachment. Cystic retinal tufts may be located within or posterior to the vitreous base, at the equator, or in all quadrants. It may be avulsed by vitreous traction with or without posterior vitreous detachment, which may cause retinal breaks or holes.

A **noncystic retinal tuft** is a bilateral, short, pointed internal projection of the retina located almost always within the vitreous base. Often appearing in clusters, the tuft is surrounded by a nonspecific retinal degeneration and pigment dispersion. It may break off, producing small spherical fragments that may float in the vitreous. The tuft extends from a vitreous attachment to a base that is less than 0.1 mm in diameter. *It is smaller than is the cystic tuft* and produces no retinal breaks or retinal detachment.

A **zonular traction retinal tuft** is a unilateral or bilateral, single, internal, anterior projection of the retina toward the zonule. The tuft appears as a thin strand that often overhangs the pars plana. It is not present at birth. Usually, the tuft is caused by the tractional forces of the zonule. Commonly, it is located within the vitreous base, particularly in the nasal quadrant, and is attached to the retina less than 0.5 mm posterior to the ora serrata. This tuft follows an acute sharp angulation toward the ciliary body. Anteriorly, it may be surrounded by microcystic retinal degeneration and, posteriorly, it splays. At the tuft base, the retina may demonstrate trophic or tractional alterations, including small, round, partial- or full-thickness peripheral retinal holes, that occur mostly at the time of cataract surgery. The tuft may join the zonular fibers at the apex and may vary in length and thickness.

Histopathology

Histologic examination reveals retinal tufts that have an irregular surface and a layer of dense-staining glial cells that partially surround the microcysts. Strands of fibroglial tissue appear, and there may be glial cells with dense cytoplasm and (occasionally) epithelial cells on the inner surface of the tuft. The disorder may produce a degeneration of neurons and pigment dispersion into the deeper layer. The outer retina beneath the tuft may show marked degeneration of the photoreceptors. The vitreous over the tuft may be distorted, and a coarse bundle of vitreous fibrils may be present. Noncystic tufts are composed of altered cells and proliferating glial tissue.

Treatment

Treatment includes observation. Possible interventions are cryopexy and laser photocoagulation.

Enclosed Ora Bay

Enclosed ora bay (also known as *ring tooth* or *hole in a tooth*) is a peripheral retinal degeneration—a developmental abnormality of the pars plana—in which a portion of its nonpigmented epithelium remains completely (or nearly completely) isolated by two ora teeth. It unites and forms the structure called *enclosed bay*. It has no clinical significance.

Enclosed ora bay appears as a small, yellowish brown, depressed oval island of the pars plana. The island is surrounded by normal retina and is formed by two broad dentate processes. These processes converge anteriorly toward a prominent ciliary process of the pars plicata and may join to enclose a bay. It is located immediately behind the ora serrata, at about 1.8 mm.

The differential diagnosis includes retinal tears.

Histologic evaluation reveals that the pars plana epithelium is thinned and is surrounded by a normal sensory retina. There may be typical cystoid degeneration.

Treatment is not required.

Melanocytosis

Melanocytosis (*bilateral diffuse uveal melanocytic proliferation*) is a benign, bilateral melanocytic infiltration. It is a *paraneoplastic syndrome* associated with systemic carcinoma and usually occurs in the macula. This occurs more frequently in older women. It does not metastasize.

Melanocytosis may be caused by a common oncogenous stimulus—a *cellular growth factor*—secreted by a visceral primary tumor, most often an adenocarcinoma of the pancreas, or by a tumor of the esophagus, lung, ovary, colon, or gallbladder, or by a cervical carcinoma. Additionally, this proliferation of normal uveal melanocytes at the level of RPE may be produced only in the presence of anomalous melanocytes, before the onset of the malignancy. Further, it may be due to a toxic or an immune-mediated process as a result of a melanocytic proliferation. Finally, it may be caused by interaction of a systemic malignancy and the RPE.

Melanocytosis is considered to have five ocular cardinal signs that may accompany the vision loss: (1) multifocal, faintly visible round or oval, red, **subretinal patches** with prominent hyperfluorescence seen during the early phase of fluorescein angiography; (2) multiple pigmented and nonpigmented **uveal melanocytic tumors** that are slightly elevated (up to 2 mm); (3) diffuse **thickening of the choroid**; (4) exudative **retinal detachment**; and (5) a rapid progression of **cataract**.

Melanocytosis appears as a serous macular detachment. It may have multiple round or oval, red, yellow-orange, or creamy patches and is located in the perifoveolar region and at the posterior pole. Usually, the foveal reflex is hazy. The disorder produces a diffuse nonpigmented thickening (perhaps 0.5 mm) of the choroid at the macula and lightly pigmented nodules (perhaps 1 mm in height) that decrease gradually toward the periphery. Also visible at the posterior pole may be small choroidal nevuslike pigmented masses that may enlarge and coalesce slowly. Sometimes, a few pink flecks may appear in the papillomacular area. Occasionally, there may be a moderate anterior uveitis. Severe progression of cataract also may occur. Occasionally, bullous sensory retinal detachment may develop, accompanied by shifting of the subretinal fluid.

Symptoms

The predominant symptom of melanocytosis is visual disturbance that often takes the form of severe vision loss.

Diagnosis

Fluorescein angiography may reveal multifocal areas of early hyperfluorescence that corresponds to the pigmented patches. These areas may enlarge progressively and produce a reticular hyperfluorescent pattern. ERG may show a normal photopic response or a severe scotopic response. The results of the EOG may be borderline.

Differential Diagnosis

Considerations for differential diagnosis include uveal effusion syndrome (choroidal detachment), ocular lymphoma (reticulum sarcoma), metastatic carcinoma, leukemia, choroiditis, acute posterior multifocal placoid pigment epitheliopathy, sympathetic ophthalmia, sarcoidosis, posterior scleritis, rhegmatogenous retinal detachment, and Vogt-Koyanagi-Harada syndrome.

Histopathology

Histologic analysis demonstrates a serous macular detachment with degeneration of the photoreceptors. Melanocytosis results in an infiltration of small polyhedral, and fusiform plump spindle cells that are lightly pigmented and demonstrate a well-delineated cytoplasm and small round nuclei. A few nucleoli, without mitotic figures, advance into the choroid and focally into the sclera. Foci of spindle B and epithelioid cellular differentiation may be evident. The disorder may result also in pigmented nodules, which have a necrotic center and a basophilic nucleus located centrally (but lacking nucleoli), comparable with melanocytoma cells. The RPE usually is degenerated and depigmented, with variable zones of total necrosis, melanocytic proliferation, hyperplasia, and metaplasia.

These RPE alterations may decrease in severity in a centrifugal fashion: The older lesions are located centrally and are larger (perhaps 500 μm) and most are confluent; the younger lesions are located peripherally and are much smaller. An exudative retinal detachment may be evident.

Treatment

Treatment for melanocytosis is similar to treatment for early visceral carcinoma.

Solar Retinopathy

Other names for solar retinopathy are *photic retinopathy*, *eclipse retinopathy*, *welding-arc maculopathy*, *foveomacular retinitis*, and *actinic macular RPE degeneration*. Solar retinopathy is a photochemical retinopathy—an actinic burn or phototoxic lesion of the macula—that occurs after direct gazing at the sun, either inadvertent or intentional (as part of religious or fanatic cult worship). Solar retinopathy can result from myriad types of exposure to intense light (e.g., watching a solar eclipse without adequate filter protection, casual sunbathing, looking at a welding-arc light or a nuclear fireball, using an unprotected operating microscope in cataract extraction, experiencing a hypoglycemic insulin reaction, or even among military personnel assigned to outdoor duty in the tropics).

The disorder is due to a **mechanical**, **thermal**, or **photochemical** effect of light to the retina. Mechanical injuries usually result from an intense, ultrashort, high-irradiance, Q-switched laser exposure, which produces retinal photodisruption. Thermal injuries result from an intensive brief exposure to light, which increases the retinal temperature to 10°C or greater, such as occurs in photocoagulation. Photochemical injuries result from a retinal uptake by the macular **xanthophyll pigment** of unfiltered high-energy short-wave blue-light infrared (750–1,400 nm) or ultraviolet radiation (320–400 nm). Such injury occurs also (as in phototoxic injuries) from the release of free radicals and lysosomal enzymes that damage the photoreceptor membrane. Light is absorbed by **melanin** of the RPE, is converted to heat, and produces retinal damage in the RPE and surrounding layers.

Solar retinopathy appears as a bilateral, often asymmetric, reddish yellow discoloration. The circular lesion is well demarcated and is surrounded by a mild macular edema. Accompanying it may be a small central macular pit located in the inner retina and often adjacent to the foveola. In time, the lesion may become darker, with mildly pigmented edges that may fade in approximately 2 weeks.

After a more prolonged period of light exposure, a sharply circumscribed lamellar macular hole may develop and may become permanent. A fibrous metaplasia or a mottled irregular scar may occur. Fine hemorrhages or macular cysts also may develop.

Symptoms

A prominent symptom of solar retinopathy is brow ache. Users of video display terminals may experience such symptoms as transient color vision changes or chromatopsia (such as erythropsia) that may last for several hours, albeit without anatomic or physiologic damage. Minimal or considerable decreased vision may ensue, an effect that may revert partially or totally to normal visual acuity in 4–6 months.

Diagnosis

Fluorescein angiography may be normal or may reveal small window defects in the center of the foveolar avascular zone or an area of hyperfluorescence surrounding a hypofluorescence and corresponding to the lamellar hole. An Amsler's grid test may be normal. The visual field may reveal a persistent juxtafoveolar scotoma.

Differential Diagnosis

The basic consideration in the differential diagnosis is adult foveomacular dystrophy.

Histopathology

Histologic evaluation reveals a focal loss of rod and cone nuclei in the outer layers of the foveolar area. There may be RPE depigmentation and thinning, but otherwise an intact RPE remains. Bruch's membrane and the choriocapillaris are normal.

Treatment

No treatment for solar retinopathy exists. Corticoids may help in the early stages of the disorder. Sunglasses are highly recommended.

Radiation Retinopathy

Radiation retinopathy is a slowly progressive ischemic vaso-occlusive retinopathy. Sometimes it occurs after a long period (18 months to 3 years) of external proton-beam radiation, such as *teletherapy* with 1,500–3,500 cGy. The disorder also may result from localized plaque of ^{125}I, such as *brachytherapy*, or after roentgenograms of the skull. Other precipitating factors include radiation therapy with ^{60}Co or radon seeds for retinal capillary hemangioma, retinoblastoma, choroidal melanoma, orbital lymphoma, orbital pseudotumor, intracranial metastatic central nervous system tumor, thyroid disease, paranasal sinus disorders, or skin tumors of the eyelid and face. Occasionally, radiation retinopathy may occur in newborns after therapeutic radiation therapy of a pregnant mother with as little as 10 cGy in the first trimester of gestation. The disorder may be exacerbated by chemotherapy as well.

Radiation retinopathy appears as superficial and deep intraretinal hemorrhages, cotton-wool spots, microaneurysms, telangiectasia, vascular sheathing, macular edema, hard exudates, neovascularization of the disc or neovascularization elsewhere, RPE alteration, and vitreal hemorrhages.

Less commonly, radiation retinopathy may demonstrate central retinal vein and artery occlusion. Also, after delayed radiation damage to the blood vessels, a retinal vascular incompetence may develop. Papilledema and optic atrophy also may occur. Occasionally, neovascular glaucoma may result after external-beam irradiation.

Mechanisms

Radiation retinopathy is produced by electromagnetic radiation of almost any wavelength to the retina by the following mechanisms: *ionizing*, *phototoxicity*, or *ultraviolet light effect*. The **ionizing** effect is caused by radiation doses from 1,500 to 10,000 cGy, which produce immediate damage to retinal neural cells and photoreceptors. The **phototoxicity** effect is produced, as in solar retinopathy, by the release of free radicals and lysosomal enzymes, which damage the photoreceptors. The **ultraviolet light** effect is due to ultraviolet light with a wavelength form of 10–400 nm, which produces CME in aphakia or produces denaturation of the collagen matrix and, subsequently, a shrinkage of the vitreous or a retinal degeneration.

Symptoms

Radiation retinopathy mildly decreases visual acuity—which may improve spontaneously over several months—or results in total vision loss.

Diagnosis

Fluorescein angiography may reveal areas of variably sized capillary nonperfusion (from 0.25 dd to large confluent areas), microaneurysms, and dilatation and tortuosity of the disc capillaries.

Differential Diagnosis

Diabetic retinopathy should be considered in the differential diagnosis. Additional possible diagnoses are hypertensive retinopathy, branch retinal artery occlusion, and telangiectasia from other causes.

Histopathology

Histologic analysis reveals possible intraretinal blood located in the inner retinal layers or in the vitreous. Eosinophilic deposits may be found in the outer plexiform layer and in the inner nuclear layer. The number of ganglion cells may be reduced or completely absent. Retinal vessels may have thickened or hyalinized walls.

Treatment

No treatment is totally effective for radiation retinopathy. Focal and grid laser photocoagulation may be beneficial for clinically significant macular edema. Panretinal photocoagulation should be performed in the treatment of neovascular glaucoma. Laser photocoagulation can be used for high-risk neovascularization. Interventions include pars plana vitrectomy. Hyperbaric oxygen may be administered, although it might exacerbate the disease.

Wagner's Disease

Wagner's disease (also called *hereditary hyaloid retinopathy*) is a rare, bilateral, slowly progressive, hereditary, autosomal dominant degeneration of the vitreous. It also may affect the retina and the choroid with juvenile retinoschisis and lens opacity. It may precipitate a moderate or severe myopia. Usually, it is not associated with any systemic disorders, and its etiology is unknown.

Wagner's disease appears as a massive vitreal liquefaction, an optically empty cavity in the center and posterior vitreous, except for whitish free-floating vitreous fibers, veil-like opacities, and translucent, fenestrated, avascular, dense, and grayish white preretinal membranes located at or near the equator. The disorder may cause vitreous strands attached to the retinal surface. It produces focal areas of irregularly disposed striae of chorioretinal atrophy. There are also zones of ill-defined retinal pigmentation, which most commonly are perivascular. Retinal vessels may be sclerotic, narrowed, and irregular in caliber, with peripheral vascular sheathing that is obliterated and occasionally dragged to the optic disc. There may be extensive retinal areas that exhibit the white with pressure phenomenon, usually due to the pressure exerted by the vitreous membranes. Lattice degeneration, radially oriented and located postequatorially, may be present. Peripheral cystoid degeneration also is seen frequently. Marked retinal meridional folds may occur. There may be a vitreous syneresis and juvenile retinoschisis, with large lacunae or dehiscences in the vitreous gel. *No posterior vitreous detachment results.* Mild lens opacity in childhood can occur and may progress to a mature cataract by the age of 35–40 years.

Symptoms

Wagner's disease may be asymptomatic. It is known to result in decreased vision and night blindness.

Diagnosis

The ERG may be abnormal. Dark adaptation is normal. Visual field testing may reveal contraction.

Differential Diagnosis

Goldmann-Favre vitreoretinal degeneration should be considered in the differential diagnosis. Other diagnoses include congenital retinoschisis, Turner's syndrome, snowflake degeneration, Stickler's syndrome, congenital cataract, Marfan's syndrome, myopia, Ehlers-Danlos syndrome, and retinitis pigmentosa.

Histopathology

Histologic assessment may reveal evidence of areas of RPE thinning, with pigment proliferation. Peripheral retinal vessels are decreased in number, have thick walls, are narrowed and sheathed, and occasionally are obliterated. There is a chorioretinal atrophy, which is heavily pigmented. Optic nerve atrophy is evident. A preretinal membrane, possibly with a fine network of capillaries, also may be seen. Vitreous liquefaction in the central and posterior gel is present.

Treatment

Treatment includes cryopexy and photocoagulation.

Goldmann-Favre Syndrome

Also called *vitreotapetoretinal dystrophy* or *vitreoretinal degeneration*, Goldmann-Favre syndrome is a rare, bilateral, congenital degenerative disease. It is autosomal recessive and affects the choroid, retina, vitreous, and lens in young children.

The disorder appears as a pigmentary retinopathy, with pigment clumping along the retinal vessels, in a bone-spicule pattern, unevenly located at the equator and at the posterior pole. There is central and peripheral retinoschisis that appears lacelike or as small holes in the inner retinal layers. Vessels appear thinned and irregular, particularly at the peripheral fundus. Also at the periphery there may be a glial proliferation in a wormlike pattern that extends beneath the retinal inner layers. Usually, the vitreous is liquefied, with large optical empty spaces that may contain fine fibrous strands surrounded by semiliquid gel with loosely plated membrane. The outer layers of the vitreous cortex are condensed, resembling a preretinal membrane. Occasionally, there may be posterior vitreous detachment. The macula may display microcystic changes that resemble **beaten copper**.

Symptoms

This disorder triggers symptoms of poor central and peripheral visual acuity. Night blindness may result. Progressive vision loss is possible and may lead to blindness. Another symptom is progressive cataract.

Diagnosis

Fluorescein angiography may reveal fairly symmetric, diffuse window defects but no staining of the cysts. The ERG is flat and nonrecordable. Also, the EOG may be markedly abnormal. Visual field testing shows a central scotoma. Color vision testing may show predominantly blue-yellow defects in the Farnsworth-Munsell 100-hue test and red-green defects with Ishihara's pseudoisochromatic plates.

Differential Diagnosis

The differential diagnosis should consider retinitis pigmentosa, Wagner's vitreoretinal degeneration, Stickler's syndrome, juvenile hereditary retinoschisis, and cystoid macular edema.

Histopathology

Histologic evaluation will confirm a splitting in the nerve fiber layer.

Treatment

No treatment is satisfactory for Goldmann-Favre syndrome. Genetic counseling is indicated.

Refsum's Syndrome

Refsum's syndrome (also called *phytanic acid storage disease*, *heredopathia atactica polyneuritiformis*, and *hereditary motor and sensory neuropathy type IV*) is a congenital hereditary retinal dystrophy. The disorder is an autosomal recessive trait that triggers **phytanic acid** accumulation in RPE cells. The onset occurs in childhood, although the diagnosis usually is delayed until middle age. It is associated with cerebellar ataxia, peripheral neuropathy, deafness, cardiomyopathy, ichthyosis, epiphyseal dysplasia, and anosmia.

Refsum's syndrome is caused by an enzymatic block in the degradation of phytanic acid occurring in dairy fat and cattle fat and is due to a deficiency of *phytanic acid alpha-oxidase.* That enzyme normally is present in rhodopsin metabolism, wherein vitamin A is esterified to palmitic acid, which subsequently is metabolized to phytanic acid.

The disorder appears as a pigmentary retinopathy, with clump pigmentation and bone spicules at the periphery. There is a macular degeneration. Retinal vessels may be attenuated, and optic atrophy may be present. Remissions are possible. Exacerbations are triggered by fever, surgery, or pregnancy.

Symptoms

Symptoms include night blindness, miosis, poor pupillary reaction, ophthalmoplegia, nystagmus, dry skin, progressive lower eyelid weakness, and progressive restriction of ocular motility. Additional symptoms are hypotonia, deafness, hepatomegaly, mental retardation, chronic polyneuritis with paresis and atrophy of distal extremities, drop foot, loss of deep tendon reflexes, cerebellar ataxia, intention tremor, posterior subcapsular cataract, and ectopia lentis. Corneal epithelial and stromal edema may be seen, with vascularization and guttate lesions.

Diagnosis

The cerebrospinal fluid protein level is increased, without pleocytosis. Visual field testing reveals progressive severely constricted fields and ring scotomas. Dark adaptation is abnormally marked and elevated. The ERG may reveal abnormalities involving cones and rods or may be extinguished. Assay of phytanic acid in blood, urine, and tissues shows an increased level. Low plasmogens may be evident. Cultured fibroblasts may show an absence of phytanic acid. Motor and sensory conduction velocity is markedly reduced. Electromyography reveals a denervation in the affected muscles. An elevated level of pipecolic acid, very-long-chain fatty acids, and bile intermediates are evident. Peroxisome and peroxisomal enzymes and functions are deficient. Electrocardiography may show nonspecific changes.

Differential Diagnosis

The predominant consideration for differential diagnosis is retinitis pigmentosa.

Histopathology

Histologic analysis reveals an atypical degeneration of the sensory retina. There is a loss of photoreceptor cells and a pigmentary migration. An accumulation of fatty acids, such as tetramethyl hexadecanoic acid, may exist in the outer retinal layers. Atypical retinal degeneration may be seen, and lipid deposits may occur in the perivascular accumulation of pigmented cells.

Treatment

No treatment is totally effective for Refsum's syndrome. Genetic counseling is advised. Low-vision aids are beneficial. IOL implantation is a viable intervention. Another possible treatment is a diet low in phytol (a precursor of phytanic acid), which requires long-term exclusion of dairy products, animal fats, green leafy vegetables, and fish oils.

Suggested Reading

Borruat FX, Othenin-Girard B, Regli F, Hurliman J. Natural history of diffuse uveal melanocytic proliferation. Ophthalmology 1992;99:1698–1704.

Bressler SB. Age-related macular degeneration. Focal Points 1995;3:3–10.

Brown GC. Radiation Therapy. In W Tasman, EA Jaeger, MM Parks, et al. (eds), Duane's Clinical Ophthalmology, vol 3. Philadelphia: Lippincott–Raven, 1996;36A:1–4.

Byer NE. Lattice degeneration of retina. Focal Points 1989;5:2–10.

Carr RE. Primary Retinal Degeneration. In W Tasman, EA Jaeger, MM Parks, et al. (eds), Duane's Clinical Ophthalmology, vol 3. Philadelphia: Lippincott–Raven, 1996;25:1–16.

Cavender JC, Everett A, Lee ST. Hereditary Macular Dystrophy. In W Tasman, EA Jaeger, MM Parks, et al. (eds), Duane's Clinical Ophthalmology, vol 3. Philadelphia: Lippincott–Raven, 1996;9:10–29.

Chen HC, Kohner EM. Endocrine Disease and the Eye. In W Tasman, EA Jaeger, MM Parks, et al. (eds), Duane's Clinical Ophthalmology, vol 5. Philadelphia: Lippincott–Raven, 1996;21:12–13.

Foster CS. The Eye in Skin and Mucous Membrane Disorders. In W Tasman, EA Jaeger, MM Parks, et al. (eds), Duane's Clinical Ophthalmology, vol 5. Philadelphia: Lippincott–Raven, 1996;27:17–32.

Gass JDM, Giesr RG, Wilkinson CP, et al. Bilateral diffuse uveal melanocytic proliferation in patients with occult carcinoma. Arch Ophthalmol 1990;108: 545–550.

Glascow BJ, Foss RY, Yoshisumi MO, Straatsma BR. Degenerative Diseases of the Peripheral Retina. In W Tasman, EA Jaeger, MM Parks, et al. (eds), Duane's Clinical Ophthalmology, vol 3. Philadelphia: Lippincott–Raven, 1996;26:1–8.

Guerry RK, Ham WT, Mueller HA. Light Toxicity in the Posterior Segment. In W Tasman, EA Jaeger, MM Parks, et al. (eds), Duane's Clinical Ophthalmology, vol 3. Philadelphia: Lippincott–Raven, 1996;37:8–15.

Guyer DR, Mukai S, Egan KM, et al. Radiation maculopathy after proton beam irradiation for choroid melanoma. Ophthalmology 1992;99:1278–1285.

Heckenlively JR, Rodriguez JA, Daiger SP. Autosomal dominant sectorial retinitis pigmentosa. Arch Ophthalmol 1991;109:84–91.

Jakobiec FA, Jones IS. Vascular Tumors, Malformations, and Degenerations. In W Tasman, EA Jaeger, MM Parks, et al. (eds), Duane's Clinical Ophthalmology, vol 2. Philadelphia: Lippincott–Raven, 1996;37:33–36.

Kliffen M, Mooy CM, Luider TM, et al. Identification of glycosaminoglycans in age-related macular deposits. Arch Ophthalmol 1996;114:1009–1014.

Leys AM, Dietrich HG, Sciot RM. Early lesions of bilateral diffuse melanocytic proliferation. Arch Ophthalmol 1991;109:1590–1594.

Lim IJ, Lam S. A retinal pigment epithelium tear in a patient with angioid streaks. Arch Ophthalmol 1990;108:1672–1673.

Marmor MF. Long-term follow-up of the physiologic abnormalities and fundus changes in fundus albipunctatus. Ophthalmology 1990;97:380–384.

McDonald HR, Schatz H, Johnson RN, Madeira D. Acquired Macular Diseases. In W Tasman, EA Jaeger, MM Parks, et al. (eds), Duane's Clinical Ophthalmology, vol 3. Philadelphia: Lippincott–Raven, 1996;23:3–27.

Richards JE, Kuo C, Boehnke M, Sieving PA. Rhodopsin Thr 58 Arg mutation in a family with autosomal dominant retinitis pigmentosa. Ophthalmology 1991;98:1797–1805.

Smith D, Oestreicher J, Musarella MS. Clinical spectrum of Leber's congenital amaurosis in the second to fourth decade of life. Ophthalmology 1990;97:1156–1161.

Van der Schaft TL, Mooy CM, Brujin WC, et al. Histologic features of the early stages of age-related macular degeneration. Ophthalmology 1992;99:278–286.

Yannuzzi LA, Bird A, Guyer D, et al. Retinal specialists weigh in on ARMD treatment options. Ophthalmol Times 1997;3:10–18.

7

Macular Disease

Central Serous Chorioretinopathy

Variously known as *central serous retinopathy*, *central serous choroidosis*, *serous disciform detachment of central retina*, *central angiospastic retinopathy*, and *central serous degeneration*, central serous chorioretinopathy is a unilateral serous detachment of the macular sensory retina. It occurs more frequently in young men and in pregnant women, but it sometimes also appears in the elderly (older than 60 years). Its etiology is unknown, but the disorder is self-limited and carries a good prognosis for vision recovery. It is not associated with a retinal tear or hole.

Central serous chorioretinopathy may be caused by allergy; the toxicity of alcoholism, nicotine, or indomethacin; infections; such inflammatory bowel diseases as Crohn's disease or ulcerative colitis; and by stress in the type A personality. A possible role is played by the adrenomedullary system with a higher plasma catecholamine level, by a localized angiospasm, or by the effect of glucosteroids in hypercortisolemic states (e.g., endogenous Cushing's syndrome). The disorder may be produced by a local leakage in the retinal pigment epithelium (RPE) from the choriocapillaris, in which the fluid may seep through Bruch's membrane, causing an asymptomatic small detachment of the RPE.

The disorder's appearance is that of a circumscribed, somewhat round, shallow detachment of the macula, as large as 6 dd. It is a spherical, milky, translucent blister with fuzzy ill-defined borders that form an irregular white reflex line. Initially, the foveal reflex is missing, and the center of the macula becomes cloudy. Later, the macula appears elevated by 1 or 2 D, producing a transient hypermetropia. Small, yellow-white spots (fine subretinal precipitates, probably *lipoidal macrophages* or *fibrin*) may appear in the center of the macula. Retinal vessels may bend upward. In perhaps 8–10 weeks, the detachment resolves without vision loss or scarring, usually leaving residues of yellowish deposits or mounds of pigment proliferation. In chronic cases, telangiectasis, cystoid macular edema (CME), or pigment migration may be present. Rarely, the retinal detachment becomes bullous, with shifting turbid subretinal fluid and multiple areas of RPE detachments. Alternately, retinal detachment may occur anywhere at the posterior pole. Occasionally, a secondary cystoid degeneration of the macula may develop.

Symptoms

Central serous chorioretinopathy is characterized by decreased, slightly blurred vision, with micropsia. This symptom typically improves by use of a +1-D lens. Metamorphopsia, as shown by Amsler's grid testing, is typical. Other symptoms are darkening of the visual field, increased hypermetropia, and color-vision defects.

Diagnosis

Indirect funduscopy is performed for diagnosis. Other diagnostic tools include biomicroscopy, contact fundus lens of 20, 60, or 90 D, and red-free photography. In the early phase, fluorescein angiography may reveal focal disturbances of the outer retinal barrier, window defects in the sub-RPE area called *beacons of light*. In the late stage, there is an extension of the fluorescence into the subretinal space, which may appear as a hyperfluorescent pinpoint, called *smokestack*; as an *umbrella*; or as a localized hyperfluorescence, called *ink blot*, at the central point, representing the site of origin of leakage from RPE. Digital indocyanine green angiography may reveal multiple RPE detachments, with their characteristic late central hypofluorescent area, surrounded by a rim of hyperfluorescence, or may show a choroidal hyperpermeability around the active sites of leakage. The visual field may show central scotoma, and plasma catecholamines are increased. The photostress test is positive.

Differential Diagnosis

Considerations for the differential diagnosis are congenital optic pit and age-related macular degeneration (ARMD).

Histopathology

Histologic analysis shows a defect in Bruch's membrane or in the choriocapillaris. The junctional complexes between adjacent cells are enlarged and separated. Fluid accumulated between the RPE and photoreceptors may elevate the macula. Occasionally, a retinal arterial macroaneurysm may be present.

Treatment

Observation is indicated, as recovery may take place in 3–6 months, with mild visual distortion, faint scotomas, or color-vision defects. Argon laser photocoagulation of the leak may be beneficial, particularly if the site of leakage is extrafoveolar. *Corticosteroids are not indicated, as the disease is not inflammatory.*

Central Areolar Choroidal Dystrophy

Central areolar choroidal dystrophy (*central areolar choroidal sclerosis*, *central areolar choroidal atrophy*, *central angiosclerosis*, or *central senile choroiditis*) is a familial hereditary, autosomal dominant (or autosomal recessive) disorder. It occurs in adults, with the onset at 20–40 years of age, and is slowly progressive. The disorder also may be a variant of ARMD, initially affecting the macula and extending with time. Usually, it is not associated with any systemic disorders, but it may be caused by a dystrophic process of the choroidal vessels.

In its early stage, central areolar choroidal dystrophy appears as a mild depigmented macular granularity. In the later stage (sometimes after many years), more advanced, round or oval lesions appear and may enlarge and eventually form punched-out central atrophic lesions. There is extensive loss of the retina and the choroid and RPE and choriocapillaris atrophy, more frequently paramacular, which in time may enlarge and eventually encompass the entire posterior fundus. Atrophy may occur in precapillary arteries and in branches of short posterior ciliary arteries (but to a lesser extent). Also, there may be a blood shunt to choroidal veins. Large choroidal vessels overlying the retina are visible, yellow-white, and thickened.

Symptoms

Central areolar choroidal dystrophy may be asymptomatic. Mild, moderate, or even marked gradual reduction of the central vision is evident, causing definite difficulty in reading. Poor dark adaptation and glare sensitivity also result from the disorder.

Diagnosis

Visual field testing may reveal a large central scotoma. Electroretinography (ERG) may appear abnormal: Possibly there will be reduction of full-field cones and rods to 60% below normal and a diminished light-to-dark ratio. However, usually an essentially normal scotopic ERG is obtained. Fluorescein angiography in the early phase may reveal faint areas of hyperfluorescence as large window defects and RPE transmission defects but, in a later phase, may show a sharply demarcated area of choroidal atrophy, with large choroidal vessels filling normally, and a hyperfluorescence of the rim of the lesion and scleral staining. Electro-oculography (EOG) may be normal to slightly subnormal, depending on the extent of RPE dysfunction. Color vision may show a moderate protan-deutan, that parallels the gradual vision loss.

Differential Diagnosis

Differential diagnosis should consider central areolar pigment epithelial dystrophy, Stargardt's disease, or North Carolina macular dystrophy. The disorder also may reflect ARMD and myopia.

Histopathology

Histologic evaluation should reveal a thinning, atrophic RPE; fibrosing scarring; and absence of the choriocapillaris and photoreceptors. Occasionally, the outer nuclear layer also may be absent. Choroidal vessels may appear with thickened walls and a narrowed blood column but present no evidence of vessel wall sclerosis.

Treatment

No known treatment exists for central areolar choroidal dystrophy.

Macular Detachment

Macular detachment, *primary* or *secondary*, is a separation of the retina at the macula and usually is unilateral. **Primary macular detachment** may occur in acute idiopathic maculopathy. **Secondary** (or **exudative**) **macular detachment** may occur in central serous chorioretinopathy, age-related macular degeneration, pregnancy, posterior scleritis, posterior multifocal placoid pigment epitheliopathy, birdshot retinochoroidopathy, and drusen of the optic disc. The disorder may appear in focal or multiple choroiditis (as in toxocariasis and histoplasmosis) or with tractional retinal detachment in diabetes.

Macular detachment appears as a yellowish, white, or gray, circumscribed, slightly elevated area of choroid infiltration in the macular region. It develops irregular margins and often appears in wedged configuration. As the detachment progresses, an RPE disturbance may appear as a small, dark, greenish-blackish macular ring with peripheral thickening. Sometimes, at this level, clusters of intraretinal hemorrhages in the detached sensory retina may be seen.

Symptoms

The symptoms of macular detachment include blurred vision and metamorphopsia.

Diagnosis

Fluorescein angiography may reveal early focal hyperfluorescence at the level of the RPE, then a complete staining of the neurosensory space as a classic *smokestack* pattern in the macular region. A slightly greater intensity of hyperfluorescence of RPE is evident surrounding pigmentary disturbances, which are comparatively hypofluorescent.

Treatment

Laser photocoagulation is the indicated treatment for macular detachment.

Macular Hole

Macular hole, either **congenital** or **acquired,** is a focal depression on the macula. It can occur variously after trauma, chronic macular edema, vascular processes, intraocular infections, choroidal melanoma, and retinal detachment. The disorder is seen also in myopia and in solar retinopathy or *idiopathic* (senile) *retinopathy*, which more often occurs spontaneously in elderly women.

Macular hole may be produced by a shrinkage of the vitreous cortex in the fovea or by an ischemia combined with a localized prefoveal cortical tangential vitreous traction. Additionally, it can result from a microcystoid degeneration that may rupture and coalesce or from a migration of Müller cells and astrocytes through the internal limiting membrane, at the posterior vitreous cortex, to form a **prefoveolar vitreoglial membrane (PVGM)**.

The disorder may appear either as a *pseudohole* or as a *full-thickness hole*. **Macular pseudohole** (or **lamellar hole**) appears in the foveola as a dark-red spot with steep slopes and crinkle macular sheen. It is caused by a condensation and tangential contraction of the PVGM, which result in a detachment of the foveolar retina.

A **macular full-thickness hole** appears as a small, red, circular, punched-out spot in the macula or as an eccentric can opener–shaped tear. Its sharply demarcated margins are bowed inward, and it is more opaque than is the contiguous retina. Initially, it measures some 200 μm; then it enlarges to the classic 500 μm (or to 0.66 dd). It forms a dark base and a grayish halo, which corresponds to a thickened rim of a subretinal detachment. Foveal reflex usually is absent. Sometimes, there is an oval distortion of the spot, owing to the existing radial retinal folds. Often, yellow deposits of perhaps 200–400 μm in diameter appear in the base of the hole. The shrinkage of the cortical vitreous may produce a thinning of the macular retina and a dispersion of the *xanthophyll* pigment to the sides, giving rise to a yellow halo having a reddish center. A possible operculum overlying the macular hole may represent a localized vitreous separation.

The **Gass classification** specifies four stages in macular hole formation.

Stage 1, the **premacular hole,** is divided into stages 1A and 1B. **Stage 1A** identifies a **yellow spot.** This central spot of xanthophyll pigment is caused by a localized traction of the precortical vitreous, which may lead to a macular detachment. **Stage 1B** designates a **yellow ring.** This ring signifies a loss of the foveal depression that may progress to macular detachment and to central retinal dehiscence. It may develop at the umbo under an intact layer of a prefoveal vitreous (an *occult hole*).

Stage 2 represents an **early eccentric hole.** This ring enlarges centrifugally and forms a fine hole, either centrally or eccentrically (or both), with or without vitreofoveal separation. It also may form a *pseudo-operculum* that contains vitreous, possible internal limiting membrane, and Müller cells, but *not rods and cones*.

Stages 3 and 4 typify full-thickness holes. **Stage 3**, the **full-thickness hole,** indicates a completely developed hole of perhaps 400 μm, with vitreofoveal separation and a pseudo-operculum. **Stage 4** represents a **full-thickness hole with vitreous detachment.** This complete macular hole has a posterior vitreous separation from the optic disc and macula. It may have also a pseudo-operculum.

Symptoms

Symptoms of macular hole include decreased vision to 20/200 or worse, visual distortion, and the appearance of a central scotoma on Amsler's grid.

Differential Diagnosis

Considerations for differential diagnosis include macular pucker and solar retinopathy.

Histopathology

Histologic evaluation shows a discontinuity of the retina at the macula, characterized by round edges and inward bowing (Figure 7-1); its floor is lined completely by RPE. Subretinal fluid may be present. Usually, cystoid macular degeneration and edema are seen. A possible glial mem-

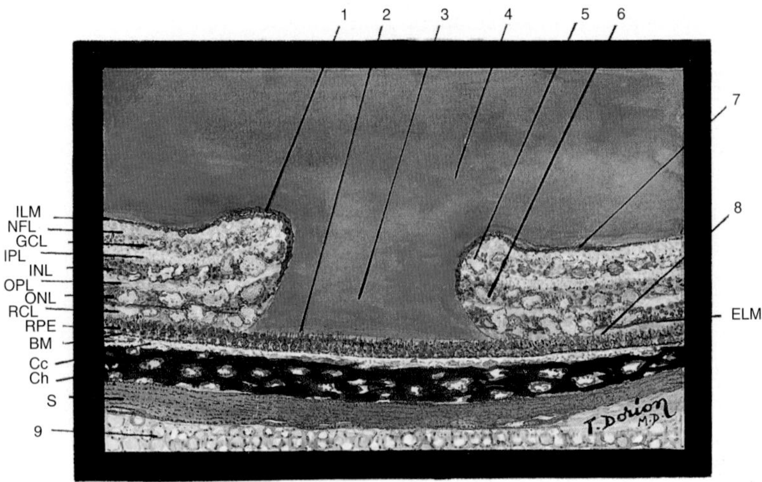

Figure 7-1. *Macular hole, full-thickness. (1) Glial membrane covering the edges. (2) Floor completely lined by retinal pigment epithelium (RPE). (3) Discontinuity of retina at the macula. (4) Vitreous. (5) Round edges bowed inward. (6) Cystoid macular degeneration. (7) Thickening of the internal limiting membrane. (8) Atrophy of rods and cones (photoreceptors). (9) Orbital adipose tissue. (ILM, internal limiting membrane; NFL, nerve fiber layer; GCL, ganglion cell layer; IPL, inner plexiform layer; INL, inner nuclear layer; OPL, outer plexiform layer; ONL, outer nuclear layer; ELM, external limiting membrane; RCL, rod and cone layer [photoreceptors]; BM, Bruch's membrane; Cc, choriocapillaris; Ch, choroid; S, sclera.)*

brane may cover the edges, and an atrophy of the photoreceptors may be present. The internal limiting membrane may be thickened, although the choroid, choriocapillaris, and Bruch's membrane appear normal.

Treatment

Macular hole is not responsive to any treatment. Observation is mandated. Interventions include pars plana vitrectomy to flatten the hole or a membrane-peeling procedure with gas-fluid exchange. Pneumatic detachment of vitreous may be performed, as may adjunctive therapy with serum, plasma, and transforming growth hormone factor beta.

Macular Edema

Also called *CME*, *Irvine-Gass-Norton syndrome*, and *vitreomacular traction syndrome*, macular edema is either a hereditary or an acquired thickening of the retina in the macula extending within 1 dd of the macular center. It usually occurs after an extracellular accumulation of fluid.

The disorder usually occurs as one of three clinical types: *focal*, *diffuse*, or *cystoid*. **Focal** macular edema occurs with a readily identifiable source of leakage. **Diffuse** macular edema is associated with multiple unidentifiable sources of leakage (e.g., capillaries or areas of nonperfusion). **CME** is typified by fluid accumulation in the outer plexiform layer and inner nuclear layer of the retina in cystoid spaces.

The disorder also can be considered etiologically: *idiopathic*, *tractional*, and *vascular* in central and branch retinal vein obstruction and retinal telangiectasia; *immunologic* and *inflammatory* in pars planitis, posterior uveitis, or sympathetic ophthalmia; *systemic* in diabetes or hypertension; *tumoral* and *degenerative* in retinitis pigmentosa; *traumatic* after cataract surgery, laser capsulotomy, laser photocoagulation, or cryotherapy; *toxic* after nicotinic acid administration; or *topical* after epinephrine or dipivefrin instillation.

Macular edema may be due to an abnormal permeability of the perifoveolar capillaries. In approximately 3–5% of cases, after an uneventful cataract extraction (more commonly intracapsular) and, to a lesser extent, in an anterior chamber intraocular lens implantation and usually after 2 months and up to 5 years, exposure to ultraviolet light may generate free radicals. This activity in turn augments the production of *prostaglandin*, which will increase the microvascular abnormality. As a result, the blood-ocular barrier will break down, and a CME or Irvine-Gass-Norton syndrome will develop.

The disorder appears as an amorphous, gray-white macula with a dull light reflex or as a petaloid, honeycomblike fluid-filled space surrounded by smaller cysts (Figure 7-2). Sometimes, an epiretinal membrane appears as a macular sheen with retinal folds and tortuous vessels or as a yellowish spot in the macula. Additionally, preretinal gliosis or involutional maculopathy may occur and, occasionally, flame-shaped hemorrhages may be present. Chronic macular edema may lead to microscopic degeneration, coalescence of cysts, and hole formation.

Clinically significant macular edema (**CSME**) is a retinal thickening or hard exudates at or within 500 µm of the center of the macula, within 500 µm of the center of the macula associated with adjacent retinal thickening that may be outside the 500-µm limit, or a retinal thick-

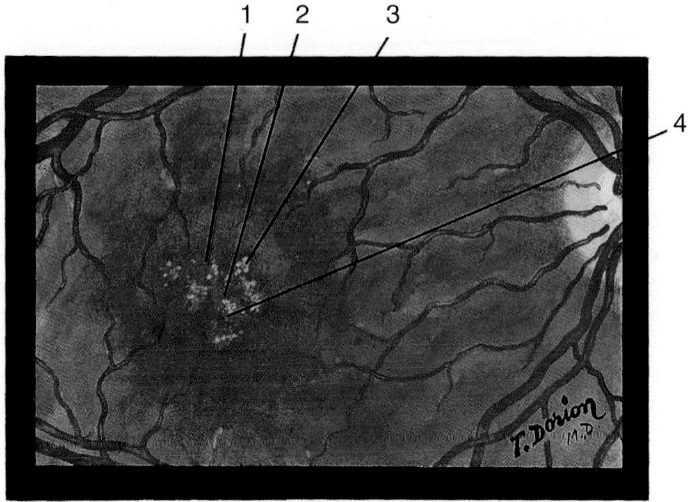

Figure 7-2. *Cystoid macular edema. (1) Petaloid honeycomblike fluid-filled spaces in a thickened retina. (2) Dull foveal reflex. (3) Yellowish spots of lipid exudates in the macula surrounding the cystoid spaces. (4) Flame-shaped hemorrhages.*

ening of 1 dd or larger, any part of which is within 1 dd of the center of the macula.

Symptoms

Rapid temporary loss of visual acuity may occur in aphakic patients, from blurred vision to as low as finger counting.

Diagnosis

Fluorescein angiography may reveal capillary nonperfusion in the early phase. This disorder may be followed by an irregularly dilated capillary and scattered microaneurysms and, in the late phase, heavy staining or accumulation of fluorescein is seen within the retinal cystoid spaces in the outer plexiform layer of Henle, giving a petaloid appearance.

Histopathology

Histologic analysis reveals a patchy loss of the RPE with pigmentary dispersion. The internal limiting membrane is virtually absent, and the retinal elements are compressed against the fiber core of Müller cells.

Treatment

Observation and encouragement are the preferred treatment for macular edema, as it may improve itself. Topical, periocular, or systemic corticosteroids are beneficial. Nonsteroidal anti-inflammatory drugs may be used to block production of prostaglandin (e.g., ketorolac [Acular] 0.5%, 1 drop four times a day, or flurbiprofen [Ocufen], 1 drop every 2 hours for 1 week, then every 4 hours for 2 weeks, then three times a day for 3 months, and then twice a day for 12 months). Other agents include fenoprofen (Nalfon), 200 mg PO four times a day; ibuprofen (Motrin), 400 mg PO four times a day; aspirin, 325 mg PO four times a day; indomethacin (Indocin), 25 mg PO twice a day; and naproxen (Naprosyn), 250 mg PO twice a day. Interventions include hyperbaric oxygen, focal laser photocoagulation (especially in CSME), vitrectomy, and lysis in incarcerated vitreous wick in aphakic or pseudophakic individuals. Treatment of the underlying disease should be supervised by an internist.

Disciform Macular Degeneration

Disciform macular degeneration (also called *Kuhnt-Junius disease*) is a progressive, exudative, proliferative macular disease. Usually, it is bilateral and is not necessarily simultaneous, although that occurs in months or years. The disorder occurs in both genders in people older than 60 years. Commonly, it is preceded by macular drusen. It may occur in patients with ARMD or in long-standing angioid streaks.

Disciform macular degeneration may be caused by a thickening of Bruch's membrane, which deprives the macular retina of its choroidal nutrition. This process leads to a local hypoxia, which releases a **neovascular factor** that in turn permits the new vessels from the choriocapillaris to invade the retina at the posterior pole. This forms a large circular lesion that in time becomes an atrophic patch. There may be either a chronic papilledema or a disciform degeneration adjacent to the optic disc occurring spontaneously or in association with tilting of the disc.

The disorder appears as a disciform, irregular thickening of the macular retina, some 3.5 mm in diameter and 0.5 mm thick. It is a fairly well-circumscribed, glassy, elevated, white-gray or white-yellow mass sometimes appearing with small cysts or schisis or as a geographic pattern. There is marked attenuation of the macular arteries and veins. Multiple yellow-white deposits arranged in a circular pattern surrounding the macula may convert to a fibrous mass. Occasionally, a prominent retinal artery may be seen over the disciform area, which dips down and disappears into the scar; this condition is called *retinal arterialization*. There is an advanced sclerosis of the retinal and choroidal vessels. The optic disc may show a senile excavation and subretinal neovascularization.

Disciform macular degeneration usually encompasses four stages: *hemorrhagic*, *edematous*, *exudative*, and *scarring*. The **hemorrhagic stage** is characterized by a choroidal neovascular growth, often horseshoe or sickle shaped, located beneath the macula and at the edges of the lesion. It may cause subretinal hemorrhages. The **edematous stage** signifies a serous RPE detachment at the macula, with a subretinal fluid accumulation, which may affect the foveal central vision but spares the extrafoveal vision. The sub-RPE space is filled with choroidal vessels, forming a *choroidal neovascular membrane*.

The **exudative stage** is represented by a slightly prominent, gray-white, connective tissue lesion called *macular pseudotumor*. It appears as a dense, white scar with an atrophic depressed center and with a circular zone of irregular depigmentation surrounding the macula. The *scarring stage* refers to a white, elevated, subretinal fibrous scar, a *burnt-out* lesion that may be mistaken for a tumor. Vessels are sometimes tortuous, course up onto the lesion, and often anastomose in its surface.

Juvenile disciform macular degeneration occurs secondary to a multifocal choroiditis such as histoplasmosis, a focal peripapillary choroiditis, a focal macular choroiditis, or toxocariasis.

Symptoms

The major symptom of disciform macular degeneration is decreased central visual acuity.

Diagnosis

Fluorescein angiography reveals an early filling of the retinal arteries, with little fluorescence and a delay in filling the rest of the retinal veins or venous collaterals on the optic disc. In the later stage, there may be an extensive submacular neovascular membrane. Finally, the scarring stage results in a staining of scar but no leakage of the dye.

Histopathology

Histologic analysis demonstrates an exudation between retina and choroid, with hemorrhage and exudative, proliferative, or atrophic changes in the RPE and retina proper (probably depending on the stage of the lesion). The exudation is located under the macula, in the perimacular area, and occasionally adjacent to the optic disc. In the early stages, the degenerative changes (partially obliterated) occur in the choriocapillaris and in Bruch's membrane, in which there are many breaks and zones of calcification manifested clinically as drusen. The disorder may progress to a serous detachment of the RPE. In a later stage, neovascularization of this macular choroidal degeneration occurs. New vessels from the choroid grow into the sub-RPE space, between the mesodermal portion of Bruch's membrane and the basement membrane of RPE. These vessels may bleed and leak; consequently, a hemorrhage (called *choroidal hematoma*) may occur in the sub-RPE space. As the hemorrhage organizes, a proliferation of RPE and a fibrous metaplasia may occur, and the ingrowth of mesenchymal tissue forms granulation tissue. The disorder is characterized by a dry macular degeneration, with fibrous or even cartilaginous degeneration, called *macular pseudotumor*. Finally, a disciform fibrous scar forms in the macula, producing massive irreversible degeneration of the RPE and sensory retina.

Sorsby's Pseudoinflammatory Dystrophy

Sorsby's pseudoinflammatory dystrophy (*Sorsby's fundus dystrophy, hereditary macular dystrophy*) is a bilateral, symmetric, autosomal dominant, slowly progressive chorioretinal dystrophy. It develops initially in the macula and then extends to a large part of the fundus (Figure 7-3). The disorder occurs mainly in middle-aged patients.

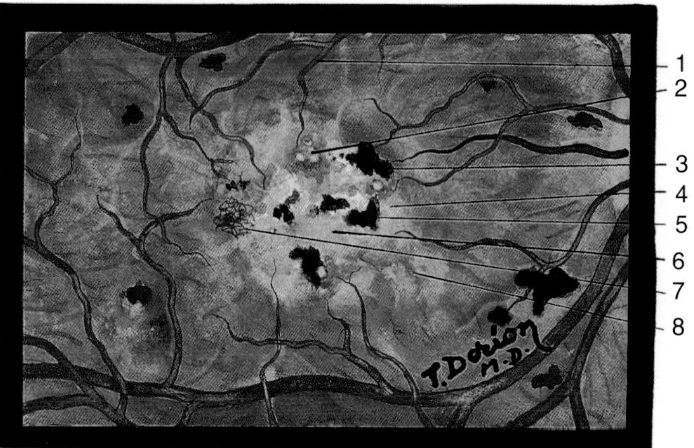

Figure 7-3. *Sorsby's pseudoinflammatory dystrophy. (1) Normal retinal vessels. (2) Drusen. (3) Heavy pigmentation. (4) Exudates. (5) Retinal hemorrhage. (6) Macular edema. (7) Choroidal neovascularization. (8) Visible choroidal vessels.*

In the early stage, it appears as a mottling of the posterior pole, then as pseudoinflammatory changes at the macula, such as edema, hemorrhage, and exudates. At a later stage, as the lesions heal, irregular heavy pigmentation and white chorioretinal atrophic scars with subretinal fibrosis occur. Drusen over wide areas and choroidal neovascularization in the macula also may be present. Choroidal vessels are visible through the atrophic scar. Optic disc and retinal vessels usually are normal.

Symptoms

The major symptom of Sorsby's pseudoinflammatory dystrophy is decreased visual acuity, sometimes since childhood.

Diagnosis

The ERG and dark adaptation initially are normal; then the ERG demonstrates subnormal imaging. Fluorescein angiography shows defects in the RPE.

Histopathology

Histologic evaluation reveals a loss of the RPE, photoreceptors, the choriocapillaris, and the outer nuclear layer. Heavy pigmentary dispersions are present in some areas. Subretinal hemorrhages, fibrosis, macular choroidal neovascularization, retinal edema, and exudation also are present.

Treatment

There is no treatment for Sorsby's pseudoinflammatory dystrophy.

Sjögren's Reticular Macular Dystrophy

Also termed *dystrophia reticularis laminae pigmentosa retinae*, Sjögren's reticular macular dystrophy is a rare, bilateral, autosomal recessive, very slowly progressive, and symmetric macular retinopathy. It is a part of **pattern dystrophies of the RPE**, which may occur at perhaps 5 years of age in children of consanguineous mates.

The disorder appears initially as a dark pigmented spot of approximately 1 dd located in the center of the macula. Then, a hyperpigmented network extends gradually toward midperiphery, with darker pigment densification at the intersections of the knots. This activity gives rise to a *fishnet*, with accumulation of a finely meshed network of polygonally arranged pigment granules. That network may appear oval at some 5 dd vertically and 7 dd horizontally. Drusen also may be present. Pigmentary and atrophic areas are located in the macula and, at a later stage, may appear as *chicken-wire* pigmentation. They may extend out of the macular area in the midperiphery and peripheral retina.

Symptoms

Although Sjögren's reticular macular dystrophy may be asymptomatic, the predominant symptom may be markedly decreased vision.

Diagnosis

Fluorescein angiography may reveal blockage of the dye, with areas of reticular hypofluorescent bands or segments surrounded by areas of non-leaking reticular hyperfluorescence, corresponding to RPE dystrophy. ERG may be normal, although EOG usually is normal to subnormal. Dark adaptation also may be normal to abnormal. Other vision tests, such as color vision or visual field examination, commonly are normal.

Differential Diagnosis

The differential diagnosis should consider Werner-Benedikt or Kingham-Fenzi-Willerson-Aaberg reticular dystrophy. Other possibilities are fundus flavimaculatus and senile reticular peripheral degeneration.

Histopathology

Histologic analysis shows an RPE dystrophy at the macular level, with hypertrophy and hyperpigmentation and RPE loss.

Fenestrated Sheen Macular Dystrophy

Fenestrated sheen macular dystrophy is a rare, autosomal dominant dystrophy of the macula with high penetrance. It is slowly progressive, starts in childhood at approximately age 4 years, and extends throughout the adult life.

The disorder begins in the early stage as a yellowish, refractile sheen over the macula. Its red fenestrations appear as tiny windows through which the underlying RPE is visible. In a later stage (in adulthood by the age of 30), an annular area of RPE depigmentation may develop, surround the central island of normal RPE, and gradually enlarge over the initial macular sheen. Adjacent to this zone, another area of hyperpigmentation may occur, giving rise to a **bull's-eye macula**. There may be abnormal RPE granulations at the posterior pole and at the peripheral retina.

Symptoms

Fenestrated sheen macular dystrophy may be asymptomatic. Central visual acuity is normal, and vision prognosis is excellent.

Diagnosis

Fluorescein angiography in younger patients is normal, but in older patients, in the arteriovenous phase it may reveal multiple punctate or large confluent annular RPE transmission window defects (with normal choriocapillaris perfusion) surrounding a central area of slight fluorescence. Visual field testing may reveal a paracentral scotoma by age 50 or older. ERG is normal in younger patients but may reveal a subnormal photopic response in adults. In children, EOG also is normal and, in older patients, may be normal to subnormal. There may be a mild red-green color defect.

Differential Diagnosis

Considerations in the differential diagnosis should include Stargardt's disease and progressive cone-rod dystrophy. Other possibilities include central areolar RPE dystrophy and central areolar choroidal atrophy.

Histopathology

Histologic evaluation demonstrates a sheen located between the RPE and retinal vessels and in the foveolar avascular zone.

Treatment

There is no treatment for the disorder, as none is necessary.

Acute Macular Neuroretinopathy

Acute macular neuroretinopathy is an acute bilateral macular disease that occurs in young (mostly female) adults. Usually, it appears after a flu-type illness or after an acute hypertensive episode or appears as an adverse reaction to an intravenous contrast media. The disorder may be produced by a virus.

It begins as subtle, reddish-brown, wedge- or tear-shaped, petaloid, retinal lesions, sometimes assuming a geographic pattern and locating itself in the macula, in the parafoveolar region, or in the deep sensory retina. Small superficial hemorrhage may be present, although retinal vessels are normal.

Symptoms

Acute macular neuroretinopathy may be asymptomatic. Mild decreased visual acuity is observed in the disorder.

Diagnosis

Visual field tests reveal scotoma. Amsler's grid testing also may demonstrate (usually paracentral) scotomas, which may become less dense in time. Fluorescein angiography may be normal.

Macular Halo

Macular halo is a retinal abnormality occurring in Niemann-Pick disease type B. The chronic form has no central nervous system involvement. The disorder is due to a defect in the lipidic metabolism in which there is a deficient *sphingomyelinase* production.

Macular halo appears as a bilateral pale discoloration—symmetric, punctate, yellow-white or gray—with scintillating crystalloid granules. They are arranged as a ring or doughnut about the macula, having a relatively sharp border on the inner edge and a ragged border on the outer edge. Multifocal deposits are located inside and outside the ring. The halo measures approximately 0.5 dd in its outer edge and may be located superficially or deep into the retina.

Diagnosis

A low sphingomyelinase level is seen in white blood cells and in cultured skin fibroblasts.

Treatment

Macular halo is not treated.

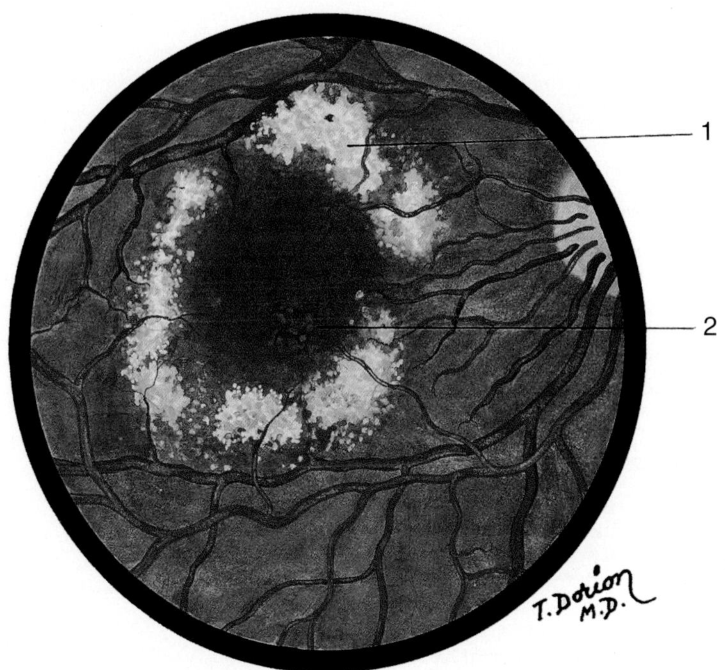

Figure 7-4. *Circinate maculopathy. (1) Hard exudates in a garland pattern. (2) Macular neovascularization.*

Circinate Maculopathy

Circinate maculopathy is a circular deposition of hard exudates at the macula and usually occurs in diabetes or secondary to an acquired arterial macroaneurysm. It is caused by an abnormal vascular permeability, which allows leakage of lipid or lipoprotein.

The disorder appears as multiple yellow-white deposits of globular, hard exudates. They are demarcated sharply, are irregularly shaped and variably sized, and are arranged in a circinate (garlandlike) pattern (Figure 7-4) as a complete or partial circle at the periphery of the macula. Sometimes, a macular edema may extend into the viable retina, so that those exudates may be considered as *edema residues*.

Diagnosis

Fluorescein angiography may reveal leakage from a previous macular branch vein occlusion.

Histopathology

Histologic analysis reveals hard exudates located in the macular retina (parafoveolar) separated by a clear zone, which includes the foveola. Also possible are subvascular exudates or neovascularization of the macula.

Treatment

Circinate maculopathy is not treated. These exudates may resolve spontaneously.

Cellophane Maculopathy

Cellophane maculopathy goes by many names: *macular pucker*, *surface wrinkling retinopathy*, *wrinkling of the internal limiting membrane*, *preretinal macular gliosis*, and various others. The disorder is a wrinkled sheen over the macula and occasionally is bilateral and either stationary or slowly progressive. It may be idiopathic, spontaneous, or secondary to a preretinal membrane, trauma, uveitis, retinal vascular disease, vitreous hemorrhage, retinal neovascularization, or retinal break. Additionally, it may result from retinal surgery (e.g., laser photocoagulation or scleral buckling for retinal detachment), cryotherapy, or diathermy. Cellophane maculopathy occurs more frequently in middle-aged patients (older than 50) or in the elderly.

The disorder may be caused by a growth of the endothelial cells or from an extension of Müller cell processes, from a fibrosis in the vascular connective tissue and a transformation of the mesenchymal cells into fibroblasts, from hyalocytes, from pigmented and nonpigmented cells of the pars plana, or from the retinal glial cells. A contraction of an epithelial membrane over the macula may be due to defects in the internal limiting membrane or to a posterior vitreous detachment.

Cellophane maculopathy appears as a gray-white, undulating, shallow, glistening, refractile opacification of the retina (an epiretinal membrane), with an increased reflex overlying the macula but usually sparing the foveola. It may vary from a minimal translucent tissue—a mild sheen or glint—to a semitranslucent membrane or an extensive, hyperpigmented, fibrous proliferation. Traction and distortion may be present in the macula, producing macular heterotopia. Also, multiple tiny, radiating full-thickness, fixed folds and vitreoretinal adhesions occur; they may wrinkle or pucker the macula, with an increased shagreen texture (like rough, untanned leather or crinkled cellophane). It may simulate a macular edema, a macular pseudohole, or a retinal hole or cyst. Vessels are straightened, irregularly dilated or displaced, tortuous, and zigzagging. Perimacular vessels are pulled toward an epicenter. Sometimes, punctate hemorrhages, striae, cotton-wool spots, or retinal detachment may be present.

Symptoms

Cellophane maculopathy may be asymptomatic. However, it can produce blurred vision, progressive vision loss, micropsia, metamorphopsia, and monocular diplopia.

Diagnosis

Fluorescein angiography may reveal a macular edema. The Amsler's grid may demonstrate distortion.

Differential Diagnosis

Differential diagnosis should include vitreomacular traction syndrome. Diabetes also is a consideration.

Histopathology

Histologic evaluation shows a wrinkling of the internal limiting membrane. Further, there is a preretinal fibrovascular proliferation. The RPE may appear as a single layer of tall pigmented cells.

Treatment

No treatment is specific for cellophane maculopathy. Surgical intervention may involve pars plana vitrectomy with surgical peeling of macular membrane.

Stargardt's Disease

Also known as *fundus flavimaculatus*, *Stargardt-Behr disease*, *Stargardt's macular dystrophy*, *juvenile macular degeneration*, and *progressive foveolar dystrophy*, Stargardt's disease comprises a hereditary bilateral group of disorders. These disorders demonstrate symmetric, progressive retinal dystrophy and autosomal recessive (and occasionally dominant or even mitochondrial) traits. Stargardt's disease occurs between ages 6 and 30.

The disorder occurs in two patterns—one with macular atrophy, the other without it—which are known as *fundus flavimaculatus*. Its comma-shaped flecks appear varied: multiple round or linear; pisciform; yellow-white; of varying shape, size, density, or outline; commonly having sharp borders; and angulated. Often, the flecks radiate on the macula and scatter diffusely at the posterior fundus. They occur initially in the perimacular area and may coalesce. New, ill-defined yellow flecks develop peripherally as the old flecks fade. The background of the fundus is vermilion.

Choroidal vessels may become visible, having a *choroidal sclerosis–like* picture. The macula usually appears reddish and is surrounded by a garland of fine, punctate, yellow-white subretinal flecks, looking like **peau d'orange** or a **snail-slime macula**. Sometimes, horizontal, oval, elliptic, or annular, sharply delineated areas of RPE atrophy are present; flecks are absent, but the areas demonstrate a tapetal-like reflex and a polychromatic appearance, giving rise to a **beaten-bronze macula**.

As the dystrophic process progresses, the choroid becomes exposed, and a pattern of marked **geographic macular atrophy** or a **bull's-eye macula** may be seen. A choroidal neovascular membrane may develop. In the early stage, the optic disc, retinal vessels, and peripheral retina may be normal. In the advanced stage, the disc becomes pale, retinal vessels are attenuated, and a reticular pattern of subretinal pigmentation in the midperiphery (or even in the macula) may be present.

Symptoms

Initially, Stargardt's disease may be asymptomatic; then it progresses rapidly to bilateral loss of visual acuity (to counting fingers) by middle age.

Diagnosis

EOG is subnormal only late in the course of the disease. ERG may be mild to moderately decreased, revealing a progressive loss of cone function and, subsequently, of rod function. Fluorescein angiography may demonstrate a generalized, fuzzy, irregular blotchy hyperfluorescence and obscuring of the choroidal vessels due to **lipofuscin** accumulation and a dark choroid called *choroidal silence*. At a later stage, as the flecks (themselves hypofluorescent) disappear, the surrounding area becomes hyperfluorescent. Visual field tests are normal.

Differential Diagnosis

Considerations for the differential diagnosis include cone dystrophy, fundus albipunctatus, drusen, and chloroquine retinopathy.

Histopathology

Histologic analysis shows marked atrophy of the RPE, which appears as irregular pisciform aggregates of giant pigment in the cells. Cytoplasm contains massive abnormal *lipofuscin* accumulation. There are phagosomes with prominent *melanin* granules and an *acid mucopolysaccharide* substance concentrated at the apex of the cells. They are surrounded by smaller, relatively normal cells. The outer nuclear layer of the retina may have cystoid degeneration and *calcium* deposition. Bruch's membrane may be thickened at its inner aspect or may have small soft drusen. The retina is thickened at the equator, and a resultant loss of the rod and cone layer (photoreceptors) occurs. The choriocapillaris is relatively preserved in the macula and in the area between the flecks.

Treatment

Treatment for Stargardt's disease is use of low-vision aids. Genetic counseling should be offered.

Butterfly Macular Pigment Dystrophy

Butterfly macular pigment dystrophy usually is a bilateral and symmetric, very slowly progressive dystrophy of the macula. It is autosomal dominant, the onset usually at between 20 and 50 years of age. The disorder appears as butterfly-shaped, irregularly branching reticular pigmentation. Sometimes, it is polymorphous, appearing as closely packed granules located in the deeper layers of macular retina. Retinal vessels course normally across it. There may be pigmentary stippling, small bone spicules, or drusenlike lesions in the peripheral retina. The foveal reflex is normal, as are the superficial retinal layers and the disc and choroid.

Symptoms

Visual acuity is normal or only slightly decreased. Metamorphopsia may be present.

Diagnosis

Fluorescein angiography may reveal a reticular hypofluorescence corresponding to the area of hyperpigmentation but does not reveal dye leakage. ERG is normal, as are color-vision tests and dark adaptation. EOG may reveal a subnormal light rise–dark trough ratio, indicating a widespread disturbance in the RPE function. Occasionally, visual field examination may reveal a relative central scotoma with normal peripheral fields.

Differential Diagnosis

Differential diagnosis should consider Steinert-Curshmann myotonic dystrophy, Best's vitelliform dystrophy, or rubella. Drug-induced macular degeneration, retinitis pigmentosa, and angioid streaks also are possible interpretations.

Histopathology

Histologic evaluation reveals that the RPE is abnormally widespread, with pigment deposits in or near it. Photoreceptors and the inner retinal layer are normal. There may be a migration of pigment in the RPE.

Geographic Areolar Macular Atrophy

Geographic areolar macular atrophy is a bilateral, degenerative lesion of the macula. It is slowly progressive, sometimes over many years, and occurs in the elderly as a part of ARMD (the nonexudative dry type).

The disorder appears as a yellow-white circular lesion. It is located in the macula, is variably sized (more commonly between 1 and 1.5 mm, or 1 dd), and is flat or mildly elevated, dry, and atrophic. It displays sharply demarcated, irregular geographic margins, which may represent a loss of pigmentation of RPE. These areas of hypopigmentation occasionally may be associated with drusen, hyperpigmentation, or metaplasia. There is choroidal atrophy in which the exposed choroidal vessels may appear white. The disorder is irreversible.

The condition is due to the progression of ARMD and may be preceded by fading drusen or RPE clumping. The RPE and choriocapillaris atrophy may produce damage to the photoreceptors, which in turn may result in vision loss. Geographic areolar macular atrophy may occur after spontaneous or laser-induced collapse of a serous RPE detachment.

Symptoms

Central vision is minimally decreased or (gradually) severely impaired to a complete vision loss. Metamorphopsia may be evident.

Diagnosis

Fluorescein angiography may reveal marked RPE window defects, with no leakage of the dye. Visual field testing may show a bilateral central scotoma. An Amsler's grid test is performed.

Histopathology

Histologic appraisal shows a macular scarring, with degeneration and total atrophy of the RPE in the affected area. Photoreceptors also are atrophic. Thinning is evident in the outer plexiform layer, which may have numerous vacuoles, and a dystrophic calcification may occur in the outer retinal layers. The inner nuclear layer usually is less affected. The outer nuclear layer appears in direct contact with Bruch's membrane, and the choriocapillaris also may be atrophic.

Treatment

No treatment is effective for geographic areolar macular atrophy. Treatment of the ARMD is undertaken.

Suggested Reading

Bouzas EA, Scott MH, Mastorakos G, et al. Central serous chorioretinopathy in endogenous hypercortism. Arch Ophthalmol 1993;111:1229–1233.

Duguel PU, Rao NA, Ozler S, et al. Pars plana vitrectomy for intraocular inflammation–related cystoid macular edema unresponsive to corticoids. Ophthalmology 1992;99:1435–1441.

Gass JDM. Advancing the classification of macular holes: the possible role of Müller cells. Ophthalmol World News 1996;5:2.

Holz FG, Evans K, Gregory CY, et al. Autosomal dominant macular dystrophy simulating North Carolina macular dystrophy. Arch Ophthalmol 1995;113:178–184.

Jaffe GJ. Cystoid macular edema. Focal Points 1994;11:1–12.

Lambert HM. Retina, Vitreous, and Posterior Segment Trauma. In Lifelong Education for the Ophthalmologist. San Francisco: American Academy of Ophthalmology, 1996;1–14.

Macular Photocoagulation Study Group. Five year follow-up of eyes of patients with age-related macular degeneration and unilateral extrafoveolar choroidal neovascularization. Arch Ophthalmol 1993;111:1189–1199.

Polk TD. Macular holes revisited. Ophthalmol World News 1996;1:23.

Schatz H, McDonald R, Johnson RN, et al. Subretinal fibrosis in central serous chorioretinopathy. Ophthalmology 1995;102:1077–1088.

Syrguin MG. No treatment for his hereditary disease (fundus flavimaculatus). Ophthalmol Times 1994;12:21.

8

Choroidopathy and Retinal Pigment Epithelium Disorders

Choroidal Necrosis

Choroidal necrosis is the death of cells or tissues within the choroid. It is caused by *ischemia* or by a *toxic* process. **Ischemic choroidal necrosis** occurs when the blood supply is reduced, causing the cytologic details to disappear, although the normal general architecture of the choroidal tissues is preserved. **Toxic choroidal necrosis** occurs when a virulent toxin causes tissue death, producing loss of tissue architecture and a prominent inflammatory cell infiltration.

Histopathologically, retinal vessels are almost entirely absent. Stroma may also disappear. There is scattered pigment or it appears in irregular clumps in the choroidal stroma. The overlying retinal pigment epithelium (RPE) is degenerated. A regional destruction of both RPE and outer segments of rods and cones (photoreceptors) may be present. There is usually a sharp transition line between the totally disrupted RPE and choroidal architecture and the partially preserved retina.

Choroidal Sclerosis

Choroidal sclerosis, alternately called *choroidal vascular atrophy*, is a hereditary, autosomal dominant or recessive disease that involves primarily the choriocapillaris and the choroidal vessels, which have thickened walls and a narrowed blood column but are not sclerosed. It may be considered to be either *benign* or *degenerative*.

Benign choroidal sclerosis is a depigmentation in situ of the retina, with an attenuated pigment in the RPE but no functional impairment. This condition usually occurs in conjunction with high myopia and aging. **Degenerative choroidal sclerosis** is an absence of the outer layers of the sensory retina, the RPE, choriocapillaris, and choroidal stroma. Functional impairment is severe. Degenerative choroidal sclerosis is usually of three types: *central*, *diffuse*, and *peripapillary.*

Central Choroidal Sclerosis

Central choroidal sclerosis (also known as *central areolar choroidal sclerosis*, *central areolar choroidal dystrophy [CACD]*, *central total choroidal vascular dystrophy*, *central choroidal angiosclerosis*, and *central senile choroiditis*) is an autosomal recessive or dominant lesion that initially involves only the macula and may remain stationary or may spread toward the periphery. It may occur in individuals as young as 15 years. Central choroidal sclerosis usually is not associated with any systemic disorders except Paget's disease (osteitis deformans).

In the early stage, a mild degree of nonspecific granularity is seen in the macula. Gradually, edema with yellowish deposits and irregular pigmented mottling of the macula may develop. At a later stage, there may be a bilateral, symmetric, sharply delineated, circular or transversely oval, yellow-white patch in the macula, representing atrophy of the sensory retina, RPE, and choriocapillaris. Choroidal vessels appear as white-yellow fine streaks and strands.

Symptoms

Among the symptoms of central choroidal sclerosis are difficulty in reading and very gradual decreased central vision to 20/200 or worse. Glare sensitivity also occurs.

Diagnosis

In the early stage of disease, fluorescein angiography may reveal faint areas of hyperfluorescence corresponding to RPE window transmission defects in the macula. RPE atrophy also may be seen. In a later stage, a sharply demarcated zone of chorioretinal atrophy, with some dye leakage but no fluorescence, is visualized. Electroretinography (ERG) may demonstrate normal to slightly subnormal photopic responses and normal scotopic responses. Electro-oculography (EOG) also may be normal or slightly subnormal. Dark adaptation usually is normal.

Color-vision testing may reveal a moderate protan-deutan defect. Visual field examination may reveal a large central scotoma but a normal peripheral field.

Differential Diagnosis

Conditions that should be considered in the differential diagnosis include uveitis, central areolar pigment epithelium dystrophy (CAPED), Stargardt's disease, Sorsby's pseudoinflammatory dystrophy, choroideremia, high myopia, and North Carolina macular dystrophy. Age-related macular degeneration (ARMD), macular coloboma, angioid streaks, gyrate atrophy, cone dystrophy, acute posterior multifocal placoid pigment epitheliopathy (APMPPE), and serpiginous choroiditis also warrant consideration.

Diffuse Choroidal Sclerosis

Diffuse choroidal sclerosis is a rare, generalized, autosomal dominant or recessive or X-linked lesion. The degree of involvement of the posterior pole usually is indicative of the duration and severity of the choroidal sclerosis. Diffuse choroidal sclerosis appears as a diffuse edema of the ocular fundus, with scattered small, white, yellow, or cream-colored spots and pigmentary migration. Choroidal atrophy, called *tigroid fundus*, is also seen. There is extensive destruction of the RPE, occasionally presenting as clumps of pigment within the RPE. Larger choroidal vessels are visible as a prominent whitish network. Also seen are complete atrophy of the choriocapillaris and surrounding tissue and exposure of the sclera.

Symptoms

Night blindness and decreased visual acuity to hand movements or worse are symptoms of diffuse choroidal sclerosis.

Diagnosis

Visual field examination may reveal central and ring scotomas or constriction of the field; alternatively, the visual field may appear tubular. ERG usually is normal in the early stage of diffuse choroidal sclerosis, but later it may become subnormal for cone and rod responses, and eventually all ERG responses may be entirely extinguished. EOG may reveal a reduced light-dark ratio. Rarely, color vision may be abnormal.

Differential Diagnosis

Choroideremia, tapetoretinal degeneration, and pigmentary retinopathies should all enter into the differential diagnosis.

Peripapillary Choroidal Sclerosis

Peripapillary choroidal sclerosis is a rare autosomal recessive disease in which the choroidal atrophy begins around the optic disc, in the area of distribution of the vascular circle. It is similar to a senile peripapillary halo. The sclerosis may be stationary or may spread toward the periphery. It appears as a lesion with diffuse, blurred margins that surrounds the disc, sometimes involving up to one-third of the fundus.

A central scotoma is the prominent sign. The differential diagnosis should include ARMD.

Histopathology

In degenerative choroidal sclerosis, choroidal arteries and veins appear decreased in caliber, as white streaks against the fundus background. Sometimes, shunt blood to choroidal veins is seen on histologic evaluation. A well-demarcated avascular zone that is atrophic and fibrotic extends from the submacular region to the disc. The outer retinal layers, together with the RPE, often are absent, and there is no glial replacement. The choriocapillaris is obliterated or completely lost. Photoreceptors usually are absent.

A fibrotic scar may be present. Bruch's membrane is generally intact, although rarely it may display secondary irregularities, ruptures, and lamellar structures.

Treatment

No effective treatment is available.

Choroiditis

Chorioretinitis, *punctate inner choroidopathy*, *progressive subretinal fibrosis and uveitis*, and *inflammatory pseudohistoplasmosis* are other names given to choroiditis. This inflammation of the choroid also may involve the retina. The condition can be *acute* or *chronic*, *solitary* or *multiple*, *localized* or *diffuse*, *congenital* (a reaction of an intrauterine inflammation) or *acquired* (consequent to infection, trauma, systemic disease [e.g., diabetes, tuberculosis, histoplasmosis], myopia, neoplasm, etc.). The inflammation may be *granulomatous* or *nongranulomatous*.

Choroiditis appears as gray-white, yellow, or tan-white; well-defined; sharply circumscribed patches measuring approximately 0.5 dd. The patches are either flat or elevated, usually are surrounded by edema, and are scattered over the fundus. They generally are round but may be polygonal or sword shaped. The patches vary in number from one to few in localized choroiditis to several hundred in disseminated choroiditis, and they are more concentrated at the periphery.

Active lesions are grayish white, have less distinct margins, and sometimes are confluent, whereas resolving lesions are yellowish white. Occasionally, instead of becoming punched-out lesions, they progress to sharply angulated bands of subretinal fibrosis. The inactive lesions are atrophic and often are surrounded by a hyperpigmented ring.

Arteries are narrowed such that the lumen may be considerably reduced to even pipe-stem width. Veins may appear darker, markedly segmented, and beaded, with a yellow-white cuffing that may occlude the blood stream or may extend along the course of the vessels in parallel sheaths. Partially obliterated choroidal vessels at the base of the scar may be present. There may be exudation along the course of arteries or veins, often in areas remote from the focus of inflammation.

The retina usually is not involved in deep choroiditis. The degree of pigmentation of the retina will vary depending on several factors: (1) *severity* of the lesion, with the most severe lesions having little pigmentation as the pigment cells usually are destroyed; (2) *duration* of inflammation; (3) *hypersensitivity* of the patient; and (4) *natural pigmentation* of the patient. Generally, *the appearance of pigmentation is an indication of the start of the healing process*. The vitreous may be full of fine, dustlike opacities.

Clinical Types

Localized or **focal choroiditis** usually appears as a small circumscribed area in which there may be tiny, glistening intraretinal dots, subretinal hemorrhages, cystoid macular edema, or serous retinal detachment. In a later stage of disease, focal choroiditis may progress to a disciform macular degeneration. The vitreous is not appreciably hazy.

Diffuse choroiditis may involve an entire quadrant or half of the fundus and flares up while another area of inflammation subsides. Peripheral pigment clumps and geographic areas of confluent scars, which may extend to the disc margins, are possible findings. Multiple active lesions may be present simultaneously. There may be a considerable haziness of the vitreous, which makes assessment of the true extent of the lesion difficult. A recurrence at the periphery of an old healed lesion, known as a **satellite** or **daughter lesion**, usually is smaller than the original lesion and is separated from the older lesion by the normal retina. Frequently, scars of repeated lesions may be present. The optic disc is usually pale and may demonstrate a mild papilledema or a peripapillary atrophy.

Symptoms

Blurred vision and metamorphopsia are common symptoms of choroiditis. Rarely, floaters, scotoma, or photopsia is seen.

Diagnosis

Diagnosis is aided by fluorescein angiography, which may reveal RPE window defects, early blockage of fluorescence followed by late staining, or a rim of hyperfluorescence in the active lesions. ERG is normal for the most part, whereas EOG is usually abnormal.

Histopathology

On histologic examination, the RPE may demonstrate areas of pigment migration that commonly do not proliferate, atrophy, or focal hyperplasia. The choroid may have mononuclear and lymphoid cell infiltration, which usually is nodular. There may be a predominance of B-lymphocytes and plasma cells as well as deposits of complement and immunoglobulin above Bruch's membrane. Chronic nongranulomatous or granulomatous infiltrates might be seen. These appear as multiple, eosinophilic, amorphous, and foamy infiltrates that stain positively for periodic acid–Schiff; they are located primarily in the inner choroid, within the choroidal vessels, or in the choriocapillaris.

Treatment

Treatment is dictated by the etiology.

Serpiginous Choroiditis

Serpiginous choroiditis (also known as *geographic helicoid peripapillary choroiditis*, *serpiginous degeneration of the choroid*, *choroidal vascular abiotrophy*, and *helicoid and central gyrate atrophy*) is a nonhereditary, usually bilateral condition (but with a unilateral onset that for several years does not involve the second eye). It is an asymmetric, progressive dystrophy of the choroid and retina of unknown etiology. Serpiginous choroiditis occurs more commonly in middle-aged, white, healthy adults, typically 30–60 years of age. It may be associated with systemic HLA-B7. The disease may be caused by a mild inflammation of the choriocapillaris and the RPE, or it may be due to an immunologic process.

Serpiginous choroiditis appears in the acute phase as multiple, fluffy, creamy, whitish-yellow lesions located usually in the temporal quadrant. In a later phase, the lesions appear pseudopodial, propellerlike, or geographic map–like, of varying sizes and with well-defined, irregular margins. They may spread in a tonguelike pattern from the peripapillary area, centrifugally toward the equator and far periphery. There may be some areas of edema. Usually, marked white-gray scars of choroidal atrophy, revealing varying degrees of fibrosis, are surrounded by a hyperpigmented rim. A subretinal neovascularization, with exudate and hemorrhage around the margin of the lesion, may be present.

As the disease progresses, the initial lesions begin to heal over several weeks up to 18 months, leaving pigmentary clumping and choriocapillaris atrophy. A relapse of new lesions may reappear sporadically as an area of grayish subretinal swelling, as APMPPE-like, creamy, contiguous lesions in the active area, or elsewhere at the border of the previous scar. After several episodes of remission and relapsing activity, lesions take on a specific *snail-like* appearance. There may be **satellite** or **skip lesions** near an old lesion. Occasionally, the serpiginous chorioretinitis may originate in the macula, not in the peripapillary area, and serous or hemorrhagic macular detachment as well as a disciform macular scar may develop in time. Rarely, there may be neovascularization of the disc, RPE detachment, or occlusion of retinal arteries or veins, possibly owing to a secondary inflammation. In the area of choroidal atrophy, choroidal vessels may be visible within the scar. Retinal vessels usually are normal, but a focal phlebitis may occasionally be seen. Vitritis, with few cells in the vitreous, may also be present.

Symptoms

Serpiginous choroiditis may be asymptomatic. Severe decreased visual acuity to finger counting may occur when the macula is involved, with irreparable loss of vision.

Diagnosis

Fluorescein angiography may reveal an early masking, followed by late diffuse leaking and retinal neovascularization. EOG and ERG usually are normal. Visual field examination may show absolute or relative central, cecocentral, or paracentral scotomas.

Histopathology

Atrophy and fibrous metaplasia of the RPE are seen on histologic assessment. The choriocapillaris may be totally absent. There is pigment clumping at the RPE and, as the lesions heal, the RPE is seen to degenerate. Hypopigmentation and scar formation may occur. There is also choroidal vascular atrophy of the posterior pole.

Treatment

No treatment is effective for serpiginous choroiditis, although laser photocoagulation may be used for subretinal neovascular membranes.

Pneumocystis carinii Choroiditis

Pneumocystis carinii choroiditis is a slowly progressive, multifocal, usually bilateral choroiditis that occurs particularly in patients with acquired immunodeficiency syndrome (AIDS) (80%). The disease is produced by infection with the opportunistic pathogen *P. carinii*, a protozoan, sporozoan, or yeastlike fungus that causes a highly contagious, epidemic interstitial plasma cell pneumonia in debilitated and immunosuppressed patients.

P. carinii choroiditis appears as discrete multiple clusters of flat or slightly elevated, sharply circumscribed, yellow-white or orange, round, oval, or large plaquelike, creamy choroidal lesions. Alternatively, they may be geographic, irregular in shape, or multilobulated and deep. The lesions are usually approximately 0.5–3.0 dd in size and are located at the posterior pole, in the midperiphery, or along the temporal arcade. *P. carinii* choroiditis may appear as solitary choroidal lesions, or occasionally, the lesions may coalesce, become confluent, or become elevated under the foveolar avascular zone. In later stages, there may be subretinal hypopigmented lesions without inflammation in the overlying retina. When the macula is involved, vision is reduced. Occasionally, a serous retinal detachment may be present.

Symptoms

Dry cough and dyspnea may be present. The patient may experience no ocular symptoms, or there may be blurring of vision.

Diagnosis

Chest roentgenograms reveal a diffuse, bilateral interstitial infiltrate. Sputum culture, bronchoalveolar lavage, and transbronchial or open lung biopsy may be necessary to confirm the diagnosis.

Differential Diagnosis

In the differential diagnosis, cryptococcal choroiditis, lymphoma, metastases, atypical mycobacterial infections, Vogt-Koyanagi-Harada syndrome, sympathetic ophthalmia, and sarcoidosis should be considered.

Treatment

Trimethoprim-sulfamethoxazole (Bactrim), 80 mg trimethoprim and 400 mg sulfamethoxazole PO twice a day; pentamidine (Pentam 300), aerosolized four times a day or 4 mg/kg/day IV for 14 days; and zidovudine (Retrovir), 100 mg PO every 4 hours or 1 mg/kg IV infused over 1 hour are treatment options.

Epstein-Barr Virus Choroiditis

Epstein-Barr virus (EBV) choroiditis is a multiple choroiditis produced by a herpesvirus (human herpesvirus 4) of genus *Lymphocryptovirus* that causes infectious mononucleosis, oral hairy leukoplakia, chronic malaise, and lethargy syndrome. It appears as panuveitis, optic neuritis, retinal hemorrhages, and exudates, or as multiple choroiditis, punctate retinitis, retinal pigment epitheliitis, and severe vitritis. EBV choroiditis may be complicated by a chiasmal neuritis.

Symptoms

Follicular conjunctivitis, nummular and stromal keratitis, iritis, convergence insufficiency, and extraocular muscle palsy may all be part of the symptom complex.

Diagnosis

In EBV choroiditis, antibody titers to EBV capsid agent (VCA), which can be detected by immunofluorescence, will be elevated. Positive heterophil antibody is diagnostic. The Paul-Bunnell test is a useful diagnostic aid.

Differential Diagnosis

Histoplasmosis may appear similar to EBV choroiditis and so should be considered in the differential diagnosis.

Treatment

Steroids are the mainstay of treatment. Initial therapy consists of prednisone, 60 mg PO, tapered for 10 months. If this regimen fails, prednisone can be given together with acyclovir, 600 mg PO five times daily for 5 months, as a combination therapy.

Jensen's Juxtapapillary Chorioretinitis

Jensen's juxtapapillary chorioretinitis is a focal inflammation of the choroid and retina adjacent to the optic nerve head. Its etiology is unknown. The disease occurs in young patients aged 20–30 years, usually after contact with cats or after eating improperly cooked meat. Jensen's juxtapapillary chorioretinitis probably is caused by the protozoa *Toxoplasma gondii*, but *Candida*, *Cryptococcus*, and *Toxocara* spp., *Nocardia asteroides*, and sarcoidosis and tuberculosis are other possible causes.

The chorioretinitis manifests as a round or oval, slightly elevated, edematous, smoky white lesion of approximately 1 dd located immediately adjacent to the disc, more commonly nasally. The lesion is pigmented and exhibits irregular margins and atrophic areas, through which bare sclera becomes visible. The optic disc may be pale and may have a remnant of exudate in the physiologic cup area.

Retinal vessels that course through the lesion are usually irregular in caliber. In a late stage, after the lesion heals, a pigmented scar and satellite lesions may develop. There may be a vitreous infiltrate and, occasionally, a posterior vitreous detachment occurs.

Diagnosis

Visual field examination may reveal a nerve fiber bundle defect as a sector-shaped field loss that extends like a comet tail from the blind spot to the periphery.

Treatment

Cycloplegic therapy includes cyclopentolate (Cyclogyl) 1%, three times a day. Corticosteroids are used either topically (prednisolone, 1% four times a day) or systemically (prednisone, 60 mg/day PO for 2 weeks).

Birdshot Chorioretinopathy

Birdshot chorioretinopathy (*vitiliginous chorioretinitis*) is an acquired, bilateral chorioretinal inflammation of the posterior pole that clinically resembles birdshot scattered from a shotgun (Figure 8-1). Of unknown etiology, it occurs more frequently in white, middle-aged women.

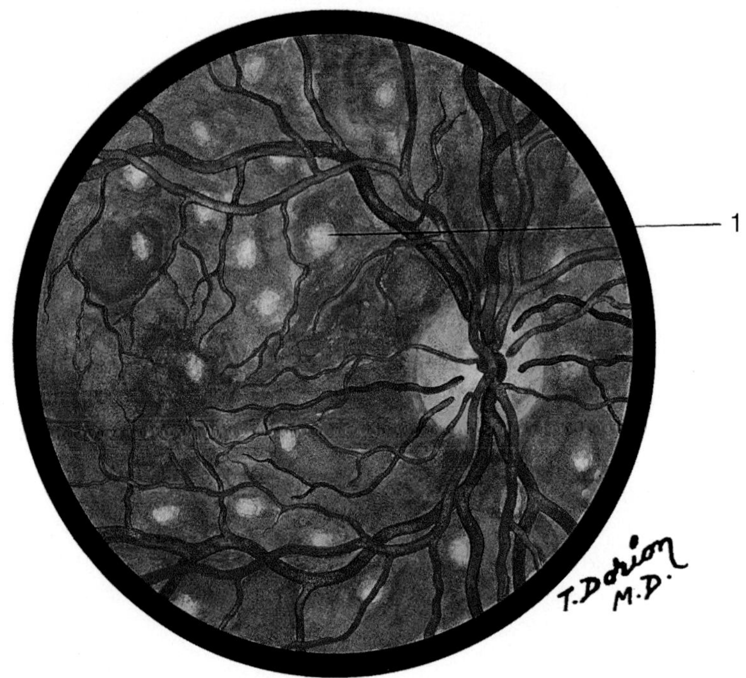

Figure 8-1. *Birdshot chorioretinopathy. (1) Multifocal choroiditis.*

Patients may experience exacerbations and remissions. No metabolic defect is present. It is usually associated with a positive HLA-29 antigen.

Birdshot chorioretinopathy may be caused by an inflammatory process of the choroid and deep retina, which also may affect the vitreous. The disorder appears as multiple choroiditis with discrete, flat, ovoid or round, uniform or irregular spots having soft, diffuse margins. The spots are depigmented, yellow-white, creamy, pink, or orange, but they do not exhibit any hyperpigmentation. Usually 0.25–1.00 dd in size, they are scattered subretinally throughout the posterior pole, located mostly beyond the equator or along the choroidal vessels. The spots may coalesce, forming large lesions that are sometimes geographic or resemble cobblestone degeneration, are radially oriented, or appear as salmon patches. Occasionally, there is a low-grade vasculitis, with narrowed vessels, perivenous sheathing, tortuosity, or localized beading.

Often complications such as cystoid macular edema, cataract, serous macular detachment, chronic vitritis, epiretinal membranes, neovascularization of the disc or elsewhere, papilledema, and optic atrophy occur. The vitreous may be hazy, syneretic, and degenerated or may demonstrate hemorrhage or debris.

Symptoms

Vision loss from macular edema or cataract may be presenting symptoms.

Diagnosis

Fluorescein angiography may show minimal changes in the RPE and some leakage of dye. Indocyanine green videoangiography may reveal hypofluorescent lesions in a vascular pattern. ERG and EOG are normal. Testing for HLA-29 antigen may be positive.

Differential Diagnosis

Retinoblastoma must be excluded in children and ocular lymphoma in adults. Fungal infections, spirochetal diseases, sarcoidosis, and tuberculosis are other considerations in the differential diagnosis.

Histopathology

On histologic examination, deep deposits are seen in the RPE and in the choroid, whereas mild cellular infiltrates may be found in the vitreous. Retinal vessels may be narrowed.

Treatment

Anti-inflammatory drugs are administered, as are corticosteroids. Effective agents include systemic prednisone, 60 mg/day PO for 1 month, and methylprednisolone (Depo-Medrol), 40 mg subconjunctivally. Cyclosporine (CyA), 2.5–5.0 mg/kg/day, alone or with azathioprine, 1.5–2.0 mg/kg/day, also is useful. Other immunosuppressive drugs may be used, but the use of acyclovir in this setting is controversial.

Choroidal Folds

Choroidal folds are known also as *fixed folds*, *striae*, and *plicae*. Choroidal folds are curved margins of the choroid that vary in size and number and occur in people of any age and either gender. They usually occur in choroidal or retrobulbar masses (e.g., orbital tumors or pseudotumors) or after trauma or scleral laceration. They also occur in intraocular tractional processes, Graves' ophthalmopathy, posterior scleritis, uveitis, diabetes, ARMD, ocular hypotony after cataract surgery, hypermetropia, and idiopathically in a normal eye.

Choroidal folds may be caused by choroidal congestion, retinal detachment, focal puckering, a subretinal fibrovascular membrane, an orbital inflammatory pseudotumor, papilledema, traction of the optic disc, or compression by an orbital tumor, which will produce folds of Bruch's membrane, the RPE, and the choroid.

The folds appear as light or dark lines, or striae, located usually in the temporal side of the posterior pole, often radiating parallel to and horizontal from the disc or concentric to the optic disc. In relation to the disc, the fold may also be vertical, oblique, or irregular and multidirectional, resembling a *jigsaw puzzle*. Sometimes, there are superimposed retinal folds. Flecks of intraretinal exudates may occasionally be present. Retinal vessels are not distorted by the underlying choroidal folds.

Symptoms

Blurring of vision, proptosis, diplopia, increased hypermetropia, and astigmatism are symptoms that might accompany choroidal folds.

Diagnosis

Amsler grid distortion will be evident. Fluorescein angiography may reveal alternating hyperfluorescent and hypofluorescent, dark and light, curvilinear streaks with bright peaks and dark valleys. Computed tomographic scan of the orbit may reveal displacement of the globe if the folds are due to an intraconal orbital tumor. B-scan ultrasonography may reveal flattening of the posterior sclera. Magnetic resonance imaging might prove useful in making the diagnosis.

Histopathology

Histologic evaluation reveals that the RPE is doubled in the valleys but normal on the crests of the folds. Bruch's membrane is folded, and the inner choroid is corrugated, undulated, and folded.

Treatment

Treatment addresses the underlying disease.

Retinal Folds

Retinal folds, like choroidal folds, may also be called *fixed folds*, *striae*, and *plicae*. They are doubling layers, curved margins, or plicae of the retina that may be *congenital* or *acquired*. **Congenital retinal folds** are usually unilateral and extend from the disc into the periphery. They are considered an anomaly of the differentiation of the retina and may occur in persistent hyperplastic primary vitreous or in retinopathy of prematurity.

Acquired retinal folds may be unilateral or bilateral. They occur more often after trauma, such as in shaken baby syndrome, in which the extreme acceleration and deceleration forces may produce lateral displacement of the sensory retina, owing to a vitreous traction or as a direct result of trauma. These folds may occur also after vitreous or retinal surgery or chronic papilledema; in diabetes; or in retinal detachment, wherein the shrinkage of glial or RPE membranes on the internal or external surfaces of the sensory retina and within the retina may produce **fixed retinal folds**. In macular detachment, a characteristic retinal folding of the outer retina, called *retinal shagreen*, may be present as a result of the edema. Also, traction of an epiretinal membrane may cause full-thickness folds called *star folds*. At the macula, the retinal folds probably are due to tight adhesions of the vitreous to the internal limiting membrane.

Retinal folds appear as white-yellow lines and grooves radiating from a point of visible pathologic process. *They are thinner than choroidal folds* and are translucent. They may have a ring-shaped configuration surrounding the macula, outside the vascular arcades, forming **circinate perimacular folds**, or they may be associated with a disciform macular scar. Often, they appear spreading horizontally from the disc; these are called *falciform folds*.

Symptoms

Symptoms of retinal folds include metamorphopsia and blurred vision.

Histopathology

Histologic assessment reveals a folding of the internal limiting membrane, caused by shrinkage *on the internal surface* of the sensory retina or by shrinkage of a subretinal membrane *on the outer surface* of the sensory retina. The fold may be separated from the rest of the retina by hemorrhage. In fixed retinal folds, striations of the retinal surface may be seen, and RPE proliferations bridge the epiretinal fibrous tissue between the retinal layers. Vitreous also may be partially separated from the internal limiting membrane or may remain focally attached to it.

Treatment

Vitrectomy may be appropriate for retinal folds. The underlying disease must be treated.

Choroidal Rupture

Choroidal rupture is a tear or a disruption of the choroid, commonly occurring after a local or distant trauma. It can be caused (1) by a contrecoup mechanism of the shock wave at the interface of tissues of differing densities, (2) by a stretching of the choroid produced by compression of the eye that expands its horizontal axis, or (3) as a consequence of posttraumatic necrosis.

Choroidal rupture appears as an oblique, hypopigmented, yellow-white linear defect that is arcuate, elliptic, crescent shaped, or curvilinear, mostly vertically oriented, and of variable length. Rarely, it is radially oriented. In *direct* or *anterior choroidal rupture*, the defect is located *parallel to the ora serrata*, whereas in *indirect* or *posterior choroidal rupture*, which is more common, the defect is crescent shaped, concentric, and *parallel to the disc margin*, between the disc and macula, thereby exposing the underlying white sclera.

Choroidal rupture occurs more frequently at the temporal side, which is more vulnerable and less protected, and often passes through or near the macula. There may be single or multiple, yellow-white fibrovascular chorioretinal scars parallel to one another. Sometimes, there is an overlying retinal tear. Choroidal hemorrhage, appearing as a dark red-blue mound with pinkish edges and usually located at the equator or near the disc, may be seen breaking into the vitreous or may produce a choroidal detachment. A surrounding area of **commotio retinae (Berlin's edema)**, which might affect the entire posterior pole, may also be present. Subretinal hemorrhage, which initially may completely or partially mask the rupture, and subretinal neovascularization or vitreous hemorrhage can occur.

After distant trauma, retinopathy occurs: If characterized by *arterial alterations*, it is called **forward retinopathy**; if there are *venous alterations*, it is called **backward retinopathy**; and if it demonstrates both alterations, it is known as **mixed retinopathy**. Areas of diffuse or patchy choroidal atrophy, surrounded by pigment, and areas of retinitis sclopetaria, fibrous intraocular proliferation, and bare visible sclera are possible. More extensive destruction may exist and is often associated with secondary glaucoma. The retina is usually thin. The macula may undergo traumatic degeneration, and the optic disc may be atrophic.

Symptoms

Choroidal rupture may be asymptomatic. Some patients suffer reduced visual acuity.

Diagnosis

Scleral retroillumination can aid in making the diagnosis. Fluorescein angiography may reveal hyperfluorescence of the RPE and atrophy of the choriocapillaris, chorioretinal vascular anastomoses, neovascular membranes underlying the macula, and blockage secondary to the hemorrhage.

Differential Diagnosis

Angioid streaks and the lacquer cracks of high myopia should be included in the differential diagnosis.

Histopathology

In choroidal rupture, a full-thickness discontinuity of the choroid is seen on histologic examination. A large gap is apparent within the RPE–Bruch's membrane–choriocapillaris complex. Blood might accumulate between the RPE and sensory retina, and RPE detachment may be found in the macula. The retina may be normal, atrophic, or ruptured.

Treatment

Cycloplegics such as cyclopentolate (Cyclogyl) 1 %, 1 drop three times per day; laser photocoagulation of any neovascularization; and surgical scleral exploration are therapeutic options.

Choroidal Coloboma

Choroidal coloboma, or *chorioretinal coloboma*, is a congenital, usually bilateral, autosomal dominant defect of the choroid and retina that also may involve the optic disc. It commonly is associated with other anomalies, such as trisomy 13, Aicardi's syndrome, Goldenhar's syndrome, or encephalocele. The coloboma is due to the embryonic fissure's failure to close.

Choroidal coloboma appears as a gray-yellow, glistening defect of the choroid (Figure 8-2). It is oval or round; measures approximately 1–3 dd; has distinct, sharply delineated margins and sometimes patchy pigmentation; and is located more frequently beneath the disc, either inferiorly or inferonasally. The coloboma often fades gradually into the surrounding normal tissues. Its surface generally is slightly depressed, completely featureless, or filled with fibroglial tissue. There may by retinal breaks or a bridge that divides the coloboma in two. A gray-green area of RPE elevation or retinal detachment may be evident. Retinal vessels course normally over the defect.

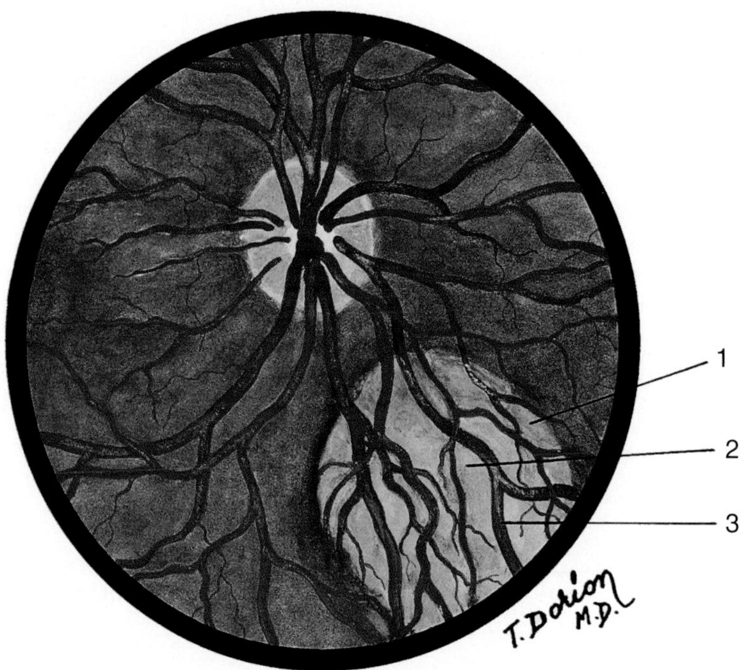

Figure 8-2. *Choroidal coloboma. (1) Choroidal and retinal defect. (2) Choroid is absent. (3) Retinal vessels course normally over defect.*

Histopathologically, the retina is thinned and appears as an ill-defined membrane. It exhibits various stages of degeneration: The inner layers (sensory retina) are undifferentiated, atrophic, or gliotic, whereas the outer layers (e.g., RPE, Bruch's membrane, and choriocapillaris) usually are absent. The choroid is absent, or a rudimentary choroid may be present. The sclera is thin and ectatic.

Multiple Evanescent White-Dot Syndrome

Multiple evanescent white-dot syndrome (MEWDS) is a rare, unilateral choroiditis, a multifocal posterior uveitis that occurs more often in young women after a viral illness. It may be associated with acute macular neuroretinitis (AMN). Its etiology is unknown, although it probably is produced by alteration of the posterior blood barrier.

MEWDS appears as multiple, faint, small (although sometimes large), deep, flecklike, creamy whitish spots, scattered throughout the posterior pole but initially inferior to the disc. A mild papilledema is present. Occasionally, there may be peripapillary atrophy with pigmentary disturbance. The macula may show granular pigmentation. In time, a darkish, brownish red, wedge-shaped perifoveolar lesion may be seen in the outer macula as an acute macular neuroretinopathy. These spots may disappear in several days or weeks, and vision might improve concurrently, but more spots may develop, usually superotemporal to the macula. Occasionally, there may be vascular sheathing and a more pronounced phlebitis. A mild vitritis too, with few cells in the vitreous, is possible.

Symptoms

Decreased central visual acuity and dim vision are usual symptoms. Unilateral photopsia also is known to occur.

Diagnosis

Visual field examination may reveal a marked loss in the entire visual field, with a giant, enlarged blind spot. In the early stage of disease, fluorescein angiography may show hyperfluorescent dots in the region of the RPE and, in a later stage, widespread leakage of the dye, with staining of the outer retina, RPE, optic disc, and occasionally, the inflamed vessels.

Histopathology

Histopathologically, there is disorganization of the outer retina and RPE and alteration of the posterior blood barrier.

Treatment

Treatment is not necessary as vision will return to normal within weeks.

Acute Posterior Multifocal Placoid Pigment Epitheliopathy

APMPPE is a rapidly progressive, bilateral, inflammatory disease affecting RPE function and the choroid, probably caused by an **adenovirus type 5**. It occurs usually in young adults, more commonly in healthy women aged 15–40 years, who may have a history of preceding flu-like illness or respiratory infection. It may develop alone or in association with cerebral vasculitis, meningoencephalitis, erythema nodosum, nephropathy, platelet abnormality, hearing loss, thyroiditis, sarcoidosis, or systemic bacterial infections.

APMPPE may be produced by a *primary* dysfunction of the RPE or by a *secondary* epitheliopathy following a multifocal choroidal vasculitis. Other causes are a focal swelling of the RPE overlying a non-perfused lobule of choriocapillaris and an immune mechanism.

In the acute phase, APMPPE appears as one or multiple, flat, pale, swollen, round areas of yellow-white, creamy, or gray, deep subretinal lesions that usually are well circumscribed. Sometimes, these lesions have fluffy, indistinct margins, are bilateral, and exhibit asymmetric RPE involvement and minimal alterations of the retina and choroid. They are located at the posterior pole, especially in the macula. They vary in size from 0.125 to 0.5 dd and often are confluent. In the late phase, when they heal, these lesions appear maplike, with new, small satellite lesions arising at the periphery of placoid patches, eventually extending anterior to the equator and becoming more pigmented. There may be periphlebitis, cells in the vitreous or vitreal infiltrates, retinal edema, diffuse vasculitis, perivascular choroiditis, hemorrhages or, very rarely, serous retinal detachment and a subretinal vascular membrane. The lesions may resolve spontaneously, within 6–8 weeks, usually with a good prognosis, leaving scattered depigmented areas of RPE atrophy and residual pigment clumping.

Symptoms

Symptoms of APMPPE include acute blurred vision, floaters, fixed spots surrounding the central visual area, and rapidly reduced vision (unilaterally or bilaterally) that improves in weeks or months and rarely recurs. Antecedent flu infection is not uncommon. Sensitivity to penicillin may be present.

Diagnosis

Cerebrospinal fluid analysis may demonstrate pleocytosis. Fluorescein angiography may reveal an early nonfluorescence or a hypofluorescence, with blockage and masking of the background fluorescence, which may be due to irregular filling of the choriocapillaris. These findings may be followed by late hyperfluorescence, with staining and leaking of the dye, which may be due to alterations of the cellular membrane's integrity and the outer blood-retina barrier as a result of ischemic injury.

Indocyanine green angiography might aid in the diagnosis of APMPPE. Dark adaptation may show a transient abnormality. ERG may reveal minimal diffuse or focal retinal damage, and EOG may reveal a permanent, severely disturbed RPE function. Visual field examination may demonstrate permanent scotomas. Blood culture for virus may reveal rising adenovirus type 5 titers.

Differential Diagnosis

Conditions that should be considered in the differential diagnosis include Vogt-Koyanagi-Harada syndrome, diffuse choroiditis (inflammatory, infectious, or neoplastic), diffuse unilateral subacute neuroretinitis (DUSN) syndrome, serpiginous choroiditis, heredomacular degeneration, and birdshot retinochoroidopathy.

Histopathology

APMPPE is a multifocal posterior uveitis. Histopathologically, there is atrophy of the RPE and choriocapillaris, retinal vasculitis, and a pigment accumulation.

Treatment

Treatment of APMPPE is controversial. No therapy has been proven to be effective. Observation is recommended, and corticosteroids such as prednisone, 60 mg PO daily, may be used.

Acute Retinal Pigment Epitheliitis

Acute retinal pigment epitheliitis (ARPE) is a rare, usually unilateral but sometimes bilateral, benign, self-limited lesion of the RPE. Its onset is abrupt, and it is probably of viral or parasitic origin. This lesion occurs mostly in men aged 20–45 years and resolves usually in 6–12 weeks, with complete recovery.

ARPE may be related to APMPPE. It may occur in EBV-associated infectious mononucleosis. ARPE may be caused by a direct action of a virus or by friction or feeding of a worm (a nematode), which may destroy the pigment granules of the RPE.

ARPE appears as one or more discrete, grapelike clusters of a few (one to four) small, round, dark-gray or black, deep lesions, some of them resembling Elschnig's spots. They are located in the macula, usually surrounded by a pale, yellow-white halo or retinal atrophy. The retina may appear slightly elevated, with some gray, black, or deep-red underlying swelling. There also may be areas of crisscrossing tracks of depigmented retina which, as they resolve, may become darker or pigmented or may fade.

Symptoms

ARPE may be asymptomatic. In other cases, there is an abrupt unilateral decrease in visual acuity, blurred vision, and metamorphopsia.

Diagnosis

Visual field examination may reveal a central scotoma. Fluorescein angiography may be normal or may reveal a hypofluorescent center with a normal or hyperfluorescent halo, granular areas of choroidal window transmission defects in the RPE that do not change in size or shape, but no leakage of the dye. Color vision may be abnormal. EOG is not definitive for ARPE as it may be normal or abnormal.

Differential Diagnosis

Central serous chorioretinopathy, rubella, acute macular neuroretinopathy, APMPPE, drusen, and fundus flavimaculatus are conditions that should be ruled out in the differential diagnosis.

Histopathology

The RPE appears attenuated and forms a linear pattern, with hypopigmented cells that are reduced in height but have *normal nuclei.* Sometimes, areas of hypertrophy and hyperplasia of the RPE are seen, which form several layers, more commonly at the site of a choroidal scar. There also may be focal atrophy of the choriocapillaris. Bruch's membrane is normal. Areas of retinal disorganization with pigmentary migration, if present, give rise to a pattern called *pseudoretinitis*. Several chorioretinal scars may be seen.

Treatment

Effective treatment is not known.

Retinal Pigment Epithelium Hypertrophy

Congenital hypertrophy of the RPE (CHRPE) is another term applied to the condition known as *retinal pigment epithelium hypertrophy*. This congenital, autosomal recessive, benign hamartoma of the RPE remains stationary, having no malignant potential. It occurs in both genders and all races and may be associated with familial adenomatous polyposis, Gardner's syndrome, and Turcot's syndrome.

RPE hypertrophy appears as solitary, unilateral (or sometimes multiple bilateral), flat, round or oval, avascular lesions that are darkly pigmented (jet black or gray-green). These irregular patches of uniform size (0.1–3.0 mm and larger at the periphery than at the posterior pole) may be angular, with well-delineated scalloped margins. They occasionally are surrounded by a narrow hypopigmented ring of RPE atrophy and are interspersed with areas of amelanotic, depigmented, yellow-orange fenestrations, or *lacunae*, giving rise to a nummular or geographic pattern. They usually occur in the midperiphery or peripheral retina but, occasionally, they may be more diffuse and may involve the macula or the juxtapapillary region. Rarely, a secondary choroidal neovascularization occurs. Lipid exudation can occur and may be massive. Sometimes, the peripheral lesions are elevated and are mistaken for choroidal melanoma. They may be clustered and give the appearance of **bear tracks**, called *grouped pigmentation*.

Symptoms

RPE hypertrophy is usually asymptomatic.

Diagnosis

Visual field examination may reveal scotomas corresponding to the lesion. Fluorescein angiography may show masking of transmission defects, a hypofluorescent area due to blockage of the background choroidal fluorescence by the greater density of pigment in a hypertrophic RPE. Colonoscopy might be a useful diagnostic tool because congenital RPE hypertrophy is often associated with familial intestinal polyposis (Gardner's syndrome).

Differential Diagnosis

Considerations in the differential diagnosis should include malignant choroidal melanoma, retinitis pigmentosa, chorioretinitis, cryopexy application scars, and cobblestone degeneration.

Histopathology

On histologic evaluation, one sees a monolayer of enlarged, taller-than-normal RPE cells that contain an increased number of giant oval melanin granules. Bruch's membrane may appear thickened. There may be degeneration or lack of the rod and cone layer (photoreceptors). RPE atrophy of or loss of pigment, as a surrounding halo, may be present.

Treatment

The patient's condition should be observed. Any associated diseases should be treated appropriately. Laser photocoagulation may be used for lipid exudation.

Retinal Pigment Epithelium Detachment

RPE detachment is a separation of the RPE from Bruch's membrane that occurs either as an isolated lesion, usually in young people as a component of idiopathic central serous choroidopathy, or in association with ARMD, angioid streaks, histoplasmosis, Vogt-Koyanagi-Harada syndrome, or tumors such as Burkitt's lymphoma. It may be spontaneous and idiopathic or may be caused by lipid deposits of hydrophobic drusen in Bruch's membrane, which becomes thickened and may resist the passage of water through the choroid. The latter problem usually is due to a breakdown of the physiologic RPE pump, so that the RPE is pushed off Bruch's membrane by the accumulated fluid. RPE detachment might also be produced by decreased hydraulic conductivity of Bruch's membrane with age, such as a loss of scotopic sensitivity and decreased choroidal perfusion. An accumulation of a fluid that derives from blood vessels growing from the RPE rather than from the choroid is another possible cause of RPE detachment. Finally, such detachment might result from production of a faulty basement membrane of the RPE or disruption of the tight junctions between RPE cells.

RPE detachment appears as a sharply demarcated, round, oval or kidney-shaped, domelike elevation of the RPE, with or without an overlying serous retinal detachment. The lesion exhibits a smooth, homogeneous surface, occasionally marked by pigmented clumping that obscures the choroidal details. The RPE detachment is approximately 0.25–3.00 dd in size and usually is located in the macula (in the subfoveolar area), surrounded by a light-colored demarcation line. Alternatively, it may be located in the papillomacular bundle. Sometimes, there is a serous RPE detachment with adjacent subretinal fluid, which appears as a polypoid subretinal lesion, more commonly located at the posterior pole, temporal to the disc.

RPE detachment may flatten spontaneously, and RPE fold, RPE atrophy, disciform macular scar, and vision loss can occur. Sometimes, there is a tearing of the RPE detachment, which may flap back under itself, with a simultaneous hemorrhage, producing a sudden loss of vision called *pigment epithelial tear* or *rip-off syndrome*.

Symptoms

A person with RPE detachment might experience decreased visual acuity, distortion, hypermetropia, decreased recovery from glare, and generalized darkening of the visual field.

Diagnosis

Fluorescein angiography usually reveals early, uniform, hyperfluorescent filling of the entire area of RPE detachment and late leakage of dye across

Bruch's membrane. An intense, bright hyperfluorescent pooling of the dye remains well demarcated and constant. Digital indocyanine green videoangiography may separate the hyperfluorescent neovascularized portion of RPE detachment from the hypofluorescent serous fluid.

Differential Diagnosis

In the differential diagnosis, Best's vitelliform dystrophy, central serous chorioretinopathy, and soft drusen should be ruled out.

Histopathology

A loosening of the adherence and a separation between the basement membrane of the RPE and the inner collagenous portion of Bruch's membrane are histologically evident. In addition, the choriocapillaris may be attenuated, and there may be choroidal scarring.

Treatment

No treatment for RPE detachment is effective. After photocoagulation, vision deteriorates.

Suggested Reading

Campbell RJ, Steele JC, Cox TA, et al. Pathologic findings in the retinal pigment epitheliopathy associated with the amyotrophic lateral sclerosis parkinsonism dementia complex of Guam. Ophthalmology 1993;100:37–45.

Coles RS. Uveitis. In A Sorsby (ed), Modern Ophthalmology, vol 4 (2nd ed). Philadelphia: Lippincott, 1972;689–746.

Foster RE, Lowder CY, Meisler DM, et al. Presumed *Pneumocystis carinii* choroiditis. Ophthalmology 1991;98:1360–1365.

Freeman WR. Infectious Retinitis. In W Tasman, EA Jaeger, MM Parks, et al. (eds), Duane's Clinical Ophthalmology, vol 4. Philadelphia: Lippincott–Raven, 1996;45:2–22.

Gopal L, Kini MM, Badrinath SS, Sharma T. Management of retinal detachment with choroidal coloboma. Ophthalmology 1991;98:1622–1627.

Holland GN, McArthur LJ, Foos RV. Choroidal pneumocystosis. Arch Ophthalmol 1991;109:1454–1455.

Howe LJ, Woon H, Graham EM, et al. Choroidal hypoperfusion in acute posterior multifocal placoid pigment epitheliopathy. Ophthalmology 1995;102: 790–798.

Jacobson MS, Gagliano DA. Choroiditis. In W Tasman, EA Jaeger, MM Parks, et al. (eds), Duane's Clinical Ophthalmology, vol 4. Philadelphia: Lippincott–Raven, 1996;49:5–16.

Lindlblom B, Anderson T. Choroidal neovascularization with retinal pigment epithelial folds. Arch Ophthalmol 1995;113:946–947.

Marin DF, Cian CC, De Smet MD, et al. The role of the choroidal biopsy in the management of posterior uveitis. Ophthalmology 1993;100:705–714.

Morinelli EN, Duguel PU, Riffenburgh R, Rao NA. Infectious multifocal choroiditis in patients with AIDS. Ophthalmology 1993;100:1014–1021.

Nozik RA. Laboratory testing in uveitis. Focal Points 1993;8:2–10.

Roper-Hall MJ. Mechanical Injuries. In A Sorsby (ed), Modern Ophthalmology, vol 3 (2nd ed). Philadelphia: Lippincott, 1972;446–449.

Schatz H, McDonald R, Johnson RN. Retinal pigment epithelial folds associated with retinal pigment epithelial macular degeneration. Ophthalmology 1990;97:658–665.

Tessler HH, Schlaegel TF. Miscellaneous Uveitis Syndromes. In W Tasman, EA Jaeger, MM Parks, et al. (eds), Duane's Clinical Ophthalmology, vol 4. Philadelphia: Lippincott–Raven, 1996;57:1–4.

Walker J, Davidof FH, Kelly DR, Doyle WJ. Laceration of the globe due to blow-up fracture. Arch Ophthalmol 1990;108:1522–1523.

Zeithahn MAZ, Bennett SR, Cameron D, Mieler WF. Retinal folds in Terson syndrome. Ophthalmology 1993;100:1187–1190.

9

Retinal Injury

Commotio Retinae

Commotio retinae (or *Berlin's edema*) is a retinal edema and hemorrhage involving the macula and sometimes the peripheral retina, usually immediately (or within 24 hours) after an ocular or orbital trauma. It is caused by the effect of the trauma, which by a contrecoup mechanism produces shock waves through the impact. The disorder traverses the fluid-filled eye and strikes the retina; consequently, an ischemia developing in a circumscribed retinal area may produce a spastic contracture and a vasoparalysis of small retinal vessels. It also results in a misalignment of the outer segments, with a widespread marked retinal edema, scattered hemorrhages, and other structural changes, especially of the rod and cone cells (photoreceptors).

Commotio retinae appears as a transient, deep retinal whitening, a pale, slightly opaque edema of the macula, with a silvery sheen or a milky-white macular circle, often located at the peripheral retina. Occasionally, it may be a perivascular sheathing of the attenuated artery that courses from the center. Choroidal vessels may be barely visible beneath the retinal edema.

Edema involving the macula is called *Berlin's edema*. The macula may appear punched-out and may exhibit parallactic displacement between the edges; its center (the foveola) might appear as a dark, bright-red spot due to a visible underlying granular choroid and is surrounded by a retinal whitening, as a small serous macular detachment. Variably sized intraretinal or subretinal hemorrhages are scattered throughout the fundus. Occasionally, in more severe injury, vitreous hemorrhage may obscure the background. In a few days or weeks, the hemorrhage subsides, the edema is absorbed, and extensive fine-pigment disorganization around the macula may be present. Sometimes, it may progress toward a cystoid macular edema or degeneration, a retinoschisis from breakdown of septa in the microcysts, an atrophic macular hole, or chorioretinal scarring. Usually, the prognosis is excellent, and vision may be recovered fully. However, possible complications that may result include traumatic anterior chamber recession, choroidal rupture, avulsion of the vitreous base, tearing of the nonpigmented epithelium of the pars plana, dialysis, or cataract.

Symptoms

Commotio retinae may be asymptomatic. However, it may result in markedly reduced central vision when the macula is involved.

Diagnosis

Visual field testing may reveal a permanent scotoma. Fluorescein angiography shows an opaque retina that blocks the choroidal background fluorescence, but no leakage occurs in mild cases. Biomicroscopy with a Hruby or contact lens should be performed.

Differential Diagnosis

Retinal detachment is one consideration in the differential diagnosis. Branch retinal artery occlusion also should be considered. White without pressure is another possibility.

Histopathology

In an early stage, histologic evaluation shows damage of the photoreceptor cells and the cell bodies in the outer nuclear layer of the retina. Retinal pigment epithelium (RPE) hyperplasia and pigment migration into the sensory retina also are present. In a late stage, multiple pyknotic nuclei appear in the outer nuclear layer. Vacuolization of the inner portion of the photoreceptors, with marked disruption of mitochondria, usually is present. At the end, sometimes microcystoid macular degeneration occurs, or a full-thickness through-and-through hole in the sensory retina is found, surrounded by a focal retinal detachment and residual pigment dispersion.

Treatment

No known treatment is effective for commotio retinae.

Retinal Detachment

Retinal detachment (also known as *ablatio retinae* or *amotio retinae*) is a separation between the RPE and the sensory retina, which comprises the remaining nine retinal layers. The disorder occurs between the RPE and sensory retina because the sensory retina only loosely adheres to the RPE by a weak bond containing an *acid mucopolysaccharide*. Retinal detachment is characterized as two clinical types: *rhegmatogenous* and *nonrhegmatogenous*.

Rhegmatogenous Retinal Detachment

Rhegmatogenous retinal detachment (*rhegma* meaning "hole, fissure") is a discontinuation of the retina and is caused by one or more full-thickness holes (Figure 9-1). It may be *congenital* via retinal degeneration or *acquired* as a consequence of vitreal traction or trauma.

Acquired retinal detachment depends on three factors: a **break**, which may be a *tear* secondary to a dynamic vitreoretinal traction, or a *hole* secondary to disintegration or atrophy of the retina; a **liquid** within the vitreous with free access to the hole; and a **force**. The disorder appears as a dark red or gray, opaque retina. Initially, it is diaphanous at the periphery and is large, bullous, and convex. It may bulge inward but may remain flat, displaying a diminished red reflex and loss of the details of the normal choroidal pattern. Its surface is dull and corrugated, lacking its transparency and its glowing red color. It trembles with each movement of the eye. Vessels are darker, distended, tortuous, and course over the retinal detachment, with almost no differentiation in oxygenation of the arteries and the veins.

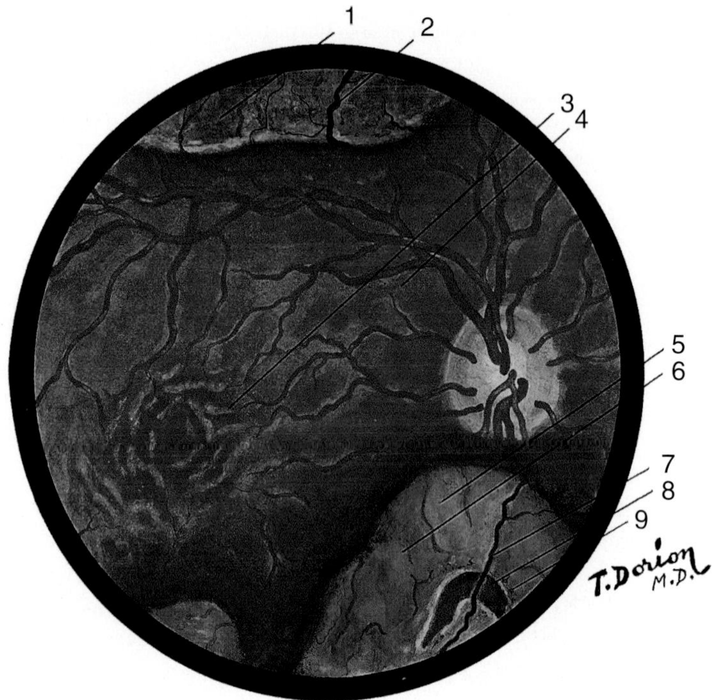

Figure 9-1. *Retinal detachment. (1) Dark gray-red, convex, opaque retina, with dull corrugated surface and diminished red reflex. (2) Vessels are darker, and arteries and veins have similar color. (3) Retinal shagreen in the outer retina. (4) Tobacco dust (Shaffer's sign). (5) Loss of choroidal pattern. (6) Fixed retinal folds. (7) Vessel bridges the tear. (8) Horseshoe retinal tear, as an arrowhead, with the tip always pointed posteriorly and the base anteriorly, having a contracted flap or operculum. (9) Flecks of hemorrhages on the margins of the tear.*

Retinal fixed folds may be evident, appearing in a radial or star formation, and do not change with the position. Macular detachment may display a characteristic retinal folding on the outer retina, called *retinal shagreen*, which results from the edema. The breaks of the retina have a bright, red reflex of the choroid shining through a grayish, opaque veil of the surrounding detached retina. Usually, the disorder is associated with posterior vitreous detachment or peripheral cystoid degeneration. It may be complicated by a cellular proliferation (called *epiretinal membrane*) on the retinal surface.

Retinal breaks usually appear in four types: (1) tractional tear with a flap (**horseshoe tear**), (2) **tear with operculum** of avulsed tissue, (3) **atrophic hole**, and (4) **dialysis.** With respect to the vitreous base, they may be located **intrabasally, juxtabasally**, or **extrabasally**; also, they may be **equatorial**, a type that usually occurs in patients older than 45 years (more commonly bilateral, in men, owing to lattice degeneration or perivascular degeneration); **oral**, which occur at the ora serrata and are due to aphakia, dialysis, or direct or indirect trauma; or **macular.**

Horseshoe tear retinal detachment may appear as a large foramen with contracted flap, or **operculum**, as a U-shaped tear, or as a V-shaped tag of the retina pulled up. It gives rise to an arrowhead type of tear and *always points posteriorly*, having its base anterior; usually it is located in the upper temporal quadrant. This tear may be small (less than one-fourth of 1 clock-hour meridian), giant, or total (extending from 90 degrees to 360 degrees), and it may be bridged by a retinal vessel.

Flecks of hemorrhage may be found on the margins of the tear, and retinal vessels course normally over it. The vitreous may exhibit RPE cells (called *tobacco dust* or *Shaffer's sign*) floating on the surface of the retina or on vitreous strands. Also, vitreous hemorrhage is present, possibly due to a constant or intermittent vitreous contraction.

Dialysis (either *congenital* or *acquired*) is a traumatic disinsertion of the retina that occurs more frequently in the young. It appears as a single, semilunar break located at the extreme periphery (mostly in the inferior temporal retina or superonasally) and is pathognomonic for blunt trauma. The sensory retina is stripped and torn away from the ora serrata, and the vitreous base is avulsed. The disorder may develop also in the vicinity of the injury or, if the vitreous loss through the wound is more severe, the dialysis may occur in the quadrant opposite the injury, due to a transvitreal traction.

Nonrhegmatogenous Retinal Detachment

Nonrhegmatogenous retinal detachment is characterized by the absence of any retinal break. It may appear as any of three types: *transudative*, *exudative*, and *tractional*. **Transudative retinal detachment** usually is caused by a transudation from the choroidal vessels to the retinal vessels. **Exudative retinal detachment** is caused by local or systemic conditions that damage the RPE, which allows passage of the choroidal fluid into the subretinal space. It may occur in scleritis, chorioretinitis, diabetes, eclampsia, sickle cell retinopathy, endocrine disease, peptic ulcer, choroidal tumor, pars planitis, choroidal detachment, nanophthalmos, Coats' disease, retinal vein occlusion, Vogt-Harada-Koyanagi syndrome, high myopia, Wagner's disease, cytomegalovirus retinopathy, rheumatoid arthritis, or in congenital abnormalities, such as morning-glory anomaly, optic pit, and choroidal coloboma.

The disorder appears as a *convex* retina bulging toward the pupil, sometimes so elevated that it may reach the lens. It demonstrates a smooth shiny surface but contains no fixed folds. The subretinal fluid shifts rapidly according to the patient's posture, and choroidal vessels commonly are dilated.

Tractional retinal detachment may result from a vitreal preretinal traction. Usually, it occurs in proliferative diabetic retinopathy, retinopathy of prematurity, toxocariasis, or sickle cell retinopathy. It appears as a *concave* retina and is immobile, exhibiting a smooth surface; occasionally, vitreous membranes pull the retina.

Retinal detachment may also be considered as *primary* or *secondary.*

Primary Retinal Detachment

Primary retinal detachment is caused almost invariably by retinal tears (e.g., those encountered in high myopia, aphakia, or pseudophakia) after vitreous loss or YAG (yttrium-aluminum-garnet) laser capsulotomy and occurs in old age. It may be associated with thinning, degeneration, retinal cysts, macular edema, peripheral neovascularization, and massive preretinal proliferation, such as proliferative vitreoretinopathy. Occasionally, there are nonpigmented and pigmented demarcation lines, called *high water marks.*

Secondary Retinal Detachment

Secondary retinal detachment may be caused by a primary or metastatic tumor (mainly choroidal melanoma or retinoblastoma) or by hypertension, toxemia of pregnancy, chronic glomerulonephritis, angiomatosis retinae, papilledema, choroidal detachment, occlusive retinal venous disease, Vogt-Koyanagi-Harada syndrome, retinal vasculitis, and (rarely) after congenital cataract surgery. The disorder may appear as a solid retinal detachment that does not regress with bed rest, does not transilluminate, has a darker color, and does not have a hole. There may be a serous fluid between the RPE and the sensory retina, and both of these structures may be elevated.

Symptoms

Symptoms of retinal detachment may be minimal. They include sudden flickering and flashing lights (photopsia), a vitreous *tadpole* (or shower of floaters), or dark floating specks. A progressive painless loss of visual field (like a dark veil, a shadow, or a black curtain) develops more often in the nasal quadrant and gradually migrates from the periphery. The continual loss can progress to light perception or to total blindness in a total retinal detachment.

Diagnosis

Relative afferent pupillary defect is noticeable. Intraocular pressure is lower than in the unaffected eye, and visual field examination may show absolute scotoma. Transillumination, binocular indirect ophthalmoscopy with scleral depression, and fundus Goldmann contact lens evaluation are useful. Electro-oculography may reveal an abnormal or absent light rise. B-scan ultrasonography may reveal thickening of the retina, high elevation of the retina, and retraction of the detached posterior hyaloid membrane, called *triangle sign.*

Differential Diagnosis

Considerations in the differential diagnosis are senile retinoschisis, choroidal detachment, choroidal malignant melanoma, juvenile retinoschisis, migraine, and vitreous hemorrhage.

Treatment

For some retinal holes, treatment may not be necessary. Surgical repair to seal the holes and to reduce the vitreous volume is recommended. External drainage of the subretinal fluid and scleral buckling with silicone sponge (*plombage*) are intervention options. Encircling polyethylene bands or tubes (*cerclage*) are beneficial. Additional interventions include indentation of the retina toward the vitreous cavity by scleral implant or explant or suprachoroidal fluid; lamellar scleral resection; pneumatic retinopexy—use of air or long-acting gases (e.g., sulfur hexafluoride, perfluoromethane, perfluoropropane, perfluoro-*n*-butane, perfluoroethane, or octofluorocyclobutane) to tamponade the retina; pars plana vitrectomy; transscleral diathermy; xenon or argon laser photocoagulation; and cryotherapy. Treatment of the underlying disease involves enucleation of tumor, radiation therapy, and chemotherapy.

Retinal Dialysis

Retinal dialysis (or *retinal disinsertion*) is a large, *congenital* or *acquired*, and traumatic retinal break. It constitutes a separation of the sensory retina from the nonpigmented ciliary epithelium and occurs at the ora serrata, mainly in young persons. It is not associated with the posterior vitreous detachment.

Congenital dialysis is usually bilateral and spontaneous and is located inferotemporally. The disorder occurs mostly in the male population, may develop in utero, and may produce a secondary, congenital, or developmental retinal detachment. **Acquired dialysis** is mostly unilateral and traumatic and is located superonasally. It may be produced by an avulsion of the vitreous base, and it may occur after a vitrectomy.

Retinal dialysis appears as a large arc of retinal tear concentric to the ora serrata and usually is less than 90 degrees long. Splitting occurs in the basal vitreous gel, so that the vitreous base is disinserted and hangs loosely in the vitreous cavity. The vitreous is attached commonly to the posterior margin of the break. The disorder is produced by a dynamic vitreoretinal traction.

Symptoms

Retinal dialysis may be asymptomatic.

Histopathology

Histologic evaluation demonstrates a separation of the retina at the ora serrata or just posterior to it. The retina appears normal or may have dysplasia. The vitreous is normal.

Treatment

Scleral buckling is the first-line treatment for retinal dialysis. With cryopexy, it is usually successful (approximately 95% of cases).

Retinitis Sclopetaria

Retinitis sclopetaria is a traumatic retinal lesion (a chorioretinopathy) that may result from an indirect blunt injury, a severe concussion, or a gunshot wound by a bullet through the orbit that ricochets off the sclera. The disorder appears as an extensive fibrous proliferation, like a membrane scar, and occupies a large part of the ocular fundus. Irregularly dispersed pigment proliferation also is evident. A choroidal rupture, which in time may produce late choroidal atrophy, may be found. The optic disc may become atrophic and often is reduced to a scarlike lesion. A vitreous hemorrhage may be present.

Symptoms

Visual acuity is decreased, depending on the site and extent of the retinal tissue destroyed.

Diagnosis

In an early phase, fluorescein angiography may reveal hypofluorescence due to a local choriocapillaris disruption. A late phase may demonstrate fluorescein leakage into a rupture of the choroid.

Treatment

Treatment for retinitis sclopetaria is surgical repair (if necessary).

Suggested Reading

Akiba J, Yoshida A, Trempe CL. Risk of developing macular hole. Arch Ophthalmol 1990;108:1088–1090.

Chitoshi O, Hidenao I, Nagasaki H, et al. Retinal detachment with atopic dermatitis similar to traumatic retinal detachment. Ophthalmology 1994;101: 1050–1054.

Sidikaro Y, Silver L, Holland GN, Kreiger AE. Rhegmatogenous retinal detachments in patients with AIDS and necrotizing retinal infections. Ophthalmology 1991;98:129–135.
Slusher MM, Pugh HP, Hackel RP. Bilateral serous retinal detachment in thrombotic thrombocytopenic purpura. Arch Ophthalmol 1990;108:744–745.

10

Vitreal Disorders

Posterior Vitreous Detachment

Posterior vitreous detachment (PVD) is a separation between the *type II collagen* of the posterior vitreous cortex and the *type IV collagen* of the internal limiting membrane; it occurs at the posterior pole and the optic disc. Usually, it is unilateral and appears more commonly in women older than age 50 and in aphakia, diabetes, myopia, or vitritis, or after trauma or surgery. The disorder may produce elevation of new vessels, vitreal contraction, retinal detachment, macular edema, macular heteropsia, or white with pressure or white without pressure lesions.

PVD may be **complete** (i.e., total, when extending to the ora serrata) or **incomplete** (localized or partial). It may be classified further as **true** or **anomalous** or as **rhegmatogenous** or **nonrhegmatogenous.**

The disorder may be caused by a contraction of the fibrovascular tissue and a shrinkage of the vitreous gel. It exhibits subsequent breaks at the posterior vitreous base, at the edges of a retinal scar, at the area of a lattice degeneration, at the site of firm vitreoretinal adhesions (as a vitreoretinal tuft or a meridional fold), or along the major retinal vessels. Conversely, it may result from rheologic vitreous changes that lead to liquefaction (**synchysis**), with weakening of the vitreous–internal limiting membrane adhesion. It may be a depolymerization of the hyaluronic acid and a dissolution of the collagen network caused by aging and by numerous pathologic, metabolic, or light-induced processes, which may produce a collapse (**syneresis**) of the vitreous.

Rhegmatogenous posterior vitreal detachment is an acute, sudden, complete PVD, in which a liquefied central vitreous passes abruptly into the retinal space through an operculated or nonoperculated hole. It may exhibit a bridging vessel or tear or break usually located at the prefoveolar area, in the posterior hyaloid membrane. As a result, a vitreous hemorrhage (sometimes peripapillary) may occur, and the retinal vessels may be torn or avulsed from the retina. The posterior surface of the vitreous, separated from the retina, may remain attached to the vitreous base or at the disc and may appear as a circle (called *vitreous peephole*) viewed against the background.

Nonrhegmatogenous posterior vitreous detachment is a slow, gradual separation of a thickened posterior hyaloid membrane from the retinal surface. It may appear as a sharply delineated area against the liquefied vitreous or as a dark, annular, glial ring (*Weiss' ring*) of vitreous collagen fibers, hemorrhage, or epipapillary glial tissue torn from the optic disc.

Symptoms

In PVD, floaters cast a shadow on the retina, which is perceived as gray *hairlike* or *flylike* structures or as *spiders*, *cobwebs*, or *threads*. Light flashes prevail (photopsia), especially in dim illumination. The disorder is characterized by blurred vision and metamorphopsia.

Diagnosis

Visual field testing may show a field defect. Slit-lamp examination with a condensing lens of 60 or 90 D or a Hruby lens may reveal a **smoke-ring** floater suspended over the posterior pole. Indirect ophthalmoscopy is performed, with scleral depression to localize the breaks.

Differential Diagnosis

The differential diagnosis should consider migraine, vitritis, retinal detachment, and vitreous hemorrhage.

Histopathology

Histologic analysis confirms that retinal inner layers may be torn. A tenting of the retina is observed, along with a traction with fibrous proliferation at the site of PVD. A fibrous membrane may line the surface of a posterior detached retina.

Treatment

There is no treatment for PVD.

Vitreoretinal Traction Syndrome

Variously termed *retinal dragging syndrome* and *vitreous adhesion syndrome*, vitreoretinal traction syndrome is a partial PVD displaying residual adhesions between the attached vitreous and macula and the optic disc. The disorder appears as one of three types: *vitreomacular*, *vitreo-optical*, and *peripheral vitreoretinal* traction syndrome.

Vitreomacular traction syndrome has the appearance of an elevated ring of the posterior hyaloid face of the vitreous (perifoveolar) or a broad 2- to 3-mm area of vitreomacular attachment (perimacular). It causes a partial PVD combined with a persistent tiny anteroposterior adherence extending to the center of the macula. As a result, there may be retinal striae, a minimal macular ectopia, or a sensory macular elevation as an uneven ridge of a macular crest. There are areas of retinal rigidity (as a gray-white cast of preretinal membranes) that may appear shrunken and produce thickened retinal folds. Exudative retinopathy and retinal detachment also may be present. Occasionally, a cystoid macular edema (called *Irvine-Gass-Norton syndrome*) may be present. Alternately, a wrinkling of the retinal internal limiting membrane (called *cellophane maculopathy*) may be evident.

The **vitreo-optical traction syndrome** may appear as a pseudoswelling of the disc and as a curvilinear area of opacified hyaloid located at the optic disc margin. The tissue may be elevated, and a ring of fibrous adherence (called *fleshy doughnut sign*) may appear at the disc surface. Occasionally, preretinal membranes pull retinal folds together to obscure the optic disc.

The **peripheral vitreoretinal traction syndrome** may appear as horseshoe-shaped tears (usually in clusters) between the equator and the posterior margin of the vitreous base, with a flap held open by a persistent attachment of the vitreous. At the ora serrata, peripheral holes or retinal dialysis may be seen. Areas of retinal rigidity, as gray-white casting of preretinal membranes, may shrink, producing retinal folds. Also, exudative retinopathy, cystic degeneration, and retinal detachment are possible.

Symptoms

The predominant symptom of vitreoretinal traction syndrome is decreased visual acuity, which may worsen gradually. Also possible are blurred vision and metamorphopsia.

Diagnosis

Fluorescein angiography may reveal a marked vasculitis and disc leakage produced by the vitreous traction.

Histopathology

Histologic evaluation reveals a massive vitreous retraction. Fibroglial membranes on the surface of the retina extend into the vitreous. The retina may appear thickened, with retinal folds, or may be detached in some areas. Fibrous and glial membranous proliferations are possible on the internal and external surface of the retina. Retinal breaks, holes, and (occasionally) cysts also may be present.

Treatment

Vitrectomy is the first-line treatment for vitreoretinal traction syndrome.

Terson's Syndrome

Terson's syndrome is a retinopathy that consists of retinal and vitreous hemorrhages associated with an acute subarachnoid or subdural hemorrhage. Frequently, the hemorrhages are bilateral and occur after a trauma or in thrombotic thrombocytic purpura, leukemia, and temporal glioma. The disorder is due to a sudden increase of the intracranial pressure, which increases the venous pressure, in turn producing a rupture of an intracranial aneurysm.

Terson's syndrome appears as multiple preretinal hemorrhages, each forming a dome-shaped accumulation of blood with a flat top and rounded bottom due to gravity. The hemorrhages are usually located within the temporal vascular arcades (or in the peripapillary region). The disorder also manifests as intraretinal or subretinal hemorrhages scattered throughout the fundus or as dispersed and often dense vitreous hemorrhages. Sometimes, the retinal details are not visible. More commonly, the preretinal hemorrhages resolve, leaving residual epiretinal membranes that may replace the posterior hyaloid face of the vitreous.

Symptoms

Terson's syndrome produces sudden, painless decreased visual acuity, which may be marked. It is accompanied also by flashing lights, black spots, headache, and relative afferent pupillary defect.

Diagnosis

Computed tomography scan may reveal a subarachnoid hemorrhage.

Histopathology

Histologic appraisal shows an accumulation of blood between the internal limiting membrane and the posterior hyaloid face of vitreous. Blood is seen progressing into the vitreous.

Treatment

A surgical alternative is vitrectomy. Treatment of any underlying condition is recommended.

Proliferative Vitreoretinopathy

Proliferative vitreoretinopathy, also called *familial exudative vitreoretinopathy*, constitutes a congenital vitreoretinal degeneration that may occur in larger and (often) full-term infants. The disorder usually is autosomal dominant or, rarely, X-linked and occurs bilaterally.

Proliferative vitreoretinopathy appears as a thickened macula, with serous fluid and lipid exudates, and as cystoid macular edema. There may be macular dragging. Retinal capillaries may be prominent and distorted. In advanced cases, an excessive subretinal exudation may occur, and vitreous traction bands and PVD may ensue. Irregular or regular folds usually are present. An epiretinal membrane (with dragging of the retinal vessels) and fibrovascular proliferation (mostly in the temporal periphery) also may be seen. Occasionally, preretinal hemorrhages and retinal detachment are present.

Proliferative vitreoretinopathy may be due to the organization or fibrosis of inflammatory exudates in the vitreous, most commonly in diabetic retinopathy. This activity may result in a pathologic growth of cells capable of forming cellular and collagenous membranes on the surface of the retina, on posterior hyaloid, in the vitreous cavity, and in the vitreous base. Such cell growth may produce traction and epiretinal proliferation, which give rise to radial retinal folds (as a star) or to large, fixed, irregular folds. The retinal pigment epithelium (RPE) may have a primary role in producing this disorder.

According to the **classification of the Retina Society**, four subgroups of proliferative vitreoretinopathy are delineated: grades A, B, C, and D. **Grade A** has pigmented clumps of RPE cells in the vitreous and on the anterior retinal surface, with cells in the vitreous and less mobile posterior vitreous face. **Grade B** demonstrates a wrinkled inner retinal surface and retinal breaks with rolled edges.

Grade C has star folds and fixed irregular folds. It is divided into six types. **Type C-1** has regular retinal folds (called *star folds*) that radiate by a tractional force centripetally toward a focal area of proliferative vitreoretinopathy, usually located in one quadrant. **Type C-2** has irregular retinal folds in the posterior pole, which radiate by a tractional force posteriorly, circumferentially, or perpendicularly and pull the retina toward the center of the vitreous, narrowing a funnel of retinal detachment over the optic disc. Usually, it is located in two quadrants.

Type C-3 has a subretinal membrane that creates an annular constriction (called **napkin ring**) around the disc in a circumferential traction with irregular folds, elevating the retina toward the center of the vitreous. Usually it is located in three quadrants. **Type C-4** has irregular folds behind the vitreous base, which creates a contraction of the adjacent posterior hyaloid and a stretching of the retina inward within the vitreous base, forming a fold in the coronal plane. Usually, it is located in all four quadrants.

Type C-5 has radial folds that pull the retina toward the center of the vitreous and contract the posterior hyaloid. **Type C-6** has an antero-posterior contraction of the hyaloid and vitreous base, which pulls the anterior retina forward.

Grade D has the funnel appearance of a retinal detachment. This grade has been eliminated in a new classification.

Diagnosis

Fluorescein angiography may reveal a disruption of the macula, with dilatation and distortion and pulling and stretching of the capillaries. Also evident are dye leakage, nonperfusion, and fibrovascular proliferation at the periphery. B-scan ultrasonography may show a *double-leaf echo* in severe proliferative vitreoretinopathy, due to a total retinal detachment with the apex at the optic disc and a transvitreal membrane (called *triangle sign*) located anteriorly, connecting the two leaves.

Histopathology

Histologic evaluation demonstrates RPE atrophy with secondary pigment migration.

Treatment

Treatment for proliferative vitreoretinopathy uses laser panretinal photocoagulation with argon diode. Surgical interventions include sclerotomy, lensectomy, vitrectomy, and membrane peeling and sectioning. Also useful are scleral buckling, fluid-gas or fluid-silicone exchange, and relaxing retinotomy or retinectomy. Further procedures are retinal tamponade with silicone oil or intraretinal gases, such as air, perfluoropropane, perfluoroethane, and sulfur hexafluoride, and retinopexy for creating chorioretinal adhesions with laser, cryopexy, diathermy, and cyanoacrylate tissue adhesive.

Persistent Hyperplastic Primary Vitreous

Persistent hyperplastic primary vitreous (PHPV) is a congenital, usually unilateral nonhereditary malformation of the primary vitreous that is present at birth. It is not associated with any systemic diseases. *It is the most common cause of a unilateral cataract in newborns.*

PHPV is due to a failure of the **primary vitreous** (composed of blood-filled branches of the hyaloid artery) to regress in utero and to a hyperplasia of the vascular meshwork of the embryonic lens (*tunica vasculosa lentis*). Normally, these vessels disappear, and their place is filled by a transparent and avascular gel (the **secondary vitreous**) present in living humans. The astrocytes and glial cells may synthesize the *fibrous* component of the PHPV. Also, there may be an abnormal metabolism that may synthesize the *collagen* fibrils in the vitreous.

PHPV may take two forms: *anterior* and *posterior*. **Anterior PHPV** appears as a pinkish, gray-yellow, retrolental mass of fibrovascular connective tissue. It will cause a white pattern of the pupil, called *leukokoria*. There may be a shallow anterior chamber, elongated and inward drawing of ciliary processes, a retrolental mass or plaque, dilated iris vessels, lens intumescence, cataract, and angle-closure glaucoma by pupillary block. There also may be spontaneous hemorrhage deep into the vitreous. A persistent hyaloid artery may hang free from its lens attachment site in the vitreous. Abundant mesenchymal fibrovascular tissue may be present just behind the opacified posterior lens capsule. Buphthalmos may develop.

Posterior PHPV appears as vitreous membranes that usually extend from the disc toward the equator, with stalks, peripapillary retinal traction folds, retinal detachment, and peripapillary fibrotic bands extending forward from the disc into the vitreous. An opaque connective tissue (called *Bergmeister's papilla*) may arise from the glial remnant of the hyaloid artery at the disc. Pearly, gray, wrinkled, and translucent congenital cysts (remnants of the hyaloid system) also may be seen. Usually, there is macular hypoplasia.

Symptoms

Symptoms include amblyopia, esotropia, and poor visual prognosis.

Diagnosis

Unilateral cataract appears in a newborn or infant.

Differential Diagnosis

Differential diagnosis should consider Norrie's disease, retinoblastoma, retinopathy of prematurity, congenital cataract, and retinal dysplasia.

Histopathology

Histologic analysis reveals a generalized hyperplasia of the retinal astrocytes. Also, the glial tissue arising from the disc is hyperplastic. There is metaplasia of the mesenchymal elements in the primary vitreous.

Treatment

Treatment consists of early surgical removal of the lens and retrolental membranes. Pars plana vitrectomy and antiglaucomatous iridectomy are other surgical interventions.

Suggested Reading

Antoszyk AN, McCuen BW II. Vitreous Surgery in Proliferative Vitreoretinopathy. In W Tasman, EA Jaeger, MM Parks, et al. (eds), Duane's Clinical Ophthalmology, vol 6. Philadelphia: Lippincott–Raven, 1996;58:22–23.

Cox MS, Hassan TS. Management of Posterior Segment Trauma. In W Tasman, EA Jaeger, MM Parks, et al. (eds), Duane's Clinical Ophthalmology, vol 6. Philadelphia: Lippincott–Raven, 1996;66:1–4.

McDonald HR, Johnson RN, Schatz H. Surgical results in the vitreomacular traction syndrome. Ophthalmology 1994;101:1397–1403.

Schultz PN, Sobol WM, Weigeist TA. Long-term visual outcome in Terson syndrome. Ophthalmology 1991;98:1814–1819.

Sebag J. Surgical anatomy of the vitreous and the vitreoretinal interface. In W Tasman, EA Jaeger, MM Parks, et al. (eds), Duane's Clinical Ophthalmology, vol 6. Philadelphia: Lippincott–Raven, 1996;51:6–29.

11

Tumors

Choroidal Nevus

Choroidal nevus, otherwise known as *benign choroidal melanoma*, is a benign tumor of the choroid located beneath the retinal pigment epithelium (RPE), more frequently posterior to the equator. It appears as a flat or slightly elevated, 3-mm wide, 2-mm thick, placoid, oval, or round tumor (Figure 11-1) with well-delineated margins. The tumor is slate gray, with pigmentation that may vary from complete amelanosis to a dense black hue. Retinal vessels course normally over it. Occasionally, overlying drusen, orange pigment, or RPE defect may be present. Secondary choroidal neovascularization or, very rarely, malignant transformation may develop.

Symptoms

Usually, choroidal nevus is asymptomatic, although an absolute scotoma is seen on occasion.

Diagnosis

Fluorescein angiography shows hypofluorescence due to a blockage by the nevus of the background choroidal fluorescence. There is no tumor circulation.

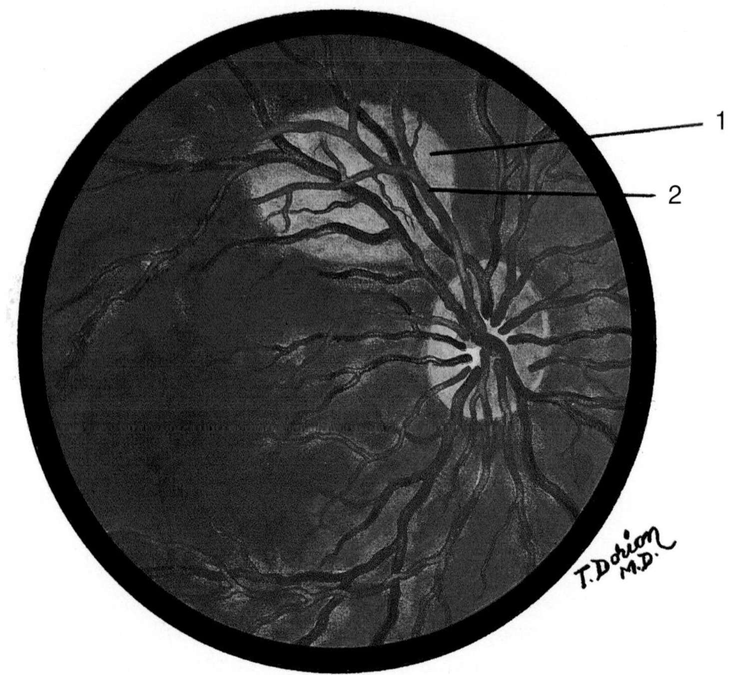

Figure 11-1. *Choroidal nevus. (1) Benign choroidal tumor underneath the retinal pigment epithelium. (2) Retinal vessels course normally over tumor.*

Differential Diagnosis

In the differential diagnosis, malignant melanoma should be considered.

Histopathology

Choroidal nevus is composed of four types of benign atypical uveal melanocytes, called *nevus cells* (Figure 11-2): (1) **plump polyhedral cells,** having small, uniform nuclei and abundant pigmented cytoplasm; (2) **slender spindle cells,** having little or no pigment; (3) **dendritic and plump fusiform cells,** which are polyhedral and have large nuclei and dendritic projections of heavily pigmented melanocytic cytoplasm; and (4) **balloon cells,** large cells with abundant foamy cyto-

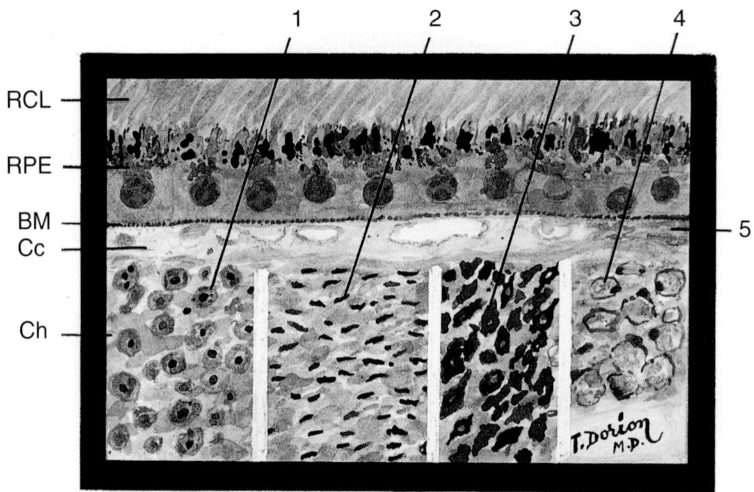

Figure 11-2. *Histopathologic findings in choroidal nevus. (1) Plump polyhedral cells. (2) Slender spindled cells. (3) Dendritic and plump fusiform cells. (4) Balloon cells. (5) Obliterated choriocapillaris. (Ch, choroid; Cc, choriocapillaris; BM, Bruch's membrane; RPE, retinal pigment epithelium; RCL, rod and cone layer [photoreceptors].)*

plasm. The choriocapillaris usually is spared, but it may be narrowed or obliterated. The overlying RPE is normal.

Treatment

Periodic observation, by way of serial photographs obtained over several months, is appropriate to determine any changes.

Choroidal Hemangioma

Choroidal hemangioma is a benign, slow-growing, progressive, vascular tumor of the choroid—a **hamartoma**, composed of mature cells and tissues that normally are present in the choroid—which exhibits blood-filled spaces. It may be either *circumscribed* or *diffuse.*

Circumscribed choroidal hemangioma appears as a sessile or slightly elevated, round or oval tumor that usually measures approximately 2–6

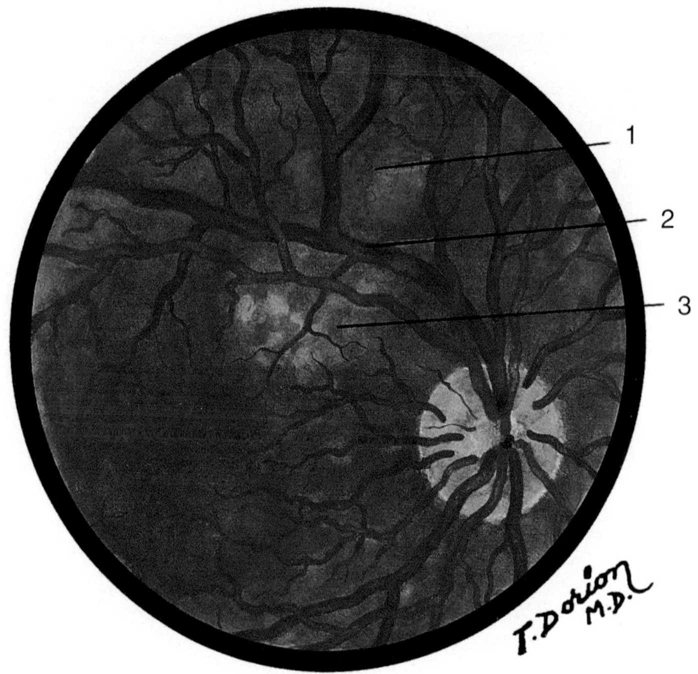

Figure 11-3. *Choroidal hemangioma. (1) Serous retinal detachment. (2) Dilated retinal vessels. (3) Placoid elevated lesion, with pigment changes at its surface.*

mm in thickness (Figure 11-3). It is red-orange but usually not pigmented and similar in color to the surrounding normal fundus; rarely, it may appear whitish. The tumor has indistinct margins and a smooth surface, which often may display pigmentary changes. Circumscribed choroidal hemangioma is located at the posterior pole, more frequently in the macula, or in the peripapillary region. The optic disc may have a pronounced cup. Pressure on the eye may produce blanching of the lesion. This hemangioma is not associated with any systemic disease.

Diffuse choroidal hemangioma is larger and flatter than the circumscribed variety, with less sharply defined borders. It varies in size to up to several disc diameters and may extend over one-half of the fundus and anteriorly to the equator. It usually is located between the disc and macula. It lacks a capsule, which may cause bleeding into the surrounding choroid and accumulation of subretinal fluid that may reach the macula, producing a central serous retinopathy or a cystoid macular edema. The retinal vessels coursing over the tumor usually are dilated or tortuous or may even have arteriovenous communications. The tumor may produce a deeper, brighter red reflex, as compared with the other eye, a condition called *tomato-ketchup fundus*. Diffuse choroidal hemangioma may be part of Sturge-Weber syndrome.

Symptoms

Choroidal hemangioma is characterized by decreased visual acuity. A secondary glaucoma may develop owing to a retinal detachment.

Diagnosis

Visual field examination may show arcuate field defects or localized scotomas. Fluorescein angiography may reveal irregular hyperfluorescence. On indocyanine green angiography, an intense hyperfluorescence of a speckled mass with stellate margins may be evident. Doppler scanning may reveal a pulsatile blood flow. A-scan ultrasonography may show high internal acoustic reflectivity from multiple changes in the tissue density, whereas on B-scan ultrasonography, an elevated choroidal lesion might be seen. Computed tomography (CT) of the skull may reveal an associated intracranial angioma with meningeal calcifications. Other potentially useful diagnostic aids include magnetic resonance imaging (MRI) of the brain and thermography.

Differential Diagnosis

Among the conditions to be considered in the differential diagnosis are malignant choroidal melanoma, choroidal nevus, RPE tumors, ocular lymphoma, subretinal hemorrhage, age-related macular degeneration, and posterior scleritis.

Histopathology

On histologic evaluation, numerous engorged, cavernous, vascular spaces filled with blood are seen (Figure 11-4), which may involve the

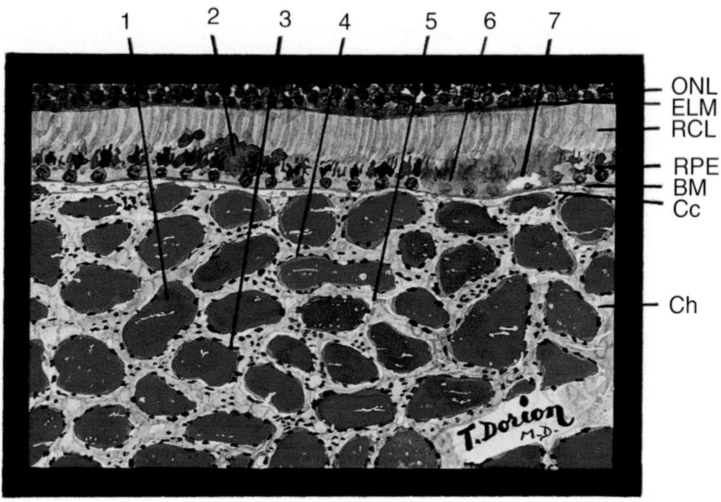

Figure 11-4. *Histopathologic findings in choroidal hemangioma. (1) Engorged cavernous vascular spaces, filled with blood. (2) RPE proliferation. (3) Endothelial cells. (4) Thin wall of new vessels. (5) Sparse connective tissue. (6) RPE metaplasia to whitish connective tissue. (7) Calcification (epichoroidal membrane). (ONL, outer nuclear layer; ELM, external limiting membrane; RCL, rod and cone layer [photoreceptors]; RPE, retinal pigment epithelium; BM, Bruch's membrane; Cc, choriocapillaris; Ch, thickened choroid [up to 10 times the normal size].)*

full thickness of the choroid. RPE proliferation and metaplasia, with dense, whitish connective tissue known as an *epichoroidal membrane*, may lead to calcification. New vessels having a thin wall and only sparse connective tissue surrounding the endothelial cells coat the red cells. The choroid may become 10 times thicker than normal owing to these newly formed vessels. There may be cystoid degeneration in the overlying retinal outer plexiform layer. Also possible is a bullous retinoschisis or, at a later time, a total exudative retinal detachment.

Treatment

Treatment of choroidal hemangioma may be not necessary. Hypermetropic amblyopia should be treated early. Laser photocoagulation and beam or plaque radiotherapy are treatment options. Surgical repair of retinal detachment may be undertaken. Secondary glaucoma should be treated appropriately.

Cavernous Hemangioma

Cavernous hemangioma is a congenital, unilateral, benign, stationary or slowly progressive retinal vascular tumor that occurs in patients of both genders and all races and that is associated with central nervous system or cutaneous cavernous hemangioma or telangiectatic vascular lesions. It may occur also in the orbit, being *the most common benign orbital tumor of adults.*

Cavernous hemangioma appears as a thin-walled, saccular tumor, composed of multiple cluster-of-grapes aneurysmal dilatations. The tumor has a fibrous capsule, is filled with venous blood, and appears dark reddish or purplish. It lies along the retinal vessels or on the optic disc or may be retrobulbar in the intraconal space. Cavernous hemangioma varies in size from approximately 2 to 6 mm, each saccule measuring between 100 and 1,500 μm. The surrounding retinal vessels are normal. There may be an extensive fibrosis or gliosis on the surface of the tumor. Sometimes, RPE hyperplasia or retinal striae, produced by indentation of the globe at the posterior pole by the muscle cone or by an epithelial membrane, macular dragging, papilledema, or optic atrophy, can be seen. Occasionally, preretinal, intraretinal, and subretinal hemorrhages may occur that resemble those in retinal arterial macroaneurysms. Vitreous hemorrhage, possibly due to traction of the vitreous strands with entrapped blood, also may be present.

Symptoms

Cavernous hemangioma may be asymptomatic. More often the tumor causes slowly progressive mild proptosis (usually less than 5 mm), extraocular motility difficulty, decreased visual acuity, blurred vision, and floaters.

Diagnosis

A-scan ultrasonography may reveal high-amplitude internal echoes, whereas B-scan ultrasonography may show smooth, contoured shadows with acoustic cystic properties. A well-encapsulated, round tumor might be seen on CT scanning. During the arterial phase on fluorescein angiography, early filling of choroidal vessels appears as a mottled pattern within the tumor, with delayed and incomplete perfusion caused by the stagnant circulation but exhibiting no vascular leakage.

Differential Diagnosis

Coats' disease and idiopathic perimacular telangiectasia should be included in the differential diagnosis.

Histopathology

Intraretinal, large, vascular aneurysmal spaces that are filled with blood are apparent histologically. The tumor is lined with flattened endothelial cells and has a clear-cut fibrous capsule at the periphery in which small dilated capillaries and vascular shunts but no feeder vessels are present. The retina is thickened by edema and large vessels in the inner retinal layers. There may be calcification, fibrosis, or hemosiderin deposits.

Treatment

Cavernous hemangioma may be observed. Treatment, if undertaken, might involve laser photocoagulation, cryotherapy, or excision by a lateral orbitotomy or posterior vitrectomy.

Angiomatosis Retinae

Angiomatosis retinae, also called *von Hippel–Lindau disease*, *retinal cerebellar capillary hemangioma*, and *hemangioblastoma*, is a congenital vascular anomaly that is autosomal dominant with incomplete penetrance. This capillary hemangioma of the retina and cerebellum, a **phakomatosis**, is a *hamartoma* formed by elements normally found in the tissue. Occasionally, it may involve the spinal cord. It occurs usually at 20–30 years of age and frequently is bilateral, or multiple lesions may appear in the same eye. Angiomatosis retinae is progressive and can be lethal. It sometimes is associated with cysts of the kidney, pancreas, adrenal glands, and epididymis, hypernephroma, pheochromocytoma, or renal cell carcinoma.

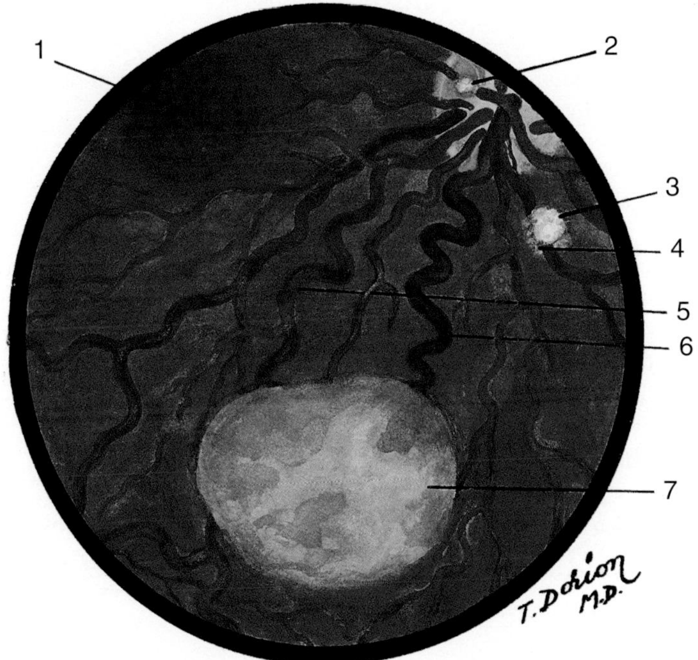

Figure 11-5. *Angiomatosis retinae (von Hippel–Lindau disease). (1) Macula. (2) Angioma of the disc. (3) Early angioma, normal vessels. (4) Lipid exudation. (5) Tortuous and dilated feeding artery. (6) Tortuous and dilated draining vein. (7) Capillary angioma, fully developed.*

Angiomatosis retinae appears initially as a small intraretinal tumor with normal vessels, located frequently temporally and inferiorly at the posterior pole (Figure 11-5). The lesion measures approximately 1.5 mm but may develop to a larger tumor of many disc diameters. It may be an oval, slightly elevated, dome-shaped, bullous, orange-red, pink, pale vascular globulus having a smooth surface. It may grow nodularly, and circinate rings of fatty exudates may surround it. The feeding arteries and the draining veins are markedly dilated, beaded, and tortuous. There may be hard exudates in the macula, cholesterol deposits, fixed retinal folds, organized fibroglial membranes, retinal edema, or retinal detachment.

Symptoms

Decreased visual acuity and, occasionally, secondary glaucoma are symptoms of angiomatosis retinae.

Diagnosis

Fluorescein angiography may show an early arterial filling of a circumscribed arterial lesion and an early discoloration of the hamartoma. MRI might be useful in making a diagnosis. Regular renal ultrasonography is appropriate.

Differential Diagnosis

Coats' disease should be considered in the differential diagnosis.

Histopathology

On histologic assessment, thin-walled capillaries are seen growing in disarray. Pericytes, endothelial cells with large, lipid-filled vacuoles, polygonal cells, endothelial cells, and stromal cells are present (Figure 11-6). There may be marked gliosis.

Treatment

Laser photocoagulation with yellow dye (577 nm) will occlude the angioma and draining vein via high absorption of hemoglobin. Cryotherapy and transscleral diathermy are treatment options. Genetic counseling should be offered.

Retinoblastoma

Also known as *glioma retinae*, retinoblastoma is a unilateral or bilateral, hereditary or nonhereditary, familial or sporadic, primary malignant tumor that may regress spontaneously and completely in 95% of cases via a toxic effect of the lymphocytes against the tumor cell, prob-

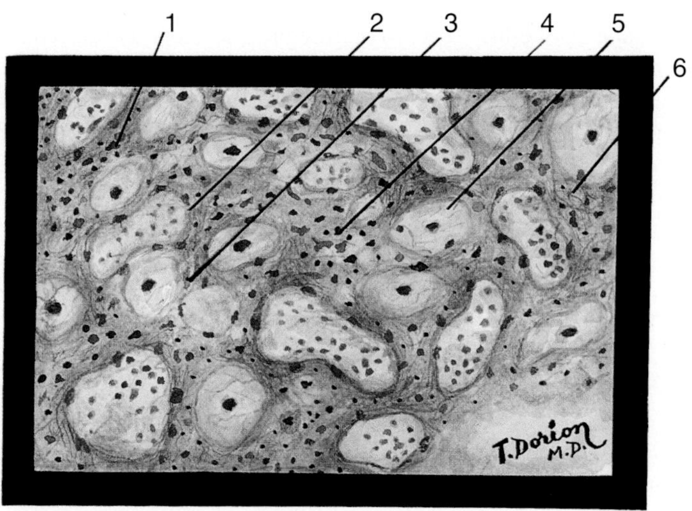

Figure 11-6. *Histopathologic findings in angiomatosis retinae. (1) Polygonal cells. (2) Thin-walled capillaries growing in disarray. (3) Interstitial cells. (4) Marked gliosis. (5) Endothelial cells with large lipid-filled vacuoles. (6) Stromal cells.*

ably through an immunologic mechanism. It may also be fatal. *Retinoblastoma is the most frequent intraocular tumor in children,* occurring in 1 in every 20,000 live births, usually before 3 years of age, but rarely in adults of 20 years or older. All the bilateral cases (approximately 6%) are attributable to a hereditary, familial, autosomal dominant trait with 90% penetrance. Retinoblastoma may spread to bone marrow or brain or directly into the orbit.

Retinoblastoma may derive from retinal photoreceptors or from the inner nuclear layer, ganglion cell layer, nerve fiber layer, and especially the outer nuclear layer. Although the exact mechanism is unknown, it is thought that its cause may be a mutation of an autosomal dominant gene due to deletion of a suppressor gene, identified on the long arm of chromosome 13; the mutation is closely associated with decreased levels of the enzyme esterase D, which encodes a phosphoprotein (pRB) that is involved in regulation of the cell growth cycle. Retinoblastoma may be produced by loss or inactivation of both normal alleles of the retinoblastoma gene (*RB1*), which may determine whether the disease is *genetic* (inherited by an offspring of an affected patient) or *somatic* (not heritable by an offspring of an affected person).

Knudson's "two-hit" theory regarding the development of retinoblastoma posits the necessity for occurrence of two separate genetic events: The first hit consists of the combination of one *defective gene*, which exists in the germinal cell that generates every retinal cell, and one *normal anticancer gene*, whereas the second hit is a *mutagenic alteration* that suppresses the function of the normal gene. Consequently, retinoblastoma develops.

Retinoblastoma usually takes one of two forms, although the two may occur in combination: *Endophytic* retinoblastoma grows from the retinal inner nuclear layer toward the vitreous, whereas *exophytic* retinoblastoma grows from the subretinal space toward the retina and retinal detachment may occur as a result.

The appearance is a white-gray or creamy pink, flat or elevated tumor on the retinal surface (Figure 11-7) or a mushroom-shaped tumor protruding into the vitreous, usually on the temporal side. The tumor exhibits well-delineated margins and numerous chalky white, sharply demarcated, glistening or occasionally translucent calcium deposits that may lie deep within the lesion or on its surface and resemble cottage cheese.

Retinoblastoma is more often located at the ora serrata or the peripheral retina, but it may also be present in the macula or optic disc. Few hemorrhages or neovascularization may be seen on its surface. The feeder vessels may be prominent. Often, there is in the tumor a vascular system, called *skeleton of the tumor vessels*, that is not part of the retina or the choroidal circulation; this system appears after most of the tumor cells have disappeared. Occasionally, there is a pigmented atrophic ring around the circumference of the tumor, which may signify spontaneous regression. Adjacent to the tumor or in the macula, some yellow fat exudates may be present. White *DNA-calcium* deposits usually are seen. Tumor cells may invade the vitreous. *Calcification of the tumor and seeding of the tumor cells into the vitreous are pathognomonic for retinoblastoma.*

Retinoblastoma metastasizes widely, primarily to the brain via the optic nerve. Often, there is a secondary glaucoma, produced by neovascularization of the iris angle structures, with formation of peripheral anterior synechiae. Occasionally, retinoblastoma may undergo spontaneous necrosis, leading to phthisis bulbi. Children may demonstrate bilateral genetic retinoblastoma associated with a primary intracranial nonretinoblastoma malignancy (e.g., such as a pinealoblastoma) called *trilateral retinoblastoma.* Rarely, an ectopic intracranial retinoblastoma may develop.

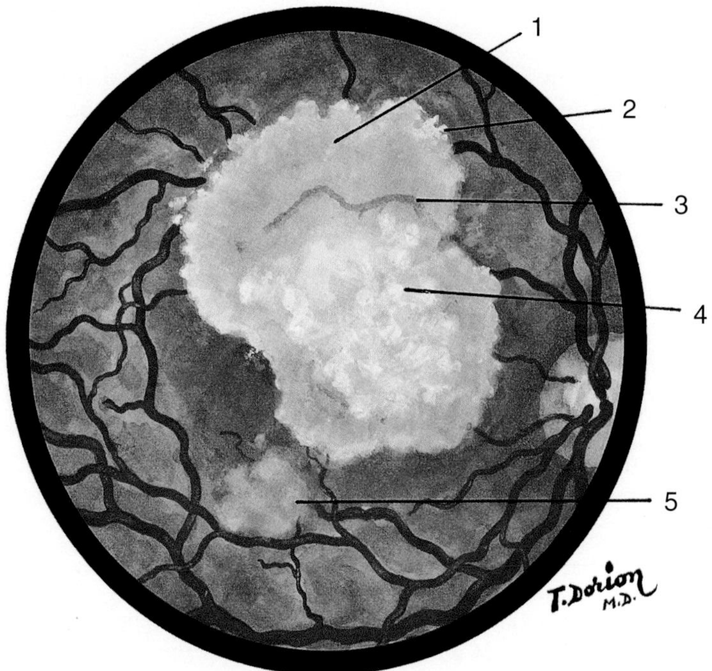

Figure 11-7. *Retinoblastoma. (1) Creamy pink, mushroom-shaped tumor, protruding into the vitreous. (2) Well-delineated margins. (3) Chalky white deposits of calcium, resembling cottage cheese. (4) Prominent feeder vessels. (5) Yellow, soft exudates adjacent to the tumor.*

Types of Regression

Four types of retinoblastoma regression can be identified: **Type 1** may be total and is the most common. It may feature cottage cheese calcification or shrunken, white fluffy tumors. **Type 2** may have *fish-flesh* tumor shrinkage, loss of vascularization, and a characteristic gray color. **Type 3** is a combination of types 1 and 2. **Type 4** is a complete elimination of the tumor, retina, and choroid, leaving a white patch of bare sclera. This type of regression occurs after treatment.

Classification

The **Reese-Ellsworth classification of retinoblastoma** delineates five groups. **Group 1** tumors carry a *very favorable prognosis.* These are solitary or multiple tumors of less than 4 dd in size, located at or behind the equator. **Group 2** tumors carry a *favorable prognosis* and are solitary or multiple tumors measuring 4–10 dd, located at or behind the equator. In **group 3** are tumors with a *dubious prognosis.* Any tumor located anterior to the equator or a solitary tumor located behind the equator and being larger than 10 dd qualifies as a group 3 lesion. **Group 4** tumors carry an *unfavorable prognosis.* They are multiple, and some are larger than 10 dd in size. Any tumor located at the ora serrata is classified in this group. **Group 5** tumors carry a *very unfavorable prognosis.* These tumors are massive—up to half the size of the retina—or exhibit vitreous seeding.

Symptoms

Strabismus, esotropia or exotropia, and squinting in sunlight are common symptoms. Leukocoria with a mid-dilated (4–5 mm) and nonreactive pupil occurs and is called **amaurotic cat's eye**. Pseudohypopyon occurs, with nodules in the iris. Redness, irritation, spontaneous hyphema, unilateral pupillary dilatation, cloudy cornea, ocular pain, tearing, irritability, heterochromia iridis, poor hand-eye coordination, floaters, secondary glaucoma, proptosis, and buphthalmos all may be present.

Diagnosis

Roentgenograms of the globe may aid in the diagnosis. B-scan ultrasonography may reveal one or more soft intraocular masses and multifocal intralesional calcifications. CT scan also may reveal calcification and may detect and fully delineate the spread of lesions outside the globe, especially into the brain and orbit. MRI may evaluate the sellar and parasellar regions of brain to rule out ectopic intracranial retinoblastoma. Paracentesis of the anterior chamber with aspiration may show an increased level of *lactic dehydrogenase (LDH)*; the ratio of *aqueous humor* LDH to *serum* LDH may be greater than 1 to 50.

Bone marrow aspiration and cerebrospinal fluid analysis are potentially useful. Fluorescein angiography may reveal hyperfluorescence.

Karyotype analysis may demonstrate the deletion in the long arm of chromosome 13, called *13q deletion syndrome*. Amniocentesis is of uncertain value in predicting retinoblastoma in a fetus.

Differential Diagnosis

Numerous conditions that can mimic the symptoms of and findings in retinoblastoma should be considered in the differential diagnosis. Among these are retinopathy of prematurity, angiomatosis retinae, persistent hyperplastic primary vitreous, pseudoglioma, Coats' disease, *Toxocara* endophthalmitis, intraocular medulloepithelioma, congenital cataract, congenital retinal folds, posterior uveitis, astrocytic hamartoma in tuberous sclerosis, vitreous hemorrhage, vitreous abscess, retinal dysplasia, choroidal coloboma, myelinated nerve fibers, retinal detachment, incontinentia pigmenti, Norrie's disease, leukemia, amelanotic melanoma, and massive retinal gliosis.

Histopathology

Retinoblastoma may be *undifferentiated* or *well-differentiated*. **Undifferentiated retinoblastoma** is composed of small, uniform, round or polygonal cells, with scant cytoplasm, numerous mitotic figures, and a large, chromatin-rich nucleus. Basophilic masses are present, but stroma is absent. Areas of calcification and necrosis liberate DNA, which is absorbed by the blood vessel walls and the internal limiting membrane.

Well-differentiated retinoblastoma (Figure 11-8) is composed of four types of lesions: (1) *Flexner-Wintersteiner rosettes*, (2) *fleurettes*, (3) *Homer-Wright rosettes*, and (4) *pseudorosettes*. **Flexner-Wintersteiner rosettes** are clusters of small, closely packed, round or polygonal cells arranged as a single layer, having large dark nuclei located away from the lumen and scant cytoplasm around a central, clear, empty lumen. *They appear to be pathognomonic for retinoblastoma.*

Fleurettes are clusters of flowerlike cell bouquets from which protrude bulbous cellular processes of ultrastructurally differentiated inner and outer segments of the photoreceptors. *Tumors composed entirely of fleurettes have a better prognosis.*

Homer-Wright rosettes are clusters of tumor cells lined up around an area that contains cobweblike neurofibrillary material, a triangle of cytoplasmic processes. There is no central lumen.

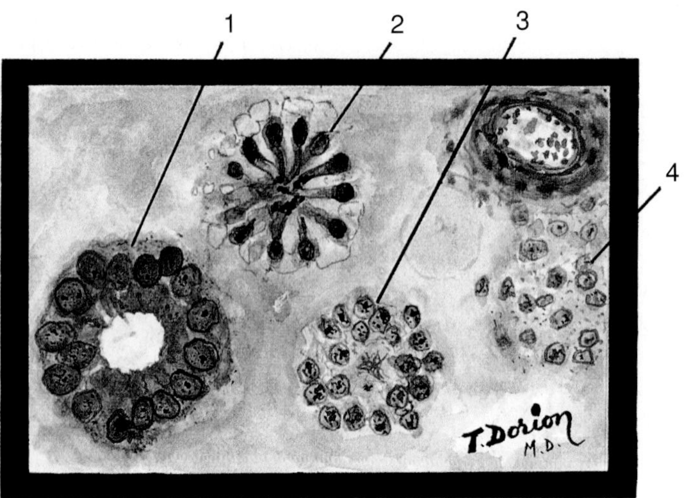

Figure 11-8. *Histopathologic findings in retinoblastoma. (1) Flexner-Wintersteiner rosettes. (2) Fleurettes. (3) Homer-Wright rosettes. (4) Pseudorosettes.*

Pseudorosettes are perivascular clusters of small, basophilic, undifferentiated neuroblastic cells that surround a central blood vessel, tumor cells located around small basophilic and granular areas of necrosis, or incompletely formed rosettes.

Calcification, necrosis, and DNA are seen around the vessels. Some tumors, called **retinocytomas** or **retinomas**, express no mitosis and are composed of photoreceptors and cells having an abundant eosinophilic cytoplasm.

Treatment

Episcleral plaque radiation therapy using an isotope ^{131}I, ^{125}I, or ^{105}Ru applicator and delivering 4,500 cGy in 2–5 days, is used. External-beam radiation therapy (EBR) with supervoltage x-rays—in a total dose of 4,500 cGy delivered through a precision lateral or oblique portal in divided doses over 4 weeks—is recommended for patients with unilateral retinoblastoma group 1–3 lesions (Reese-Ellsworth classification), for patients with bilateral retinoblastoma that is less advanced, as an alternative to enucleation, or for patients with small tumors at the posterior pole.

Chemotherapy and chemoreduction with antitumor agents, such as cyclophosphamide, vincristine, actinomycin D, carboplatin, etoposide, or doxorubicin, or sequential aggressive local therapy (SALT) may be beneficial. The **Kingston-Hungerford regimen** consists of 2-month cycles of chemoreduction, followed by EBR, 4,500 cGy to the whole eye, and two additional cycles of chemotherapy.

Cryotherapy by triple-thaw technique, using a transconjunctival retinal cryoprobe in sessions 1–3 weeks apart, is performed for lesions at the ora serrata. Small posterior primary tumors can be treated by xenon arc photocoagulation or an indirect ophthalmoscope laser delivery system. Enucleation, with removal of a long portion of the optic nerve, is recommended in unilateral retinoblastoma groups 4 and 5 (Reese-Ellsworth classification) or in bilateral retinoblastoma. Genetic counseling should be offered. Observation is mandatory.

Choroidal Malignant Melanoma

Choroidal malignant melanoma (*diktyoma*) is a slowly progressive, usually unilateral, malignant tumor that occurs more frequently in men older than 50 years. *It is the most common intraocular malignancy in the white population* and is often associated with the oculodermal melanosis or nevus of Ota. The tumor arises from melanocytes within the choroid.

Choroidal malignant melanoma appears as a solid, mottled, gray-brown, lightly pigmented, or amelanotic, lump that is either flat and diffuse or elevated (by several diopters). The lesion is dome shaped, rounded, or mushroom shaped (Figure 11-9) and exhibits discrete abnormal deposits of lipofuscin, an orange pigment, and visible large blood vessels. Alternatively, hard and soft drusen may be distributed over an uneven surface, and retinal vessels that are not associated with the retinal vasculature may be seen climbing onto this surface.

Choroidal malignant melanoma that are small (less than 6 dd) usually have a survival rate of 73%. Lesions that are much larger carry an unfavorable prognosis. Occasionally, there may be **sentinel vessels** in a large choroidal melanoma. Nonrhegmatogenous retinal detachment also may occur. Clumps of brownish cells or strands might be seen in the vitreous.

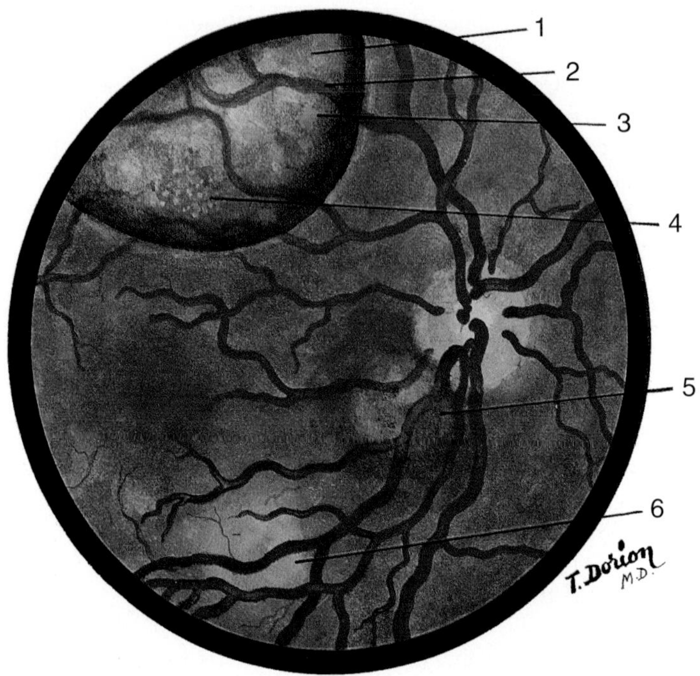

Figure 11-9. *Choroidal malignant melanoma. (1) Large dome-shaped tumor, lightly pigmented. (2) Visible blood vessels within the tumor. (3) Drusen over an uneven surface. (4) Orange pigment. (5) Peripapillary choroidal melanoma. (6) Nonrhegmatogenous retinal detachment.*

The melanoma may spread carpetlike between the sclera and Bruch's membrane, along the vortex veins or anterior ciliary arteries, rupturing the membrane and the RPE. The RPE is multilayered and forms a globular head, which may give the tumor a collar-stud or dumbbell appearance on cross-section. In *diffuse melanoma*, the lesion infiltrates the uvea without forming a bulky tumor, often extending aggressively extraocularly. It may invade the optic disc, appearing as a circumferential *peripapillary melanoma*, which may simulate optic neuritis.

Choroidal malignant melanoma may metastasize by hematogenous spread in the liver, which is by far the most common organ affected, and become invariably fatal. It also may metastasize in the lung and brain. Occasionally, a subretinal fluid is located at the posterior pole, usually on the temporal side away from both the ora serrata and vortex veins, which shifts with the patient's position, does not transilluminate, and may cause a serous retinal detachment. Cystoid degeneration of the underlying retina also is possible.

Knapp-Ronne choroidal melanoma is located near the optic disc, grows early through the retina, has both bloodless and blood-filled cavernous spaces, and may produce a massive vitreous hemorrhage, which may result in hemosiderosis bulbi and heterochromia iridis.

Symptoms

Choroidal malignant melanoma may be asymptomatic. More often there is early metamorphopsia, macropsia and micropsia, blurred or decreased vision, floaters, light flashes, and pain. Visual field examination will reveal a defect in a particular sector. A deformed pupil, photopsia, heterochromia iridis, and secondary glaucoma can occur. Prognosis is related to the type of cells and size and character of the tumor (i.e., whether it is diffuse, has mitotic activity, or displays extrascleral extension).

Diagnosis

Pupillary transillumination may help the practitioner to distinguish a pigmented tumor from a nonpigmented one. Fluorescein angiography may reveal multiple pinpoint areas of dye leakage, destruction of the RPE, irregularity of medium vessels, mixed areas of masking of choroidal fluorescence and abnormal vascular tumor channels that appear highly fluorescent. Indocyanine green angiography might also be useful. Radioactive phosphorus (^{32}P) uptake may reveal a difference of more than 100% between the counts over the tumor and those over a normal area of the same eye.

A-scan ultrasonography may reveal a solid tumor with a high initial spike and then a smooth attenuation of the medium to low internal echoes. B-scan ultrasonography may reveal a choroidal mass with a sharp anterior border, acoustic hollowness, choroidal excavation, and orbital shadowing. Chest roentgenograms and liver enzyme levels should be obtained.

Unlike other tumors, choroidal melanoma appears hyperintense on MRI T1 images and hypointense on MRI T2 images; the short T1 value is attributed to stable radicals in melanin. CT scanning of the liver, indirect ophthalmoscopy, and biomicroscopy all may contribute helpful information.

Transvitreal fine-needle aspiration biopsy may be undertaken. Detection of circulating antibodies and a positive skin reaction to a soluble extract of melanoma cells are diagnostically significant. Levels of LDH, serum glutamic oxaloacetic transaminase (SGOT) or serum glutamic pyruvic transaminase (SGPT), gamma glutamyl transpeptidase (GGT), and alkaline phosphatase should be obtained. The carcinoembryonic antigen (CEA) level also should be obtained if choroidal metastasis is to be ruled out.

Differential Diagnosis

Retinal, RPE, or choroidal detachment; choroidal hemangioma; RPE proliferation; choroidal metastases or osteoma; posterior scleritis; suprachoroidal hemorrhage (as a masquerade syndrome); pseudomelanoma (e.g., choroidal nevus, disciform macular degeneration, retinoschisis); leiomyoma; schwannoma; age-related macular degeneration; and melanocytoma of the optic nerve are all considerations in the differential diagnosis.

Histopathology

On histologic examination, the choriocapillaris may be seen to be filled with tumor and may be totally destroyed. Choroidal malignant melanoma is composed of six types of cells (Figure 11-10), defined here according to **Callender's classification: Spindle A cells** are long, narrow, spindle-shaped cells with long, slender, flattened nuclei arranged in a linear fashion parallel to the long axis of the cell, due to a nuclear membrane infolding. There is a central longitudinal dark stripe, a small, inconspicuous nucleolus, and an indistinct cytoplasm. **Spindle B cells** are oblong, oval, or spindle-shaped cells with large, plump, round or oval nuclei having prominent round nucleoli. The cytoplasm is indistinct and contains mature melanosomes, all sizes of phagosomes, and relatively normal choroidal melanocytes, intracytoplasmic filaments, a mitochondria that is elongated and partially oriented along the long axis of the cells, and mitotic figures. Both thick and thin collagen fibrils, called *reticulin*, lie between the cells. **Fascicular cells** are spindle A or spindle B cells arranged in a palisade or ribbonlike pattern. **Epithelioid cells** are

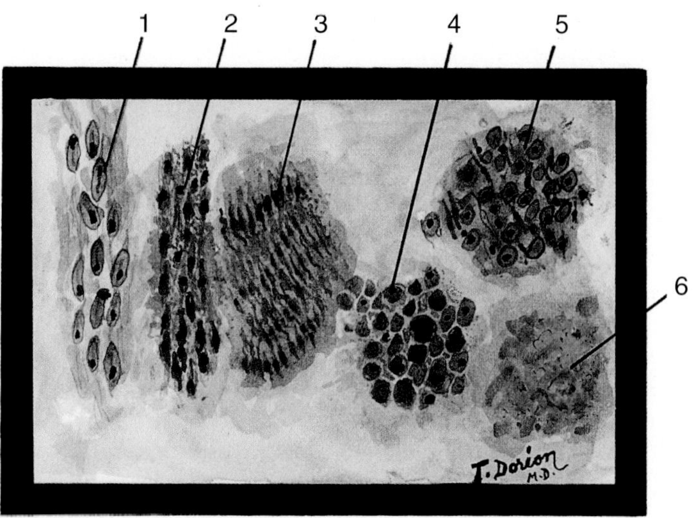

Figure 11-10. *Histopathologic findings in choroidal malignant melanoma. Callender's classification: (1) spindle A cells; (2) spindle B cells; (3) fascicular cells; (4) epithelioid cells; (5) mixed cells; (6) necrotic cells.*

large, oval or round, noncohesive cells having large nuclei, prominent nucleoli, abundant eosinophilic watery cytoplasm with mitotic figures, and a loose, nonaligned arrangement of mitochondria, but lacking cytoplasmic filaments. There is widespread dispersion of ribosomal clusters, some of which remain attached to fragments of endoplasmic reticulum called *polysomes. The epithelioid cells are the most malignant.* **Mixed cells** are the most common type, a combination of spindle cells (usually type B) and epithelioid cells. Finally, **necrotic cells** are so affected by necrosis that it is impossible to recognize cell type.

Treatment

Ionizing radiation may be applied as *brachytherapy* via episcleral application of low-energy, radioactive plaques containing gamma-emitting isotopes of ^{60}Co, ^{192}Ir, ^{125}I, or ^{106}Ru; these are left in place until 10,000 cGy is delivered to the tumor apex. Gold plaques and radon seeds are other radiation therapy options. Ion bombardment with a highly collimated beam of cyclotron-generated heavy ions, such as helium, may also be performed, as may tantalum clips attached to the sclera. Other treatment options include xenon arc photocoagulation or argon laser therapy, with injection of photosensitive *hematoporphyrin derivatives* before dye laser photoirradiation. Transpupillary thermotherapy may be administered for small choroidal melanomas near the foveola and optic disc; an infrared diode laser set at 810 nm, with a beam width of 1.2–3.0 mm, is used.

Chemotherapy might be undertaken using dimethyltriazenoimidazole (DTIC). Nonspecific immunopotentiating agents such as bacillus Calmette-Guérin (BCG) are another treatment option.

Local sclerochorioretinal resection can be performed for small- to medium-size tumors. Formerly, enucleation was the procedure of choice, but some fear exists that this measure may promote dissemination of tumor cells, according to the **Zimmerman-McLean hypothesis** that malignant cells may be pushed into large, tumor-associated vascular lumina and may be swept away from the eye to create distant metastases. Exenteration may be considered in the face of extensive extraocular involvement without metastases or in orbital recurrence after enucleation. Observation is essential.

Optic Disc Malignant Melanoma

Optic disc malignant melanoma is a very rare, slowly infiltrating, primary malignant tumor of the disc. It may arise from melanocytes located in the optic nerve substance and may simulate a melanocytoma.

Optic disc malignant melanoma appears as a slightly elevated jet-black tumor located at the upper side of the optic nerve head, measuring approximately 1.5 × 2.5 mm, and having feathery margins. It may cause venous congestion or papilledema. Occasionally, a subretinal hemorrhage may surround it.

Histopathologically, heavily pigmented neoplastic cells—usually spindle A, spindle B, and epithelioid cells—are replacing the disc's normal cells almost entirely. These replacement cells have plump, spindle-shaped nuclei laid out in a fascicular pattern and containing small nucleoli and an indistinct cytoplasm. They may have prominent nuclear folds and bear a dark stripe across the cell. Mitotic activity usually is present.

Leukemic Retinopathy

Leukemia, a systemic disease, may involve the eye in a *leukemic retinopathy*. Leukemia is a neoplasm of blood-forming tissue derived from abnormal proliferation of a leukocyte precursor. Its cause is unknown, and it may occur in all races and at any age. Leukemia may be *acute* or *chronic*. Leukemic retinopathy is more common in such acute leukemias as acute lymphoblastic, acute myelogenous, or acute monocytic leukemia. It is associated with anemia and thrombocytopenia, hepatosplenomegaly, lymphadenopathy, bone pain, fracture, ophthalmoplegia, deafness, Meniere's syndrome, meningitis, internal hydrocephalus, fever, and petechiae. There are also infections of the oral cavity, skin, and rectum.

Leukemic retinopathy may be due to blood hyperviscosity, caused by an increased number of leukemic cells and hyperproteinemia; by a hemorrhagic diathesis that may reduce the number of platelets and alter a protein involved in the clotting process; and by leukemic infiltration of the retina and choroid. Alternatively, nutrition of the capillary endothelium might be defective, secondary to poor oxygenation and to changes in the chemical composition of the blood, which may result in hemorrhage.

The most common ocular manifestation of leukemic retinopathy is hemorrhages, which are superficial, flame shaped, intraretinal and preretinal, and scattered throughout the fundus. Many of the hemorrhages have a white center of leukemic infiltrate or a platelet-fibrin embolus called **Roth's spot**. The retinal background may appear pale, varying from yellow to light pink, as a result of generalized retinal edema that is more marked over the optic disc or as macular edema. Rarely, leukemic infiltration to the fundus occurs.

Occasionally, there is mottled pigmentation of the retina, giving rise to a **tigroid fundus**, or a *leukemic retinal pigment epitheliopathy*, which appears as a **leopard fundus**. Retinal veins are irregular in caliber, dilated, darker than normal, and tortuous, with occasional parallel sheathing that appears as gray-white lines on either side of the vein. Over time, retinal arteries may become dilated and resemble the veins. In both arteries and veins, the blood column content may become yellowish owing to anemia and a high leukocyte concentration. At the arteriovenous crossings, veins may appear progressively broken up into turgid sausagelike segments. The central retinal vein may become occluded by the leukemic cells.

Microaneurysms often are seen, and neovascularization of the peripheral retina can occur. Yellow-white, hard exudates and cotton-wool spots also may be present. The choroid may be thickened and may appear gray, usually in the juxtapapillary area. In the optic disc, leukemic infiltration resembling papillitis is possible. Rarely, the disc may be swollen, with blurred margins, as in mild papilledema. There may be fuzzy, flat, white retinal leukemic infiltrates, which may be unifocal or multifocal and unilateral or bilateral. Vitreous hemorrhages often are present. Occasionally, a proliferative retinopathy similar to sickle cell disease may be seen. Sometimes, a serous retinal detachment also is present.

Symptoms

Visual acuity may be minimally decreased in leukemic retinopathy, marked by blurred or dim vision and floaters. Severe loss and blindness also occur. Iritis, secondary glaucoma, proptosis due to a leukemic orbital infiltration, orbital chloroma, dacryocystitis, spontaneous hyphema in a child, and pseudohypopyon are other symptoms of leukemic retinopathy.

Diagnosis

A complete blood cell count (with differential count) may reveal thrombocytopenia (as low as 20,000/mm^3 platelets, as contrasted to normal [150,000–400,000]) and a normochromic normocytic anemia. Auer bodies in the cytoplasm of myeloblasts or monoblasts, a low hematocrit level, circulating blast forms, and an elevated uric acid level are suggestive of the diagnosis. Roentgenograms may reveal diffuse osteoporosis. Bone marrow cytologic workup and lumbar puncture to permit cerebrospinal fluid cytologic analysis are helpful. Fluorescein angiography may reveal multiple hyperfluorescent spots and, rarely, multifocal leakage and macular ischemia. Fine-needle aspiration biopsy, pars plana vitrectomy, and anterior chamber paracentesis all can be performed to aid in making the diagnosis.

Differential Diagnosis

Conditions that present a clinical picture similar to that of leukemic retinopathy include ocular lymphoma, metastatic carcinoma, choroidal diffuse melanoma, cytomegalovirus retinitis, sickle cell retinopathy, toxoplasmosis, orbital tumor, idiopathic thrombocytopenic purpura, infectious mononucleosis, Hodgkin's disease, lymphosarcoma, and other malignancies.

Histopathology

In leukemic retinopathy, there is leukemic infiltration into the choroid and, possibly, accumulation of leukemic cells under the internal limiting membrane. The RPE may exhibit linear and stellate pigment aggregation. Another histologic finding is vitreous cells with rounded, irregular nuclei that lack cytoplasmic granules.

Treatment

Topical corticosteroids include prednisolone (Pred Forte), 1% three times daily. Chemotherapy is usually administered by the pediatric oncologist and effected with chlorambucil (Leukeran), 0.4 mg/kg as a single dose every 4 weeks for 4 months. EBR or radiation therapy with ^{32}P, 1–2 mCi IV every 2 weeks, is used in chronic myelocytic leukemia. Allopurinol (Zyloprim), 300 mg/day PO; vincristine (Oncovin), 0.05 mg/kg IV once weekly for 4 weeks; and prednisone, 1 mg/kg/day PO, are other systemic agents that have a place in the treatment of leukemic retinopathy. Marrow transplantation may be undertaken in an attempt to treat the systemic disease. Supportive treatment is vital.

Hamartoma of the Retinal Pigment Epithelium

Hamartoma of the RPE (also known as *RPE hyperplasia*, *benign melanoma of the RPE*, or *nevus of the RPE*) is a rare, congenital or acquired, unilateral or bilateral, slowly progressive, benign overgrowth of cells that normally occur in that site. The hamartoma, which has no malignant potential, is located at the margin of the optic disc or, less commonly, in the peripheral retina and occurs most frequently in young men.

Congenital RPE hamartoma appears as a solitary, usually unilateral, flat or minimally elevated, grayish, dark-brown, or jet-black lesion with moderate mottled pigmentation at its base; it may become hypopigmented over time. The hamartoma displays sharply delineated borders and variable vascularity. Retinal gliosis and traction may be seen, particularly at the macula. Congenital RPE hamartoma may be associated with Gardner's disease (familial polyposis of the colon) or von Recklinghausen's disease (neurofibromatosis type 1 [NF-1]) and bilateral acoustic neuroma (neurofibromatosis type 2 [NF-2]); the latter two diseases may occur as a result of a unique chromosomal defect.

Acquired RPE hamartoma is a combined pigment epithelial and retinal hamartoma (CPERH). It is almost always unifocal and unilateral. It occurs after an inflammation such as choroiditis; in retinitis pigmentosa, homocystinuria, diabetes, or syphilis; as senile changes; as a reactive hyperplasia secondary to trauma, inflammation, or degeneration; or after diathermy or scleral buckling surgery for retinal detachment.

RPE hamartoma appears as a slightly elevated, geographic, white gliotic lesion involving the disc, macula, and retina in the inferior and temporal quadrant. It may extend deep into the retina or subretinal layers. A gray-black pigmentation might be seen at its margins, and a grayish glial membrane on the retinal surface may overlie a portion of the disc, the vascular arcades, and the tumor itself. Retinal vessels emerging from the disc may appear pulled toward the lesion or may be markedly tortuous and angulated. Often, secondary choroidal neovascularization may develop.

Symptoms

Decreased vision, which may accompany RPE hamartoma, may be severe. Symptoms of associated diseases will prevail.

Diagnosis

Fluorescein angiography in the late phase may reveal hyperfluorescence, with leakage of dye from the abnormal capillaries.

Differential Diagnosis

Malignant melanoma should be considered in the differential diagnosis of RPE hamartoma.

Histopathology

In the presence of RPE hamartoma, the retina will be disorganized, with marked RPE proliferation, interlacing RPE cord cells, and thickened and reduplicated RPE. In addition, the sensory retina will be thickened. Glial proliferation is increased, more commonly in the juxtapapillary region. Abnormal choroidal neovascularization may be seen. The optic nerve may be elevated and distorted, with prominent tortuous vessels. Radiating retinal folds that course from the lesion toward the macula might appear at the vitreoretinal interface. Tractional retinal detachment may also be present.

Treatment

Usually, treatment of RPE hamartoma is not indicated. Laser photocoagulation may be used to eliminate neovascularization. Posterior vitrectomy is undertaken to remove vitreoretinal fibrosis.

Adenoma and Adenocarcinoma of the Retinal Pigment Epithelium

Retinal Pigment Epithelium Adenoma

RPE adenoma (or *epithelioma*) is a very rare benign tumor that may arise from the ciliary epithelium of the RPE or from a juxtapapillary inflammatory scar in a patient with ocular *histoplasmosis*. It usually is either *tubular* (papillary) or *vacuolated* (solid), but occasionally is a mixture of these two types.

It appears as a deep, lightly or heavily pigmented mass—sometimes a jet-black tumor—with a flat base, of variable size and height, located mostly between the equator and ora serrata. RPE adenoma may have a premacular membrane.

Diagnosis

A-scan ultrasonography may reveal an elevated mass that is internally heterogeneous and has a strong acoustic shadow.

Differential Diagnosis

Reactive RPE proliferation and pseudoadenomatous RPE hyperplasia are considerations in the differential diagnosis.

Histopathology

Histologic evaluation of RPE adenoma reveals polyhedral cells in the RPE, packed tightly together with heavily pigmented cells, and little or no stroma. The cells are vacuolated in the inner half and contain *sialomucin*, which may be digested by a neuraminidase called *sialidase*.

These cells are of two types: *light cells*, which contain immature melanosomes, and *dark cells*, which contain mature melanosomes and which are the only cells containing cytoplasmic vacuoles. Rarely, mitotic figures may be present.

Treatment

Pars plana vitrectomy to peel membrane located premacularly is undertaken to improve vision.

Retinal Pigment Epithelium Adenocarcinoma

RPE adenocarcinoma is a rare, low-grade malignant tumor that may mimic a choroidal malignant melanoma. Like RPE adenoma, it generally assumes one of two forms—*tubular* (papillary) or *vacuolated* (solid)—although it may also be a mixture of both.

RPE adenocarcinoma appears as a whitish, dome-shaped, moderately vascular mass that may arise from the peripapillary choroid and may involve the optic disc. Severe macular pucker with preretinal fibrosis is possible and may extend to the tumor. Areas of shallow retinal detachment lying inferior to the tumor and expanding toward the equator may be seen. There also may be extensive exudation in the sensory retina and subretinal space.

Symptoms

RPE adenocarcinoma is marked by decreased visual acuity that is slowly progressive.

Diagnosis

Fluorescein angiography may reveal hypofluorescence of the lesion. A-scan ultrasonography may show a medium-low internal reflectivity and decreased amplitude of the echoes in the mass. In contrast, B-scan ultrasonography may reveal an acoustic solidity and minimal choroidal excavation in an elevated mass.

Differential Diagnosis

Conditions that should be considered in the differential diagnosis include choroidal malignant melanoma and melanocytoma.

Histopathology

Sheets or cords of tumor are composed of uniformly heavily pigmented, polygonal or cuboidal anaplastic cells having large, pleomorphic, round or oval nuclei, which may contain prominent nucleoli. Some of the tumor cells lack cytoplasmic pigment, but others contain a variable amount of pigmented granules, especially near the base of the tumor. In addition, there are small vacuoles containing hyaluronidase-sensitive mucopolysaccharide. Within the tumor may be scattered foci of chronic inflammatory cells. The cords of tumor are separated by intercellular matrix material. Usually, tumoral invasion is absent beyond the choroid or lamina cribrosa. There is low-grade mitotic activity.

Treatment

Pars plana vitrectomy is undertaken to peel the premacular membrane.

Ocular Lymphoma

Also known as *reticulum cell sarcoma, large-cell lymphoma*, *non-Hodgkin's lymphoma*, ocular lymphoma is a malignant tumor of the reticuloendothelial system that develops in the ocular fundus, usually bilaterally and asymmetrically. It occurs more commonly in elderly patients of both genders. The tumor is lethal and may be associated with human T-lymphotropic virus type I.

Ocular lymphoma metastasizes mainly from a central nervous system tumor through the choroidal circulation rather than from a visceral tumor. It may derive from a B-cell or a T-cell lymphoma.

Ocular lymphoma appears as creamy choroidal patches having fluffy borders, which are located at the posterior pole, progress rapidly, and become confluent. Occasionally, there is a leopard-spot pattern at the peripheral retina. At the macula, the tumor may simulate a disciform scar. In addition, multiple, yellow-white, deep, irregular, flecklike, small retinal infiltrates measuring 50 μm are found along the major vascular arcades. There may be retinal edema, retinal detachment, RPE detachment, vasculitis, perivascular exudates, retinal necrosis, and retinal hemorrhages. Moderate vitreous cells, arranged in sheets as in vitritis, may be present. The optic disc may be swollen. Commonly, there is a unilateral or bilateral posterior uveitis. Rarely, a solid intraocular lymphoma may occur. Sometimes, there is proliferation of large atypical lymphocytes in the lumen of the small arteries, veins, and capillaries, as well as clusters in the choriocapillaris and large choroidal vessels, which give rise to **angiotrophic lymphoma** (also called *intravascular lymphomatosis* or *malignant angioendotheliomatosis*).

Symptoms

Symptoms of ocular lymphoma include vitreous floaters, blurred vision, diplopia, seizures, hoarseness, and unsteady gait.

Diagnosis

Failure of a uveitic eye to respond to corticosteroids signals the presence of ocular lymphoma. Neoplastic hypopyon in a quiet eye also is a sign of ocular lymphoma. Diagnostic pars plana vitrectomy may reveal in the vitreous aspirate large pleomorphic lymphocytes with pyknotic nuclei and coarse, clumping nuclear chromatin. Choroidal biopsy and sub-RPE fine-needle aspiration biopsy are useful. Fluorescein angiography may show, in the arteriovenous phase, an early accumulation of dye within these deep retinal lesions or may reveal a diffuse mottled blockage of the dye in the choroid. B-scan ultrasonography may exhibit multifocal thickening of the retina and the choroid, whereas A-scan ultrasonography may show regular, low internal reflectivity. MRI of the brain, after gadolinium injection, may reveal central nervous system lymphoma as cerebral or cerebellar masses. Cerebrospinal fluid analysis may demonstrate atypical lymphocytes. Immunophenotype and immunologic analyses should be performed.

Differential Diagnosis

Posterior uveitis, evanescent white-dot syndrome, fundus flavimaculatus, and macular disciform scar are all considerations in the differential diagnosis.

Histopathology

Large, neoplastic, lymphomatous, pleomorphic cells that are at least twice as large as the reactive lymphocytes in the choroid exhibit scant cytoplasm and round or oval, bean- or cloverleaf-shaped, hypersegmented nuclei having nuclear membrane abnormalities, prominent nucleoli, and mitotic activity. These cells always are located above Bruch's membrane. Malignant B lymphocytes may accumulate between the RPE and Bruch's membrane. Clumps of reactive T lymphocytes may be seen in the adjacent choroid, retina, or vitreous. Reticulum cells also may be seen in the vitreous. The retina is destroyed and densely infiltrated by lymphoma cells. The choroid is minimally thickened but is not involved in the lymphomatous process.

Treatment

Treatment consists primarily of irradiation with 40 Gy in 25 fractions. Aggressive intrathecal chemotherapy is also a mainstay.

Choroidal Osteoma

Choroidal osteoma, otherwise called *choroidal osseous choristoma*, is a rare, acquired, idiopathic, solitary, benign, osseous tumor of the choroid that is usually unilateral and rarely bilateral or familial, slowly progressive, and composed of cancellous, spongy, reticular bone that is normally found in the body but *not in the choroid*. It occurs more commonly in young white women 15–20 years of age.

Choroidal osteoma is produced by full-thickness replacement of the choroid by osteoblastic activity. It may resorb through the activity of the osteoclasts, stimulated by a sub-RPE hemorrhage, pregnancy, the parathyroid hormone, prostaglandins, excessive 1,25-dihydroxycholecalciferol (a metabolite of vitamin D_3), or an osteoclastic activating factor.

The tumor appears as a dense, white-yellow or orange-yellow, pearly, amelanotic, sessile or slightly elevated, irregular, coarse, bony placoid mass of approximately 3 dd in size. Often multiple, small vascular networks appear on its surface, with small pseudopodlike projections and geographic, well-defined borders that have wedge-shaped edges. Choroidal osteoma is located at the posterior pole, more commonly in a juxtapapillary or circumpapillary position. It may grow quite extensively by osteoblastic activity, extending toward the periphery.

There may be diffuse, mottled pigmentation of the underlying RPE. Subretinal hemorrhage may be present. Rarely, a choroidal neovascularization occurs, which in time may produce macular degeneration. Occasionally, choroidal osteoma may involute spontaneously, with decalcification, leaving a crater-shaped depression in the center of the osteoma.

Symptoms

Choroidal osteoma may be asymptomatic. However, if the macula is affected, decreased visual acuity ensues.

Diagnosis

Fluorescein angiography in the arteriolar phase may demonstrate an irregular hyperfluorescent tumor that "lights up." B-scan ultrasonography may reveal dense, highly reflective plaque at the level of the choroid, with soft-tissue echoes. CT scan of the orbit may reveal choroidal calcification.

Differential Diagnosis

Conditions to consider in the differential diagnosis include benign uveoscleral calcification, choroidal malignant melanoma, choroidal metastasis, and RPE metaplasia.

Histopathology

This osteoma is a choroidal tumor composed of normal, mature, latticelike bone that replaces the choroid and interconnects with narrow spaces. The osteoma is sharply demarcated from the surrounding choroid. There may be RPE hyperplasia due to osteoclastic activity. Bony material intermingled with vascular components may also be present.

Treatment

No treatment is effective. Laser photocoagulation of the neovascular membrane may be undertaken.

Optic Nerve Glioma

Optic nerve glioma (called also *astrocytic hamartoma*, *astrocytoma*, or *juvenile pilocytic astrocytoma*) is a unilateral, stationary, benign tumor of the optic disc composed of disorganized overgrowth of mature cells and tissues that normally are present at the disc. It occurs mostly in individuals younger than 20 years. It may be associated with tuberous sclerosis or neurofibromatosis. The lesion may derive from interstitial cells, astroglia, and oligodendroglia.

Optic nerve glioma appears as a pale, white-yellow, chalky white, cheesy, or even grayish, solid optic disc having blurred margins. It is elevated approximately 3–4 D, is less vascularized than normal, and protrudes into the vitreous. Retinal vessels may be concealed or deflected. Occasionally, there is a central retinal vein occlusion. Papilledema and optic atrophy occasionally are present. The rest of the ocular fundus may be normal.

Two clinical and histopathologic types of optic nerve glioma are recognized: astrocytic hamartoma and juvenile pilocystic astrocytoma. **Astrocytic hamartoma** appears as a solitary or multiple, nodular or flat, small lesions or as glistening white-gray or yellowish tumors, measuring approximately 0.56–1.00 dd and protruding into the vitreous, located at or near the disc but also in the peripheral retina. In contrast, **juvenile pilocystic astrocytoma** usually appears as papilledema followed by optic atrophy and sometimes is associated with hemorrhages and exudates.

Symptoms

Asymmetric, unilateral decreased vision usually is preceded by unilateral, minimal or massive, axial, nonpulsatile proptosis. Downward displacement of the globe occurs. The patient with optic nerve glioma may suffer paralytic strabismus, nystagmus (vertical, horizontal, rotatory, and see-saw), hydrocephalus, headache, vomiting, and convulsions.

Diagnosis

A-scan ultrasonography may reveal regular, homogeneous, low to medium reflectivity, whereas B-scan ultrasonography may show, in large optic nerve glioma, an elongated mass replacing the optic nerve void. On CT scan, smooth, fusiform enlargement of the optic nerve might be evident. MRI may reveal any involvement of intracranial optic nerve or chiasm. Visual field examination may show central scotoma or homonymous hemianopsia.

Differential Diagnosis

Conditions that should not be overlooked in the differential diagnosis include optic nerve drusen, retinoblastoma, myelinated nerve fibers, toxocariasis, toxoplasmosis, Coats' disease, other retinal telangiectasias, tuberous sclerosis, and neurofibromatosis.

Histopathology

On histologic assessment, findings in **astrocytic hamartoma** include uniform spindle cells having small oval nuclei and long cytoplasmic processes located in the retinal nerve fiber layer. **Juvenile pilocytic astrocytoma** may take three forms: *transitional*, *reticular*, and *astrocytic*. The **transitional** form appears as numerous, large, disorganized glial cells with giant nuclei, intermingled with the normal optic nerve tissue. The nerve bundles may appear enlarged. There may also be necrotic areas with macrocystoid spaces, called **protoplasmatic astrocytoma**.

In the **reticular** form, small cells having ill-defined margins, small nuclei, and interlacing cytoplasmic processes are seen. Oblong, ovoid, fibrillar, coarse reticular and myxomatous areas marked by microcystoid spaces within the tumor, probably secondary to a tumor necrosis, characterize **fibrillar astrocytoma.**

The **astrocytic** form appears as giant spindle cells with intracytoplasmic, astrocytic, eosinophilic degenerated fibrils called *Rosenthal fibers*. There may be a reactive hyperplasia of the meningeal tissue in the nerve sheath. The optic nerve usually is replaced by neoplastic astrocytes. Also seen are small cells (called *oligodendrocytes*) with round nucleoli, clear cytoplasm, and a distinct membrane, which sometimes give rise to a honeycomb appearance. This type of juvenile pilocytic astrocytoma is known as **gigantocellular astrocytoma**.

Treatment

Optic nerve glioma may be observed. Surgical excision might be considered. Ventricular shunting is appropriate to relieve hydrocephalus. Radiation therapy and chemotherapy have a role in the treatment of this lesion.

Tuberous Sclerosis

Sometimes referred to as *Bourneville's disease* or *Pringle's disease*, tuberous sclerosis is a *phakomatosis*, a hamartoma of the disc or peripheral retina consisting of tissue that normally is found in the involved site. It occurs as a heredofamilial disease in association with mental retardation, sebaceous adenoma, and epilepsy.

Tuberous sclerosis appears as multiple, smooth, superficial, translucent or semitransparent, elevated nodular lesions that are homogeneous, granular, and avascular. The lesions, whose margins are irregular, usually measure 0.5–2.0 dd. Tuberous sclerosis has been compared with *tapioca grains*, *fish eggs*, and *mulberries*. The young hamartoma is smoother, spongy, has fuzzy borders, and is gray-white, whereas the old hamartoma is wrinkled, whitish, and irregular. The lesions may be located in an epipapillary, peripapillary, or peripheral location in the retinal nerve fiber layer, through which the retinal vessels may be seen; alternatively, the lesions may protrude into the vitreous. Sometimes, round hyaline bodies, called **giant drusen**, are seen on, within, or near the disc; these may undergo calcification in elderly patients. They usually are located anterior to the lamina cribrosa and may be mistaken for a swollen disc (i.e., pseudopapilledema).

Histopathologically, an astrocytic hamartoma is located in the nerve fiber layer, with oval, globular, sometimes vacuolated, large cells, in which there is cytoplasm at the periphery. An old hamartoma may exhibit white deposits (called **calcospherites**) usually next to the optic nerve, which may replace the full thickness of the retina. The young hamartoma is composed of glial cells without calcospherites.

Optic Disc Melanocytoma

Disc melanocytoma is also known as a *magnocellular nevus of the disc*. It is a rare, benign tumor of the optic nerve head, with a densely pigmented, atypical nevus that is stationary or slowly progressive, has low malignant potential, and occurs more commonly in nonwhites, in dark-skinned persons, and in people with dark eyes. It is engendered at the optic disc from uveal melanocytes. It appears as a jet-black, evenly pigmented, uniform tumor that sometimes is markedly elevated. The lesion generally covers the inferior and temporal part of a large disc, with fuzzy, fibrillated margins, but it may extend over the entire optic disc or anywhere in the uveal tract in addition to the disc—into the adjacent choroid, retina, or macula or, rarely, bulging into the vitreous. It may even spread out behind the lamina cribrosa. Rarely, choroidal neovascularization develops at its margins. Disc melanocytoma is not known to metastasize. It occasionally is associated with papilledema, peripapillary hemorrhages, or hypopigmentation.

Symptoms

Disc melanocytoma may be asymptomatic, although slightly impaired vision may persist for months or years.

Diagnosis

Visual field examination may reveal concentric constrictions, central and cecocentral scotoma, or enlargement of the blind spot. Fluorescein angiography may demonstrate hypofluorescence and a sharply delineated tumor that lacks intratumoral circulation.

Differential Diagnosis

Malignant choroidal melanoma and RPE adenoma should be considered in the differential diagnosis.

Histopathology

Disc melanocytoma is composed of intensely pigmented, large polyhedral nevus cells having abundant cytoplasm, giant melanosomes, and uniform, small, round or oval, pale nuclei, and scant nucleoli. Mitotic figures are absent. The cells may be of two types: round, differentiated, *metabolically inactive cells* (so-called benign cells), which contain heavy melanin pigment, and fusiform, small, less pigmented, *metabolically active cells*, which contain large nuclei, many mitochondria, excessive endoplasmic reticulum, and free ribosomes. There is no cellular invasion of the disc tissue and no juxtapapillary retinal detachment.

Treatment

No treatment is necessary.

Optic Disc Meningioma

Disc meningioma is a tumor of the optic nerve head. It is of mesenchymal origin and is more common in middle-aged women (35–45 years) and less common in children. The tumor arises usually from the cranium itself and, rarely, from the optic nerve sheath. It may be *primary* or *secondary.*

Primary optic disc meningioma arises from the optic nerve sheath and then spreads and infiltrates the subarachnoid and subdural space, compressing the nerve. It may be located also at the sphenoidal ridge, producing sclerosis and thickening and narrowing of the superior orbital fissure from infiltration of the greater and lesser wings of sphenoid and of temporal bone, with displacement of the temporal fossa. Primary optic disc meningioma may extend into the cavernous sinus.

Secondary optic disc meningioma arises intracranially from arachnoidal villi, spreads into the middle cranial fossa and orbit, and invades the subdural space through the optic canal and superior orbital fissure. It appears as a pale, round or irregularly shaped, sometimes swollen disc with blurred margins; multiple cilioretinal collateral vessels shunt the blood from an obstructed central vein to the choroidal circulation. There may be chronic papilledema and optic atrophy as a result of slow strangulation of the optic nerve fibers. Secondary optic disc meningioma may expand between the optic nerve sheath and the optic nerve and may appear as a circumferential growth. There may be juxtapapillary detachment of the sensory retina and accumulation of subretinal fluid. The optic disc may be elevated as a result of direct infiltration of the tumor and may protrude into the vitreous. Rarely, this tumor may demonstrate a potential malignant sarcomatous transformation.

Symptoms

Progressive decreased vision; mild, unilateral, irreducible, slowly progressive axial proptosis; and headache are known to accompany optic disc meningioma.

Diagnosis

Fluorescein angiography may reveal multiple optociliary shunt vessels between the venous vessels within the retina. CT scan of the orbit may show thickening of the optic nerve, sometimes with calcification, or an increased contrast of the periphery of the nerve, called *railroad tracks*. MRI with gadolinium may reveal a typical fusiform thickening of the optic nerve as well as the extent of the tumor and, eventually, infiltration of the cavernous sinus, the extraocular muscles, or the sclera. A central scotoma or a nasal step defect may be a evident on visual field examination.

Differential Diagnosis

In the differential diagnosis, glioma and neurofibromatosis should be considered.

Histopathology

Optic disc meningioma may be of four types: *syncytial*, *mixed*, *fibroblastic*, or *angioblastic*. **Syncytial** optic disc meningioma, or meningoendotheliomatous, is the most frequent. The **mixed**, or transitional, type displays nervous tissue with whorls of fibroblasts and collagenous concretions of calcium and iron located in highly cellular areas, called *psammoma bodies*. **Fibroblastic** optic disc meningioma is composed of elongated spindle cells. In the **angioblastic** type, there is a conspicuous network of capillaries. The optic nerve is compressed. The subarachnoid space may be obliterated by sheets of meningoendothelial tumor cells.

Treatment

Optic disc meningioma should be observed. Surgical exploration, complete excision, orbital exenteration in children, and optic nerve decompression carry the risk of intraorbital spreading of tumor or of further visual deterioration and ocular motor nerve damage. Radiation therapy may be performed.

Neuroblastoma

Neuroblastoma (*sympathicoblastoma*) is a malignant tumor of the paraspinal ganglion chain or of medulla or adrenal glands and may involve the optic disc. *It is the most common metastatic orbital solid tumor in childhood.* Neuroblastoma occurs in children younger than 6 years, is rapidly fatal (in less than 3 years), and may metastasize to the orbit, lung, liver, and bones.

It arises from the primitive neuroblasts, or **sympathoblasts**, of the sympathetic system, most commonly from the retroperitoneal adrenal medulla, followed by thorax, cervix, and pelvis. Two types of neuroblastoma are recognized: **pepper type**, which metastasizes locally, and **Hutchinson type**, which metastasizes early in the skull, long bones, and orbit.

Neuroblastoma may appear as a papilledema or as optic nerve atrophy.

Symptoms

Proptosis may occur abruptly and usually is bilateral. Ecchymosis of the lower eyelids may be unilateral or bilateral. Periorbital edema, globe displacement, and subconjunctival hemorrhage are known to occur in neuroblastoma. Other symptoms are myoclonic encephalopathy or opsomyoclonus, characterized by nonrhythmic horizontal and vertical oscillations of the eyes (called *dancing eye syndrome*). Horner's syndrome secondary to mediastinal involvement, tonic pupil, and heterochromia iridis, with hypochromia of the ipsilateral iris, are reported. Truncal ataxia, an abdominal mass, diarrhea, vomiting, pallor, weight loss, and hypertension also characterize this condition.

Diagnosis

In metastatic neuroblastoma, CT scan may reveal a poorly defined lytic area of bony destruction and lucency secondary to necrosis, usually in the superotemporal part of the orbit and in the zygoma. Levels of vanillylmandelic acid (VMA) will be increased owing to catecholamine secretion by the tumor. Orbital biopsy should be performed extraperiosteally, because an intact periorbita may be a barrier to tumor extension.

Differential Diagnosis

Among conditions that should be considered in the differential diagnosis are trauma, orbital cellulitis, orbital tumors that develop rapidly (e.g., rhabdomyosarcoma, Ewing's sarcoma, medulloblastoma, Wilms' tumor) and esthesioneuroblastoma.

Histopathology

On histologic examination, small cells having minimal cytoplasm and hyperchromatic nuclei often are arranged in a rosette fashion around a central mass of fibrils. Among these dark-staining cells are **embryonal ganglion cells**, which are large and round and contain pale vesicular nuclei. Massive necrosis and Homer-Wright pseudorosettes may be seen.

Treatment

Treatment usually is palliative. Local or total body irradiation, followed by bone marrow rescue, may be undertaken. Aggressive systemic chemotherapy involves use of such agents as cisplatin, doxorubicin (Adriamycin), cyclophosphamide, vincristine, carmustine, or melphalan. Surgical removal of the primary tumor and autologous bone marrow transplantation are indicated.

Neurofibromatosis

Neurofibromatosis, also known as *von Recklinghausen's disease*, is a generalized, hereditary, familial, multiple hamartomatosis that occurs with equal frequency in both genders. The disease, an autosomal dominant disorder with incomplete penetrance, also may occur sporadically, usually at 10 years of age. It is characterized by neuroectodermal tumors that involve the eye, skin, nervous system, endocrine glands, and bones. Neurofibromatosis usually is stationary or slowly progressive over a long period. It may be associated with retinoblastoma.

Basically, two clinical forms of neurofibromatosis are identified: **NF-1**, von Recklinghausen's disease, the most common, and **NF-2**, bilateral acoustic neurofibromatosis. Some other types that have been described are **NF-3**, segmental neurofibromatosis, and **NF-4**, multiple café au lait spots only.

Neurofibromatosis may appear as a diffuse choroidal involvement or, rarely, as small whitish lesions in the retina, hemispheres placed against a refractile, white, slightly uneven base that often have secondary dystrophic calcification. The latter are called *astrocytic hamartomas* and may resemble the lesions of tuberous sclerosis. Peripheral retinal vascular occlusions also are seen. An anastomotic loop may be present that obliterates the arteries and veins. The arteries are markedly narrowed and sheathed. Retinal ischemia is possible, in association with widespread preretinal proliferation. Islands of nonperfused retina are seen in the posterior pole, extending toward the center of the macula, and in the periphery. There may be a fibrotic pucker and proliferative vascular changes, with tortuosity. Multiple pigmented lesions in the fundus, mottling, or an appearance similar to retinitis pigmentosa may be demonstrated. Nonspecific cystoid degeneration of the sensory retina can occur, as can retrobulbar neuritis. Ischemia of the optic nerve with subsequent papilledema and optic atrophy may develop. Occasionally, there may be photoreceptor degeneration.

Neurofibromatosis may be due to a distinct chromosomal abnormality in NF-1, a gene located on the long arm of chromosome 17 at locus 17q11.2, and to a totally different gene in NF-2, located on the long arm of chromosome 22 at locus 22q12. It may arise from the sheaths of the peripheral nerves.

Symptoms

If the macula is affected in neurofibromatosis, decreased vision is likely, although otherwise the condition may be asymptomatic. In **NF-1**, café au lait spots (six or more) measuring more than 1.5 cm in diameter appear on the skin. Affected persons may exhibit peripheral dermal and neural tumors of various sizes, in the central nervous system, cranial nerves (particularly the eighth nerve), vestibulocochlearis, and spinal nerve. Eyelid plexiform fibroma may be present, featuring a lazy, S-shaped configuration of the upper eyelid and appearing on palpation as a **bag of worms**. Elephantiasis neuromatosa of the disc, pedunculated skin fibroma molluscum, inguinal and axillary freckling, prominent corneal nerves, ectropion uveae, and unilateral ptosis due to orbital involvement of the tumor are other reported symptoms.

NF-1 also may be marked by the occurrence of pulsating exophthalmos due to defects in the greater wing of the sphenoid with cerebrospinal fluid pulsations, although a bruit is not associated. Rarely, enophthalmos due to sphenoid wing dysplasia occurs. Other symptoms include pseudoarthrosis of the tibia, acquired scoliosis, facial asymmetry with partial hemiatrophy, short stature, mild cognitive impairment, unilateral congenital glaucoma, bilateral Lisch nodules of the iris, optic nerve glioma, and gaze-evoked amaurosis caused by optociliary shunt vessels.

The symptoms of **NF-2** include deafness, bilateral acoustic neuroma, and symptoms related to other disorders such as cerebellopontine angle syndrome, multiple neurofibromas, meningioma, glioma, schwannoma, ependymoma, myelinated nerve fibers, bone cysts, spheno-orbital encephalocele, pheochromocytoma, scoliosis, and hydrocephalus. The condition may progress to malignant degeneration, which may lead to peripheral fibrosarcoma, neurofibrosarcoma, or malignant schwannoma.

Diagnosis

CT scan and T2-weighted MRI may reveal asymmetric widening of the optic nerves and thickening of the optic chiasm. Visual evoked potentials should be assessed to determine optic nerve function and monitor possible involvement of the chiasm. Visual field examination may be normal.

Differential Diagnosis

Retinitis pigmentosa and tuberosis sclerosis should be considered in the differential diagnosis.

Histopathology

Histopathologically, the choroid may be slightly or massively involved, in which case it appears thickened by diffuse placoid lesions that contain nonpigmented spindle-shaped cells, such as Schwann cells and fibroblasts, oriented randomly or in palisades. The number of ganglion cells is increased. Sometimes, numerous plump dendritic melanocytes are seen. The choriocapillaris usually is spared. Nerve fibers often course through the tumor. A mixture of hamartomatous neural and nevus elements or a glial hamartoma might be evident.

Treatment

Symptomatic tumors should be surgically excised. Plastic surgery of the eyelid may be undertaken. EBR, growth hormone replacement, and chemotherapy are other therapeutic options. Genetic counseling should be offered. Glaucoma and amblyopia should be treated appropriately.

Choroidal Metastases

Choroidal metastases are rapidly growing malignant tumors that spread to the choroid from a distant primary neoplasm. *They are the most common intraocular malignancies.* In female patients, they metastasize more frequently from breast and lung carcinoma, whereas in male patients, they spread from lung and bronchus or gastrointestinal or prostate cancer. Less commonly, they may spread from other primary lesions in the kidney, pancreas, testicle, skin, pharynx, thyroid, ovary, uterus, bladder, or adrenal gland. Additional primary tumors include atrial myxoma, lymphoma, fibrosarcoma, neuroblastoma, osteosarcoma, Ewing's sarcoma, choriocarcinoma, and choroidal melanoma of the opposite eye. Occasionally, choroid metastases present before the primary tumor; in this case, the tumor is part of visceral malignancy and has an inevitably lethal outcome.

Choroidal metastases appear as solitary or multiple, multifocal, multinodular, more commonly bilateral, circumscribed, moderately elevated (3–4 mm), depigmented, pale, creamy white or yellow-gray, placoid or dome-shaped, oval masses, sometimes with ill-defined borders. They measure approximately 2–4 dd and are located mostly at the posterior pole, between the vascular arcades, usually within the macula. They may overlie RPE alterations.

Tumors usually have greater vascularity than does the surrounding choroid. They rarely penetrate the vitreous. Mottled brown pigment clumping or scattered orange pigment may be seen on the tumor surface, giving rise to a pattern called *leopard spots*. Often, there is a secondary, extensive, nonrhegmatogenous serous retinal detachment with sharply abrupt delineation and subretinal fluid but no retinal breaks. Retinal vessels may be attenuated, and choroidal congestion may be present.

Symptoms

Choroidal metastases may be asymptomatic. Symptoms that can occur include blurred vision, distortion, painless decreased visual acuity, floaters and flashes, a peripheral field defect, and photopsia.

Diagnosis

Fluorescein angiography initially may reveal hypofluorescence with delayed choroidal filling and, in a later phase, hyperfluorescence of the increased vascularity and multiple points and collection of dye in the subretinal space. Digital indocyanine green videoangiography may reveal a relative hypofluorescence without angiographically apparent tumor vascularity. A-scan ultrasonography may demonstrate an elevated retina, with a bumpy or lobulated surface and an irregular internal structure with predominantly moderate to high reflectivity but no acoustic shadowing. MRI, spectroscopy, CT scan of the orbit and abdomen, and routine chest roentgenograms all may contribute to making the diagnosis. Vitreal fine-needle aspiration biopsy might be useful. The plasma CEA level may be elevated. Visual field examination may reveal dense scotoma with steep borders.

Differential Diagnosis

In the differential diagnosis, amelanotic choroidal melanoma, choroidal hemangioma, choroidal osteoma, choroidal neovascularization with a disciform scar, posterior scleritis, ocular lymphoma, and granulomatous uveitis should be considered.

Histopathology

The primary tumor usually is evident. Histologic evaluation will reveal atrophy of the RPE and retinal detachment.

Treatment

Palliative radiation therapy is generally performed. Use of EBR, in which ^{60}Co or an electronic beam is employed as the energy source, is preceded by use of a *treatment simulator* for radiographically defining the tumor volume that requires radiation. Chemotherapeutic agents that are useful include dactinomycin (actinomycin D, Cosmegen), 0.04 mg/kg/week IV, and doxorubicin (Adriamycin), 60 mg/m^2/week IV. Hormonal therapy includes the administration of tamoxifen (Nolvadex), 20 mg/day PO, in breast cancer. In prostate cancer, diethylstilbestrol,

1–5 mg PO three times a day, or luteinizing hormone–releasing hormone antagonists may be administered.

Optic Disc Metastasis

Optic disc metastasis is an exceptionally rare metastatic lesion that usually occurs as a direct extension to the disc of a choroidal malignancy, a distant renal cancer, bronchogenic carcinoma, breast cancer, meningeal cancer, or skin cancer. It appears as a solid, cauliflower-shaped, amelanotic tumor having multiple prominent papillae on its surface, each of them enclosing a central, ill-defined space or a vessel. It is usually located either in the juxtapapillary region or in the disc, which may be hyperemic, edematous, or atrophic, enlarged, chalky white, or elevated over most of its surface, with a slightly lobulated contour. There sometimes is a surrounding choroidal infiltration, which may appear as leopard-spots pigmentation. Optic disc metastasis may simulate an optic neuritis or an acute anterior ischemic optic neuropathy. Retinal vessels may be tortuous and dilated. Rarely, retinal vein occlusion occurs. Occasionally, hemorrhage is present. The vitreous commonly is clear, but linear arrays of vitreal spherules emanating from the disc may also be present.

Diagnosis

Fluorescein angiography may reveal punctate hyperfluorescence of the disc.

Differential Diagnosis

Optic neuritis and anterior ischemic optic neuropathy should be included in the differential diagnosis of optic disc metastasis.

Histopathology

On histologic examination, the normal neural tissue of the disc may be seen to be replaced entirely by the tumoral mass. There also may be cystic spaces.

Treatment

No treatment is effective. Any optic disc metastatic tumor is lethal.

Suggested Reading

Blodi FC. Tumors. In A Sorsby (ed), Modern Ophthalmology, vol 3 (2nd ed). Philadelphia: Lippincott, 1972;351–427.

Buettner H. Spontaneous involution of a choroid osteoma. Arch Ophthalmol 1990;108:1517–1518.

Char D. Intraocular Masquerade Syndrome. In W Tasman, EA Jaeger, MM Parks, et al. (eds), Duane's Clinical Ophthalmology, vol 4. Philadelphia: Lippincott–Raven, 1996;53:11–16.

Collaborative Ocular Melanoma Study Group. Accuracy of diagnosis of choroidal melanomas. Arch Ophthalmol 1990;108:1268–1273.

Destro M, D'Amico DJ, Gragoudas ES, et al. Retinal manifestations of neurofibromatosis. Arch Ophthalmol 1991;109:662–666.

Ellsworth RM, Boxrud CA. Retinoblastoma. In W Tasman, EA Jaeger, MM Parks, et al. (eds), Duane's Clinical Ophthalmology, vol 3. Philadelphia: Lippincott–Raven, 1996;35:1–19.

Erzurum SA, Jampol LM, Territo C, O'Grady R. Primary malignant melanoma of the optic nerve simulating a melanocytoma. Arch Ophthalmol 1992;110: 684–686.

Glaser JS. Infranuclear Disorders of the Eye Movement. In W Tasman, EA Jaeger, MM Parks, et al. (eds), Duane's Clinical Ophthalmology, vol 2. Philadelphia: Lippincott–Raven, 1996;12:25–30.

Harbour JW, De Potter P, Shields CL, Shields JA. Uveal metastasis from carcinoid tumor. Ophthalmology 1994;101:1084–1090.

Jakobiec FA, Jones IS. Neurogenic Tumors. In W Tasman, EA Jaeger, MM Parks, et al. (eds), Duane's Clinical Ophthalmology, vol 2. Philadelphia: Lippincott–Raven, 1996;41:1–45.

Katz SE, Rootman J, Goldberg RA. Secondary and Metastatic Tumors of the Orbit. In W Tasman, EA Jaeger, MM Parks, et al. (eds), Duane's Clinical Ophthalmology, vol 2. Philadelphia: Lippincott–Raven, 1996;46:41–42.

Kilmarin DJ, Mooney DJ, Acheson RA, et al. von Hippel–Lindau disease and familial polyposis coli in the same family. Arch Ophthalmol 1996;114:1294.

Kincaid MC, Cunningham RD. Retinopathy of Blood Dyscrasias. In W Tasman, EA Jaeger, MM Parks, et al. (eds), Duane's Clinical Ophthalmology, vol 3. Philadelphia: Lippincott–Raven, 1996;18:1–18.

Landau K, Dossetor FM, Hoyt WF, Muci-Mendoza R. Retinal hamartoma in neurofibromatosis 2. Arch Ophthalmol 1990;108:328–329.

Leys AM. The Eye and the Renal Diseases. In W Tasman, EA Jaeger, MM Parks, et al. (eds), Duane's Clinical Ophthalmology, vol 5. Philadelphia: Lippincott–Raven, 1996;31:5–30.

Murphree AL, Villablanca JG, Deegan WF II, et al. Chemotherapy plus local treatment in the management of intraocular retinoblastoma. Arch Ophthalmol 1996;114:1348–1356.

Nevin S, Kiloh LG. Organic Affections. In A Sorsby (ed), Modern Ophthalmology, vol 2 (2nd ed). Philadelphia: Lippincott, 1972;447–508.
Nork TM, Millecchia LL, De Venecia GB, et al. Immunocytochemical features of retinoblastoma in an adult. Arch Ophthalmol 1996;114:1402–1406.
Orcutt JC. Neuro-Ophthalmic Aspects of Orbital Disease. In W Tasman, EA Jaeger, MM Parks, et al. (eds), Duane's Clinical Ophthalmology, vol 2. Philadelphia: Lippincott–Raven, 1996;37:1–15, 33–36.
Pollock SC, Awh CC, Dutton JJ. Cutaneous melanoma metastatic to the optic disc and vitreous. Arch Ophthalmol 1991;109:1352–1354.
Ridley MD, McDonald R, Sternberg PA, et al. Retinal manifestations of ocular lymphoma (reticulum cell sarcoma). Ophthalmology 1992;99:1153–1161.
Roseman RL, Gass JDM. Solitary hypopigmented nevus of the retinal pigment epithelium in the macula. Arch Ophthalmol 1992;110:1358–1359.
Sahel JA, Pesavento R, Frederick AR, Albert DM. Melanoma arising de novo over a 16-month period. Arch Ophthalmol 1988;106:381–384.
Sandgren O. Ocular amyloidosis, with special reference to the hereditary forms with vitreous involvement. Surv Ophthalmol 1995;40(3):173–192.
Schanzer MC, Font RL, O'Mailey RE. Primary ocular malignant lymphoma associated with acquired immune deficiency syndrome. Ophthalmology 1991;98:88–91.
Schlaegel TF Jr. Differential Diagnosis (Masquerade Syndrome). In W Tasman, EA Jaeger, MM Parks, et al. (eds), Duane's Clinical Ophthalmology, vol 4. Philadelphia: Lippincott–Raven, 1996;60:1–6.
Shakin EP, Shields JA. The Eye and Ocular Adnexa in Systemic Malignancy. In W Tasman, EA Jaeger, MM Parks, et al. (eds), Duane's Clinical Ophthalmology, vol 5. Philadelphia: Lippincott–Raven, 1996;34:1–4.
Shields JA. Tumors of Uveal Tract. In W Tasman, EA Jaeger, MM Parks, et al. (eds), Duane's Clinical Ophthalmology, vol 4. Philadelphia: Lippincott–Raven, 1996;68:1–5.
Shields JA, Eagle RC, Barr CC, et al. Adenocarcinoma of retinal pigment epithelium arising from a juxtapapillary histoplasmosis scar. Arch Ophthalmol 1994;112:650–653.
Shields JA, Shields CL, De Potter P, Belmont JB. Progressive enlargement of a choroidal osteoma. Arch Ophthalmol 1995;113:815–820.
Steuhl KP, Rohrbach JM, Knorr M, Thiel HJ. Significance, specificity and ultrastructural localization of HMG-45 antigen in pigmented ocular tumors. Ophthalmology 1993;100:208–215.

12

Parasitic Retinopathy

Toxoplasmosis

Toxoplasmosis is a congenital or acquired chorioretinopathy caused by an intracellular protozoan parasite, *Toxoplasma gondii*, passed on to humans through contact with infected cats, rabbits, rats, and fowl, or through eating undercooked meat. It occurs more commonly in white (especially teenage) girls but rarely in the elderly and frequently is seen in patients with the acquired immunodeficiency syndrome (AIDS). It may be associated with microcephaly, internal hydrocephaly, necrotizing encephalitis, cerebral calcifications, myocarditis, atypical pneumonia, hepatosplenomegaly, and deafness.

Congenital toxoplasmosis is the most common form (Figure 12-1). It appears as a bilateral chorioretinitis located between the equator and the posterior pole and often in the macula and disc. In the macula, usually a large (sometimes up to 3–4 dd), sharply demarcated, irregular, yellow-green scar is surrounded by variably sized, black pigmentation called *rosette focus of François*. Occasionally, the macula appears as a **pseudocoloboma**, or it may be surrounded by border pigmentation called *ink spot of Pillat*. The choroid appears with pigment dispersion as a necrotic lesion that seems to be pathognomonic for congenital toxoplasmosis. Vessels course over the choroidal scar. Also, multiple gray-white retinal lesions involve the outer retina and, in time, may form punctate dots, called *salt-and-pepper* fundus. Sometimes, the background has a peculiar tessellated appearance of **tigroid fundus**. The sclera often is visible beneath the healed choroidal lesions. The disc

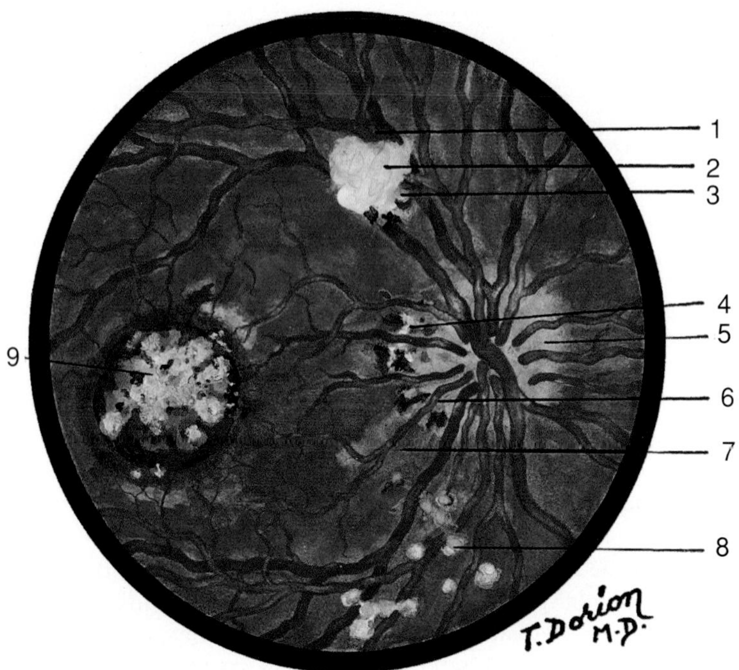

Figure 12-1. *Toxoplasmosis. (1) Retinal hemorrhage. (2) Satellite lesion. (3) Old necrotizing lesion. (4) Choroidal scar. (5) Swollen disc. (6) Vessels coursing over the scar. (7) Nerve fiber defect. (8) Retinal infiltrates. (9) Rosette focus of François.*

may be congested and elevated, with blurred margins; in later stages, it may become atrophic. The vitreous may appear with inflammatory grapevines, covered by **wet-snow** microabscesses.

Acquired toxoplasmosis usually is a reactivation of congenital toxoplasmosis. It may remain quiescent for a long period. In acute stages, the retina appears slightly translucent and gray. Onset is followed by chorioretinal lesions that commonly are solitary and fluffy white or yellow-brown, having indistinct margins. The variably sized lesions are elevated moderately and are surrounded by recurrent hemorrhage or retinal edema. Usually, acquired toxoplasmosis is located at the posterior pole, but it also can be found at the equator or anteriorly. Precipitates may be seen along the peripheral vessels. At a later stage, chorioretinal scars may develop. Often, new chorioretinal lesions (called *satellite lesions*) occur next to an old scar.

Generally, the macula is spared in acquired toxoplasmosis. Involvement of the macula results in a large amount of edema (called *central exudative retinitis of Rieger*). An epithelial membrane of the macula also may be present. The disc may be congested, and a nerve fiber bundle defect or even optic atrophy may be present. Occasionally, a bright solitary lesion (*chorioretinitis of Jensen*) is located in the peripapillary region. The vitreous may exhibit a dense accumulation of cells in clumps over the disc; vitritis; or exudates that appear as a **headlight in the fog.**

Tractional retinal detachment may accompany onset. The arteries may display refractile deposits and segmental arteritis, or an arterial occlusion may form. Periphlebitis, sheathing (with or without venous occlusion), and secondary hemorrhages may be seen. Several punched-out pigmented choroidal lesions may occur, through which the sclera may become visible and which may lead to full-thickness retinal necrosis. Also, there may be subretinal neovascularization.

Symptoms

Symptoms of toxoplasmosis are usually floaters and blurred vision.

Diagnosis

The Sabin-Feldman dye test is positive, with the antibody titer rising from 1 to 64 to 1 to 128. The complement fixation test, skin test, and serum enzyme immunoassay index for anti-*Toxoplasma* IgG and IgM antibodies usually are positive. A fluorescent treponemal antibody absorption test should be performed. Diagnosis is supported by the human immunodeficiency (HIV) test, enzyme-linked immunosorbent assay (ELISA), complete blood cell count and platelet count, chest roentgenogram, and aqueous polymerase chain reaction assay (PCR). Fluorescein angiography shows dye accumulation in the foci, representing areas of active toxoplasmosis retinochoroiditis.

Differential Diagnosis

The differential diagnosis should consider toxocariasis, syphilis, tuberculosis, uveitis, and tumors.

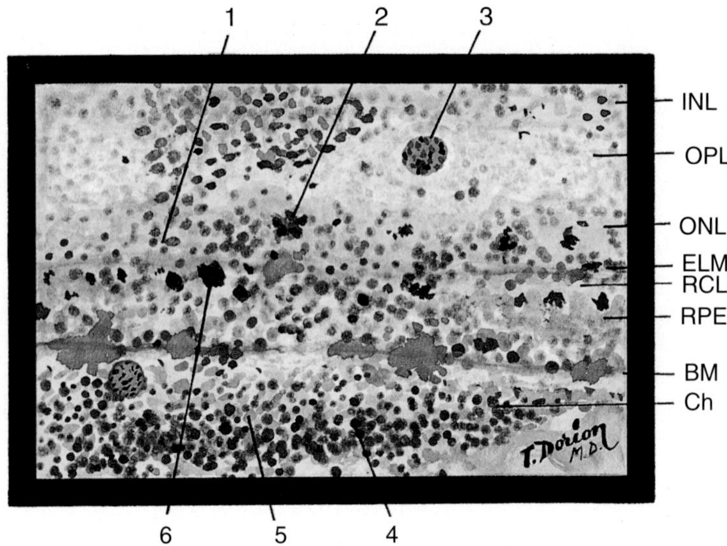

Figure 12-2. *Histopathologic findings in toxoplasmosis. (1) Destruction of the retinal layers by a coagulative necrosis. (2)* Toxoplasma gondii *as a free active form (tachyzoite). (3)* Toxoplasma gondii *as a cystic inactive form (bradyzoite). (4) Lymphocytic infiltration of the choroid. (5) Epithelioid infiltration. (6) Macrophages. (INL, inner nuclear layer; OPL, outer plexiform layer; ONL, outer nuclear layer; ELM, external limiting membrane; RCL, rod and cone layer [photoreceptors]; RPE, retinal pigment epithelium; BM, Bruch's membrane; Ch, choroid.)*

Histopathology

Histologic analysis shows a necrotizing retinitis mostly in the inner retinal layer (Figure 12-2). The retinal pigment epithelium is destroyed in some areas, with white-grayish or black pigment in others. A granuloma with a central zone of necrosis may be located in the inner layers of the retina. Epithelioid cells, macrophages, and lymphocytic infiltrations are present. The protozoan toxoplasma may be seen as a free, active, multiplying form (called *tachyzoite* or *endozoite*) and as a slow-growing, comma-shaped, cluster form enclosed by an irregular wall (called *bradyzoite*) in a coagulative necrotic area of the retina or in areas adjacent to a chorioretinal scar. Cell accumulation also may be present in the vitreous.

Treatment

Treatment relies on topical and systemic corticosteroids such as prednisolone 1% (Pred Forte), OU 1 drop three times a day, and prednisone, 60 mg PO daily. Topical cycloplegics are also used: homatropine 2% or scopolamine 0.25%, OU twice a day; antimalarial pyrimethamine, 1 g PO four times a day; or sulfadiazine, 25–100 mg/day PO. Other agents include folinic acid, 10 mg/day PO for 4 weeks; erythromycin or tetracycline, 250 mg PO four times a day; clindamycin, 1.8–2.4 g/day PO in divided doses; trimethoprim-sulfamethoxazole tablets (Bactrim DS), 80 mg trimethoprim and 400 mg sulfamethoxazole, PO twice a day for 2 weeks; spiramycin, 3–4 g/day PO in pregnancy continued until delivery; leukovorin, 10–15 mg/day PO for 6 weeks; dapsone, 50 mg PO four times a day; and atovaquone, 750 mg PO three times a day. Anticonvulsants such as phenytoin (Dilantin), 5 mg/kg/day PO in divided doses, are given to children. Other options are vitrectomy, photocoagulation, and cryotherapy. Observation is recommended.

Toxocariasis

Toxocariasis is a unilateral retinochoroidopathy (Figure 12-3) caused by the larva of a roundworm of the dog, a nematode parasite (*Toxocara canis*). The disorder may occur as two clinical types: *granuloma* and *endophthalmitis. Ocular toxocariasis is not associated with the systemic toxocariasis disease* exhibiting fever and hepatosplenomegaly and called *visceral larva migrans*.

Toxocariasis granuloma appears in a quiet eye as a hemispheric, whitish, slightly elevated solitary mass (approximately 1 dd). It is located more commonly in the macula as a full-thickness macular granuloma, in the maculopapillary bundle, in the midperiphery, or peripherally anterior to the equator. The mass may display a glistening white core and long, straight, grayish strands that may extend into the vitreous. Possible retinal striae (called *tension lines*) and fibrous bands that radiate from the granuloma may cause vitreous traction, exudative retinal detachment, disciform macular detachment, or a dragged disc. Sometimes, the larva of the parasite may be seen as a darker crescentic area in a yellow-white mass. This granuloma may grow rapidly and may be mistaken for a retinoblastoma.

Toxocariasis endophthalmitis appears as a diffuse exudative process in the peripheral retina, with inflammatory cells and large connective bands extending into the vitreous. The disorder is more advanced after

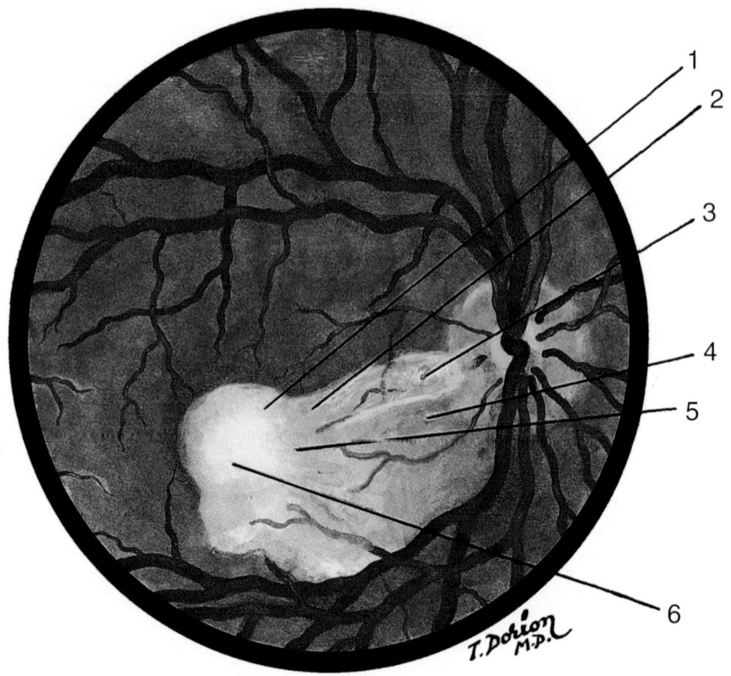

Figure 12-3. *Toxocariasis. (1) Solitary granuloma. (2) Retinal folds. (3) Fibrous bands, emanating from the disc. (4) Exudative retinal detachment. (5) Vitreous traction. (6) Gliotic mass.*

the larva has died. There may be preretinal and vitreous hemorrhages and, rarely, papillitis or vitreous abscess. Retinal artery occlusion, exudative retinal detachment, and heteropsia of the macula also may be present. Usually, fibrous bands emanate from the disc, and whitish-yellow fibrous scar tissue forms. Occasionally, there are visible tracks across the fundus; these tubular structures beneath the retina represent a previous passage of the parasite *T. canis*. Retinal folds, glial proliferation, and scars also may be present.

Symptoms

The disorder exhibits unilateral blurred vision and leukokoria.

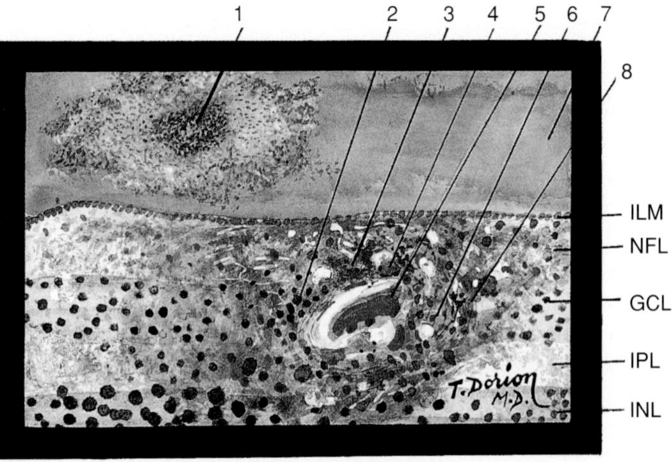

Figure 12-4. *Histopathologic findings in toxocariasis. (1) Eosinophilic abscess in the vitreous. (2) Lymphocytic infiltration. (3) Hemorrhagic necrosis. (4) Foreign-body giant cells. (5) Tracks of migrating second-stage larva. (6) Fibrin. (7) Vitreous. (8) Epithelioid cells. (ILM, internal limiting membrane; NFL, nerve fiber layer; GCL, ganglion cell layer; IPL, inner plexiform layer; INL, inner nuclear layer.)*

Diagnosis

Paracentesis of the anterior chamber is undertaken to detect eosinophils. The serum ELISA test is positive, and fluorescein angiography may show leakage.

Histopathology

Histologic appraisal shows a possible retinochoroidal granuloma (or eosinophilic mass of fibrin), lymphocytes, epithelioid cells, and foreign-body giant cells (Figure 12-4). A larva of some 30 μm in diameter and 250 μm long may be present. Hemorrhagic necrosis, multiple infiltrations of eosinophils, neutrophils, and lymphocytes, and the tracks of the migrating larva may be seen. Occasionally, a vitreous abscess also may be present.

Treatment

Treatment for toxocariasis is supportive and focuses on the disorder's symptoms.

Cysticercosis

Cysticercosis is a usually unilateral exudative retinitis that occurs as a parasitic infection by a bladder worm, *Cysticercus cellulosae*, the larval form of the pork tapeworm (*Taenia solium*). The disorder is endemic in all countries and continents except Australia and usually is associated with central nervous system involvement.

Cysticercosis is produced by eating raw or inadequately cooked pork, as the pig is the intermediate host of *T. solium*. The parasite may remain harmlessly in the human small intestine for years, attaining a length of 2–7 feet. It hatches and remains there until emerging *oncospheres* penetrate the wall of the intestine and disseminate throughout the body through hematologic spread via posterior ciliary arteries. It develops to a mature larva of *C. cellulosae* and localizes (most frequently subcutaneously) in the intermediate muscular tissue, eye, and brain. That cyst may migrate and break the retina, producing a hole or a tear, retinal and vitreous hemorrhage, retinal detachment, fibrous proliferation, and inflammation. It is seen floating into the vitreous or in the subretinal space, but it may be present also subchoroidally.

Cysticercosis appears as a whitish, round vesicle up to 20 mm in size, with protruding *scolex*, sucker, and hooks. It undulates in a slow, pendulumlike movement, retracts into a white mass and, as stated earlier, may break the retina. The retina may exhibit areas of atrophy, and a macular star may be present. Additionally, the optic disc may be swollen.

Symptoms

Cysticercosis may be asymptomatic. However, symptoms include subcutaneous, painless nodules; such neurologic disorders as seizures, mental deterioration, personality disturbances, and intracranial pressure; and internal hydrocephalus with headache, giddiness, nerve palsies, meningitis, or transverse myelitis. In Finland, anemia is the predominant symptom.

Diagnosis

B-scan ultrasonography may identify the cyst. The excised cyst is microscopically examined. Diagnostic tools include computed tomography scan of the brain; roentgenograms of skin, orbit, and brain may reveal calcified lesions. Enzyme electrophoresis of glucose phosphate isomerase is performed. Cerebrospinal fluid analysis may reveal an increased number of mononuclear cells and an increased pressure.

Differential Diagnosis

Considerations for the differential diagnosis include retinoblastoma and epilepsy.

Histopathology

Histologic examination reveals a granulomatous reaction (frequently surrounded by a fibrous capsule) in the vitreous or retina. A calcified cyst with a collapsed wall and a spindle-shaped body with scolex and numerous hooklets also may be present.

Treatment

Treatment includes praziquantel, 10 mg/kg PO (only one dose) or, in neurologic disturbances, 50 mg/kg in three divided doses for 15 days; niclosamide for adults, four tablets (2 g) chewed thoroughly and swallowed with water (only one dose in the morning before eating), followed after 2 hours by a purge with magnesium sulfate, 15–30 mg PO to eliminate the cysts (for children, two to three tablets, according to weight); dichlorophen, 75 mg/kg, to a maximum 6 g (one dose); and mebendazole, 300 mg PO twice a day for 3 days. Oral corticosteroids also are useful. Surgical excision is an additional intervention.

Lyme Disease Choroiditis

Choroiditis may be part of a systemic disease, Lyme disease, that is caused by the spirochete *Borrelia burgdorferi*. Lyme disease is transmitted by the deer tick vector *Ixodes dammini*, reported for the first time in Old Lyme, CT, in 1975. This tick may harbor another pathogen, *Ehrlichia bacterium*, which produces a human granulocytic ehrlichiosis that usually is fatal. The disorder occurs more frequently in New England and the Middle Atlantic states, especially in persons who are camping outdoors.

Lyme disease appears as a diffuse bilateral choroiditis with papilledema, vitritis, exudative retinal detachment, and even panophthalmia. Exudates are found in the macula, and the disorder is associated with pars planitis, anterior ischemic optic neuropathy, acute idiopathic optic neuritis, retinal hemorrhage, optic atrophy, and pseudotumor cerebri.

Symptoms

Symptoms occur in three stages that usually begin in the summer. The **first stage** is associated with skin lesions, such as erythema chronicum migrans, or with rash. Myalgias, headache, fatigue, chills, low back pain, and arthralgias and stiffness of the neck also ensue.

The **second stage** is characterized by meningitis, peripheral radiculoneuropathies, hemiparesis, and cranial nerve palsies (nerves III, IV, or VI). This stage also produces numbness of the tongue and fingers, palpitations, cardiac manifestations (e.g., atrioventricular block), or myopericarditis. Blurred vision, decreased vision (up to hand motion), relative afferent pupillary reflex, optic neuritis, papilledema, and ischemic optic neuropathy also result. Additional effects are diplopia, pseudotumor cerebri, exposure keratitis, retinal detachment, iritis, and panophthalmia.

The **third stage** exhibits migratory oligoarthritis, synovitis, joint effusion, lymphadenopathy, splenomegaly, orchitis, hepatitis, and pharyngitis.

Diagnosis

Serum Lyme titer for *B. burgdorferi* may be positive (1:256 for IgM, and 1:600 for IgG) along with a positive T-cell blastogenic response to the parasite. Indirect fluorescent antibody and ELISA should be performed. Visual field examination may reveal a paracentral scotoma and an inferior defect. Impairment of color vision is noted on Ishihara pseudoisochromatic plates. Magnetic resonance imaging of the brain may show multiple areas of demyelinization in the periventricular areas, in the brain stem, and in the cortex. For syphilis, serum rapid plasma reagin and fluorescent treponemal antibody absorption tests should be performed. A lumbar puncture may show a cerebrospinal fluid pleocytosis. A history of tick bite is relevant in diagnosis.

Differential Diagnosis

The differential diagnosis should include considerations of syphilis, acute rheumatic fever, rickettsiosis, and rheumatoid arthritis.

Treatment

Treatment includes the administration of ceftriaxone, 2 g/day IV for 2 weeks; doxycycline, 100 mg PO twice a day; tetracycline, 250 mg PO four times a day; penicillin VK, 500 mg PO four times a day for 2 weeks; erythromycin, 250 mg PO four times a day for 2 weeks; and amoxicillin, 250 mg PO three times a day for 2 weeks.

Corticosteroids administered topically include prednisolone 1%, 1 drop, or dexamethasone 0.1%, 1 drop, four times daily. For mydriatic-cycloplegic therapy, homatropine 2% or scopolamine 0.25% twice daily are useful.

Rift Valley Fever Retinopathy

Rift Valley fever retinopathy occurs in patients with a noncontagious, acute viral febrile infection from sheep and cattle. The disorder is transmitted to humans by the bite of the mosquitoes *Aedes*, *Culex*, and *Erethmapodites* and occurs in Kenya and Egypt and throughout Southern and Eastern Africa.

Rift Valley fever retinopathy appears as cotton-wool spots disseminated throughout the posterior pole. Hard exudates, usually as a **macular star**, also are present.

The disorder produces nonspecific influenzalike symptoms. Severe cases result in acute prostration, fever, low back pain, arthralgias, gastrointestinal distress, and hepatitis.

Treatment for this retinopathy is not effective.

Suggested Reading

Fish Rh, Hoslins JC, Kline LB. Toxoplasmosis neuroretinitis. Ophthalmology 1993;100:1177–1182.

Johnson MW, Greven CM, Jaffe GJ, et al. Atypical severe toxoplasmic retinochoroiditis in elderly patients. Ophthalmology 1997;104:48–57.

Lasser RI, Kornmehl EW, Pachner AR, et al. Neuro-ophthalmic manifestations of Lyme disease. Ophthalmology 1990;97:699–706.

Ridley H. Metazoan Infections. In A Sorsby (ed), Modern Ophthalmology, vol 2 (2nd ed). Philadelphia: Lippincott, 1972;213–228.

Schlaegel TF Jr, Knox DL. Uveitis and Parasitoses. In W Tasman, EA Jaeger, MM Parks, et al. (eds), Duane's Clinical Ophthalmology, vol 4. Philadelphia: Lippincott–Raven, 1996;52:1–17.

Tessler HH. Diagnosis and treatment of ocular toxoplasmosis. Focal Points 1989;3:2–11.

13

Metabolic Retinopathy

Gyrate Atrophy

Gyrate atrophy is a metabolic, congenital, autosomal recessive, progressive, diffuse chorioretinopathy. Usually, it is associated with high myopia, cystoid macular degeneration, cataract, or vitreous degeneration.

The disorder is caused by a deficiency of the enzyme *ornithine ketoacid aminotransferase*, resulting in a markedly elevated level of the amino acid **ornithine** (as much as 10 or 20 times normal) in blood, urine, cerebrospinal fluid, and aqueous humor.

Gyrate atrophy appears as numerous, sharply delineated, punched-out patches of choroidal atrophy (Figure 13-1). Usually, they are large, polygonal, scalloped, irregular, and garland-shaped and are located at the equator and surrounded by normal retina. These patches may extend anteriorly and continuously, as a confluent, arcuate, full-thickness chain of peripheral lesions, to the ora serrata, where dense bands of clumped pigment may be present. *These lesions totally spare the central retina* between the two vascular arcades. The fundus between the lesions is normal, and retinal vessels and larger choroidal vessels course normally through these areas. As the disease progresses, a velvetlike pigmentation and glistening crystals may be seen. At a later stage, a total chorioretinal atrophy may develop, involving also the choriocapillaris and the larger choroidal vessels, and bare white sclera becomes visible.

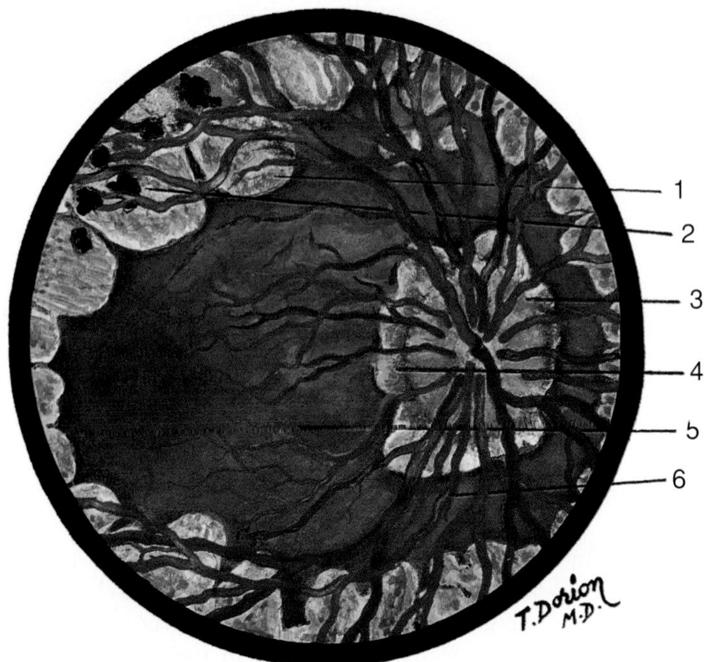

Figure 13-1. *Gyrate atrophy. (1) Midperipheral chorioretinal atrophy. (2) Pigment clumps. (3) Normal optic disc. (4) Peripapillary chorioretinal atrophy. (5) Normal retina. (6) Normal retinal vessels.*

Symptoms

Gyrate atrophy causes decreased visual acuity, night blindness, and tunnel vision.

Diagnosis

Constricted visual fields confirm the disorder. Electroretinography (ERG), electro-oculography, and dark adaptation are abnormal to nonrecordable.

Differential Diagnosis

Considerations for differential diagnosis include myopia, choroideremia, paving-stone degeneration, and thioridazine (Mellaril) toxicity.

Histopathology

Histologic evaluation reveals circumscribed areas of chorioretinal and choriocapillaris atrophy at midperiphery and at the peripheral and peripapillary fundus. An abrupt transition occurs between normal and atrophic areas. The choroid and outer retinal layers are absent, although the central retina, the optic disc, and the retinal vessels are normal.

Treatment

Treatment for gyrate atrophy is primarily a reduced protein diet with restriction of dietary arginine. Augmentation with supplemental vitamin B_6 (pyridoxine), 20–500 mg/day, and dietary lysine is helpful.

Amyloidosis

Also called *hyaline choroidal degeneration*, amyloidosis is a bilateral metabolic chorioretinopathy with deposition of an insoluble extracellular protein, called *amyloid*. The disorder may be primary or secondary and localized or generalized.

Primary amyloidosis, a systemic disease, may be nonfamilial or familial and autosomal dominant or idiopathic. **Secondary amyloidosis** may be caused by chronic infections, multiple myeloma, or neoplasia.

Amyloidosis appears as small, globular, waxy, sheetlike particles or as yellow-white clusters on the retina. They are located periarterially or in the vessel walls, producing vascular occlusion, or may be found along the optic nerve or in the choroid. They may appear in the vitreous as a proteinaceous material coating the retrolental fibrils (called *pseudopodia lentis*) first in the cortex adjacent to the retinal vessels and later in the anterior vitreous. In aphakic eyes, they may simulate an endophthalmitis. Initially, these opacities are granular, dull, and fibrillar and exhibit wispy fringes that may form strands attached to the retina or to the posterior face of the lens by thick footplates. Later, they appear as dense veil-like opacities with an irregular and waxy contour, resembling glass-wool.

Diagnosis

Diagnosis is confirmed by serum protein electrophoresis. Biopsy should be performed, and a diagnostic vitrectomy is recommended.

Histopathology

Histologic examination shows starlike amyloid structures, with a dense fibrillar center (approximately 5–10 µm in diameter) but longer in the vitreous (10–15 µm). The structures are filamentous, pale, eosinophilic, dichroic, and birefringent and are located in the vessels, in the perivascular region, and in the vitreous. The retinal and choroidal vessels are thickened.

Bietti's Crystalline Dystrophy

Bietti's crystalline dystrophy (*Bietti's tapetoretinal degeneration* or *Bietti's crystalline retinopathy*) is a bilateral, metabolic, autosomal recessive chorioretinopathy. Usually, this chorioretinopathy is associated with crystalline corneal dystrophy. The disease is probably due to a systemic abnormality of **lipid** metabolism.

The disorder may present in either a *regional* or a *diffuse* form. It appears as multiple fine dots (ranging from tiny to somewhat larger) that form as yellow-white, sparkling, glistening intraretinal crystals scattered throughout the posterior pole (Figure 13-2). Occasionally, clumps of retinal pigment, areas of chorioretinal atrophy, or sclerosis may be present.

Diagnosis

Fluorescein angiography may show a regional or diffuse loss of the retinal pigment epithelium (RPE) and of the choriocapillaris. ERG may be severely abnormal early in the disease.

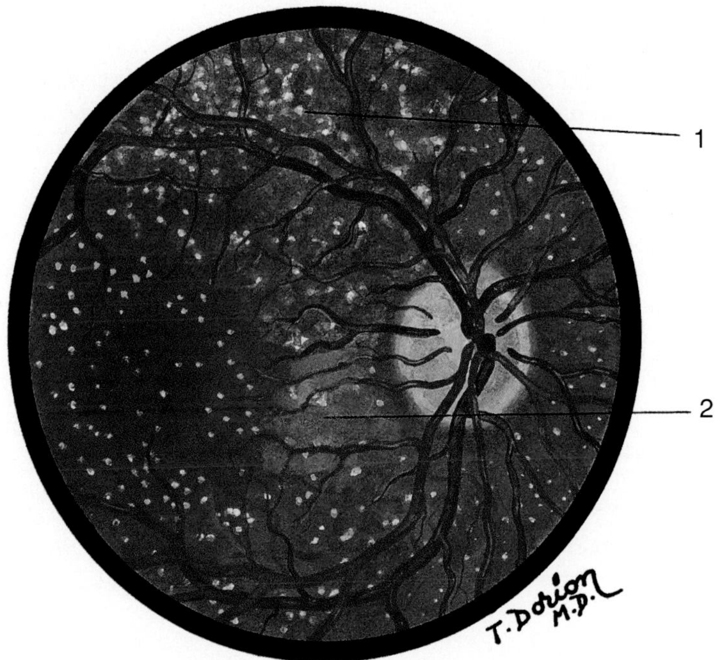

Figure 13-2. *Bietti's crystalline dystrophy. (1) Intraretinal crystalline deposits, scattered throughout the posterior fundus. (2) Area of chorioretinal atrophy.*

Symptoms

Symptoms of the regional form of Bietti's crystalline dystrophy may include reduced central visual acuity and pericentral scotoma that cause difficulty at near vision. In the diffuse form of the disease, poor night vision and impaired visual acuity at distance are accompanied by loss of peripheral vision.

Histopathology

Histologic evaluation reveals conglomerations of crystalline lipid material deposited in the RPE. The disorder also may signal atrophy of the RPE, the choriocapillaris, and the choroid.

Krabbe's Disease

Krabbe's disease also is called *globoid cell leukodystrophy*, *infantile diffuse cerebral sclerosis*, and *galactosyl ceramide lipidosis*. The disorder is a hereditary, bilateral, metabolic condition and is autosomal recessive. This sphingolipidosis, due to a deficiency of the enzyme *beta-galactosidase*, normally is concentrated in the myelin sheet and degrades galactosyl ceramide resulting from myelin turnover. As a result, lack of the enzyme produces an accumulation of **ceramide galactosidase** (*galactocerebroside*) in the tissues, with rapid central nervous system degeneration and diffuse cerebral sclerosis. Krabbe's disease appears as pallor of the disc with a decreased nerve fiber layer.

Symptoms

Symptoms of Krabbe's disease include irritability, motor and mental deterioration, nystagmus, deafness, and blindness. The disorder can be fatal by the age of 2 years because of ensuing emaciation.

Histopathology

Histologic examination demonstrates a bilateral atrophy of the retinal nerve fiber layer and of the ganglion cell layer. Globoid cells are found in the demyelinated regions.

Lipemia Retinalis

Variously known as *hyperlipoproteinemia type I*, *Burger-Grütz disease*, and *hyperchylomicronemia*, lipemia retinalis is a metabolic vascular disease in which the retinal vessels appear yellow (Figure 13-3). Usually, it occurs in familial or secondary hyperlipoproteinemia or in diabetes. The disorder is caused by a metabolic lipoprotein defect resulting in an elevated **triglyceride** serum level exceeding 2,000 mg/dl (normal, 165 mg/dl) and in increased **low-density lipoproteins**.

Lipemia retinalis appears as a lightened background and exhibits a marked diffuse discoloration of the hue of the blood column. The color is related to the level of the triglycerides and ranges from salmon pink to yellow, creamy, ivory, or white. The retinal vessels appear to be filled by a milky yellow fluid. They may have perivascular cuffs of lipid infil-

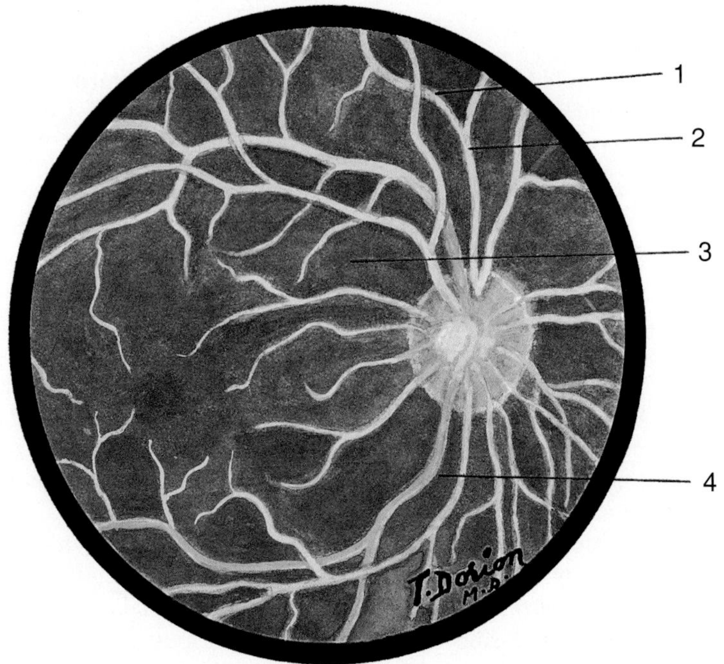

Figure 13-3. *Lipemia retinalis. (1) Perivascular infiltrates. (2) Milky, creamy, and ivory retinal vessels. (3) Lightened background. (4) Engorged vessels.*

tration, are dilated and engorged, and may lack the central-stripe light reflex. The choroidal vessels appear pinkish rather than red. The periphery is affected first.

Diagnosis

The diagnosis of lipemia retinalis is confirmed by increased levels of triglycerides, cholesterol, and low-density lipoproteins.

Histopathology

Histologic analysis reveals dilated retinal vessels with perivascular lipid infiltration. Usually, the retina, macula, and disc are normal.

Treatment

Treatment should be administered by an internist. Treatment includes a fat-restricted diet (10–20 g/day). Hypolipidemic drugs are useful for this disorder.

Fabry's Disease

Also known as *angiokeratoma corporis diffusum universale*, *alpha-galactosidase deficiency*, or *glycosphingolipid lipidosis*, Fabry's disease is a metabolic sphingolipid storage abnormality that is hereditary and X-linked recessive. It may involve the conjunctiva, the cornea, and the optic disc, may produce renal failure, and may be lethal at 30–40 years of age. It may be *primary* or *secondary* to systemic hypertension or to renal failure.

The disorder is due to a deficiency of the enzyme *alpha-galactosidase*, which may cause a progressive accumulation of the glycosphingolipid **trihexosyl ceramide** in the vascular endothelial cells. Fabry's disease appears as clusters of punctate, dark-red spots of dilated small vessels (usually veins) scattered over the fundus and displaying corkscrew tortuosity, segmentation, and dilatation. Kinked vessels and saccular telangiectases may be present at the posterior pole. The arteries also may be tortuous and may exhibit sheathing and generalized or localized dilatations. Occasionally, a retinal artery occlusion may be present and, in time, ischemic optic neuropathy, papilledema, or optic atrophy may develop.

Symptoms

A minimal decrease of visual acuity results from Fabry's disease. Pain occurs in the extremities, and fever is a common symptom. Angiokeratomatous skin lesions may appear, more frequently on thighs and genitalia. Posterior cataract in a spokelike pattern is possible. Corneal whorl-like vertical epithelial opacities, radiating white lines, or a fingerprint pattern also are seen.

Diagnosis

Diagnosis is confirmed by the appearance of a low level of alpha-galactosidase activity in tears, serum, urinary sediment, leukocytes, and cultured fibroblasts or in cultured amniocytes by amniocentesis. An elevated level of trihexosyl ceramide is seen in urine. Fluorescein angiography may reveal a low-normal, accentuated vessel tortuosity, but no staining. Conjunctival biopsy is performed.

Differential Diagnosis

The differential diagnosis should consider drug-induced vortex keratopathy (*cornea verticillata*) after the use of quinacrine, chlorpromazine, chloroquine, amiodarone, amodiaquine, and indomethacin.

Treatment

Treatment usually is not necessary. A galactose-free diet is recommended, as is genetic counseling. Surgical intervention includes kidney transplantation to reverse the renal failure and to increase the enzyme activity.

Farber's Disease

Farber's disease (or *lipogranulomatosis*, *ceramide deficiency*, or *ceramide lipidosis*) is a rare metabolic, liposomal storage disease. It is an autosomal recessive retinopathy that begins in the first weeks of life and is accompanied by widespread deposition of **glycosphingolipids** in the retinal ganglion cells and in the vascular endothelium, around joints, and in the larynx, bones, brain, heart, lungs, and kidney. Usually, cardiac and renal failure render it lethal by 4 years of age.

The disorder is caused by an inborn error in ceramide metabolism due to lack of the enzyme *ceramidase*. Farber's disease appears as a subtle, diffuse, pale grayish, peppery pigmentation of a large portion of the retina, mostly in the paramacular region. The macular also appears abnormally gray, and a few small cherry-red spots occasionally may be present. The vessels are tortuous but otherwise normal, and the optic disc is not affected.

Diagnosis

The disorder's diagnosis is confirmed by the presence of elevated levels of ceramide in leukocytes and cultured fibroblasts. GM_3 ganglioside is present in the neuronal tissue. Amniocentesis may reveal low to absent ceramidase glucosidase A activity in cultured amniocytes.

Symptoms

Symptoms include irritability, vomiting, severe hoarseness, macroglossia, aphonia, and brownish desquamating dermatitis. Also symptomatic are the failure to thrive, painful swollen joints, and subcutaneous nodules at the ankle and elbow joints. The disorder is confirmed also by accompanying lymphadenopathy, angiokeratoma, hypotonia, diminished deep-tendon reflexes, and systolic murmur. Visual function is normal, although conjunctival xanthomalike growth and subepithelial corneal whorl-pattern opacities and spokelike posterior lens opacities are present. Psychomotor retardation is evident.

Histopathology

Histologic examination reveals a granuloma containing foam cells filled with material that stains positively with periodic acid–Schiff and is extractable with lipid solvents. There are birefringent glycolipid crystals in the retinal ganglion cells but no extracellular deposits of lipid in the retina.

Niemann-Pick Disease

Niemann-Pick disease is otherwise termed *sphingomyelin-sterol lipidosis* or *sea-blue histiocyte syndrome*. It is a rare, hereditary (autosomal recessive) neurodegenerative sphingomyelin lipidosis characterized by excessive storage of phospholipids in the eye, spleen, liver, bone marrow, brain, lungs, and other tissues. This storage abnormality occurs also in the reticuloendothelial system and is encountered more frequently in Jewish children.

Niemann-Pick disease is caused by a deficiency in formation of the lysosomal enzyme *sphingomyelinase* and in cholesterol esterification. This deficiency may cause an accumulation of **sphingomyelin** and **cholesterol** in the reticuloendothelial tissue.

The disorder comprises five clinical types: *A*, *B*, *C*, *D*, and *E*. **Type A**, the **acute infantile** type, is neuropathic. *It is the most common and severe form,* resulting in advanced retarded psychomotor developmental symptoms, and is lethal in 2–3 years. It may display **cherry-red spot** in the macula, which is brown-red and less pronounced. Also, multifocal white spots may be scattered throughout the fundus, and usually the anterior lens capsule is discolored.

Type B (**chronic** or **sea-blue histiocyte syndrome**) is not involved neurologically. It is the mildest form of the disorder, exhibiting a **macular halo** and appearing as a symmetric, pale discoloration in the perimacular region. This white-gray, doughnut-shaped crystalloid ring measures approximately 0.5 dd at its outer margin. Often, yellow-white scintillating granular opacities about the macula may form a relatively sharp border on the inner edge and a ragged border on the outer edge of the ring.

Type C is the **subacute juvenile** form and demonstrates no ocular signs. Clinically, it occurs as a **DAF syndrome** (an acronym designating *d*owngaze paralysis, *a*taxia-athetosis, and *f*oam cells in the spleen, liver, and bone marrow). It typically shows a marked neurologic involvement and invariably is fatal.

Type D, the **adult** or **Nova Scotia syndrome**, occurs without ocular signs and is more benign, whereas **type E** may cause a **cherry-red spot.**

Symptoms

Niemann-Pick disease may be asymptomatic. However, visible symptoms may include poor feeding, mental retardation, abdominal distension, hepatosplenomegaly, and lymphadenopathy. Diffuse pulmonary infiltration is evident, as are skin lesions, thrombocytopenia, gastrointestinal bleeding, and fever. The skin pigmentation is noticeably yellow-brown. Epilepsy, ataxia, convulsions, dementia, and nystagmus are possible symptoms.

Diagnosis

Niemann-Pick disease may be diagnosed through culture of skin fibroblasts, which may reveal sphingomyelin and unesterified cholesterol. White blood cells may demonstrate sphingomyelinase deficiency. Amniocentesis is performed, and bone marrow biopsy may show sea-blue histiocytes.

Histopathology

Histologic analysis demonstrates numerous vacuolated, foamy, sphingomyelin-laden cells containing membranous pleomorphic cytoplasmic bodies. In many organs and tissues, they appear as birefringent crystalloid opacities located in the parafoveolar region, in the retinal ganglion cell layer, in amacrine cells, or in the RPE. They may be found also to a lesser extent in the inner plexiform, outer plexiform, and rod and cone layers.

Treatment

No treatment for Niemann-Pick disease is effective. Genetic counseling is recommended.

Tay-Sachs Disease

Also known as *infantile cerebromacular degeneration*, *ganglioside lipidosis*, *amaurotic familial idiocy*, and *GM_2 gangliosidosis type 1*, Tay-Sachs disease is a rare, bilateral, hereditary, autosomal recessive, systemic metabolic lipid storage disease. This sphingolipidosis occurs more frequently in Ashkenazi Jews who have emigrated from Northeastern Europe or in patients of French-Canadian descent. Onset of the disorder occurs in the first year of life and is fatal by the age of 2 or 3 years. Usually, it is associated with progressive, severe neurologic disorders.

Tay-Sachs disease is caused by a deficiency of the enzyme *hexosaminidase A*, which leads to the accumulation of *GM_2 ganglioside* in the ganglion cells. It may occur in two forms: **infantile** or **juvenile** (Spielmeyer-Vogt-Batten-Mayou disease, which is described separately). Two variants are delineated: **A** and **B** (in which the serum level of hexosaminidase is not increased).

Tay-Sachs disease appears as a whitish gray ring around the macula, where the ganglion cell layer is thickest. There may be a cherry-red spot in the macula, due both to an accumulation of ganglioside in the ganglion cells in the paramacula and perimacular areas and to the absence of the lipid deposit in the foveola (a ganglion cell–free area), which allows the normal red choroid to become visible. A white, opaque, slightly elevated parafoveolar halo (approximately 1.5 dd) is evident; the outer borders are less delineated than are the inner borders, which are sharper. The retinal vessels may be narrowed markedly, and the optic disc may be white, atrophic, and well demarcated.

Symptoms

Tay-Sachs disease may cause loss of vision up to blindness, in addition to strabismus, hypotonia, increased startle reflex, and hyperacusis (an increased reaction to sound). Myotonic jerk and seizures may ensue. Progressive motor and mental deterioration are evident, as are dementia, spasticity, and a state of decerebrate rigidity.

Diagnosis

Visual evoked responses (VERs) can no longer be elicited. ERG is normal. The *doll's-head maneuver* revels absence of conjugate vertical eye movements. Prenatal amniocentesis can confirm diagnosis.

Histopathology

Histologic examination shows an accumulation of glycolipid storage material (a GM_2 ganglioside) in the retinal ganglion layer, in the bipolar cells, and in the amacrine cells in the inner nuclear layer. Ganglion cells are swollen and fat-laden and exhibit a nucleus located eccentrically and a cytoplasm filled with membranous, whorl-pattern laminated bodies. Extracellular birefringent deposits are present. The photoreceptors are destroyed completely and sometimes are replaced by glial proliferation and pigment accumulation. The nerve fiber layer is thin, and the optic nerve may be atrophic.

Treatment

Treatment for Tay-Sachs disease is not available. Genetic counseling is recommended.

Spielmeyer-Vogt-Batten-Mayou Syndrome

Spielmeyer-Vogt-Batten-Mayou syndrome (or *juvenile amaurotic familial idiocy*, *neuronal ceroid lipofuscinosis*, or *Kufs disease*) is a hereditary lipid storage disease. This autosomal recessive pigmentary retinopathy is the juvenile form of amaurotic familial idiocy; the infantile form is Tay-Sachs disease. The disorder occurs in children 4–15 years of age and is lethal before age 20 from progressive neurologic disease. It is caused by an uncertain lipid metabolic defect and associated with internal hydrocephalus.

Spielmeyer-Vogt-Batten-Mayou syndrome appears as a waxy yellow disc with slightly blurred margins and a mild papilledema and may progress to a secondary optic atrophy. The macula is affected severely, its center appearing as gray white and capable of extending slowly (enlarging as much as 2 dd). The macula is surrounded by a reddish area and fine scattered pigment dispersion, often like **bone spicule**; frequently, it may exhibit a **bull's-eye** configuration but *no cherry-red spot*. At the periphery, areas of pigmentation and depigmentation (dark and light spots similar to the **salt-and-pepper** fundus) may occur, and the retinal arteries are narrowed and attenuated.

Symptoms

Spielmeyer-Vogt-Batten-Mayou syndrome produces symptoms of loss of central vision, seizures, and ataxia. Mental deterioration and progressive dementia are evident.

Diagnosis

Fluorescein angiography may show a bull's-eye maculopathy with a round area of hyperfluorescence surrounding the macula (due to a window defect) corresponding to the RPE atrophy. ERG may reveal a severely attenuated response. A complete blood cell count may demonstrate vacuolization of the peripheral lymphocytes and reveal leukocytes with characteristic abundant azurophilic granules. A skin biopsy may show metachromasia of fibroblasts in the cell culture. A rectal biopsy may reveal ceroid lipofuscin accumulation in the tissue.

Differential Diagnosis

The predominant consideration for differential diagnosis is retinitis pigmentosa.

Histopathology

Histologic evaluation reveals an accumulation of **ceroid lipofuscin** in various tissues, in the RPE, in the central nervous system, or in the rectum. There is a loss of outer retinal layers (and, partially, of the RPE). Pigment-filled macrophages may migrate into those outer retinal layers. Their cytoplasmic granules are irregularly shaped and membrane-bound, and the content may appear membranous. In the macula, the retina retains fewer ganglion cells and exhibits cytoplasmic inclusions and irregular membranes (e.g., multilaminar cytosomes) but *no lipid deposits*. Lysosomal inclusions may be detected on electronic microscopy. The photoreceptors persist in the inner layers as darkly outlined and coated with acid mucopolysaccharides whereas, in the outer layers, they are degenerated. There may be a nonspecific reformation of the external limiting membrane by the glial Müller cells. These cells have apical villi, which occupy much of the subretinal space and frequently interdigitate with the apical villi of RPE cells. In some areas, the external limiting membrane is present near the RPE, and the internal limiting membrane is wrinkled. The choriocapillaris usually is normal.

Gaucher's Disease

Gaucher's disease (or *glucosyl ceramide lipidosis*) is a metabolic sphingolipidosis, a lysosomal storage disease, and an autosomal recessive retinopathy. It occurs in infants, teenagers, and adults, mostly in Jews of Eastern European origin.

The disorder is caused by a defect in the enzyme *glucosyl ceramide beta-glucosidase*, which defect may produce an accumulation of **glu-**

cocerebroside in the reticuloendothelial system and in the liver, spleen, lymph nodes, bone marrow, alveolar capillaries, and eye.

Gaucher's disease comprises three types: *adult*, *infantile*, and *juvenile*. **Type I**, the **chronic nonneuropathic** (or **adult**) form, occurs in adult life at any age. It produces bleeding, hypersplenism, thrombocytopenia, jaundice, anemia, bone fractures, yellow skin pigmentation, and intermittent infections but no neurologic signs.

Type II (the **acute neuropathic** or **infantile** form) occurs in infancy before the age of 6 months. It causes widespread severe neurologic disturbances, failure to thrive, mental retardation, spasticity, progressive hepatomegaly, dysphagia, retroflexion of the head, and pseudobulbar palsy. It is lethal in the first year of life, usually from intercurrent infections.

Type III, or the **subacute neuropathic** (**juvenile**) form, represents clinical findings of both types I and II and follows a longer survival course (2–20 years). This disorder produces splenomegaly, lymphadenopathy, spontaneous bone fractures, and pancytopenia. The neurologic features are milder. Large yellow-brown pingueculae, with the base at the cornea and capable of enlarging and becoming yellow, also may be seen.

Gaucher's disease appears as discrete, superficial white spots on the retinal surface. They are scattered in clusters and sometimes in a semicircular pattern at the posterior pole but more frequently along the inferior vascular arcade. Their size varies from minute (and barely visible) to 0.1 mm, some of them partly covering the retinal vessels. Occasionally, there may be cherry-red spots; often, small, grayish retinal areas (called *grayness of the retina*) may involve the macula. The remainder of the fundus, the disc, and the retinal vessels are normal.

Symptoms

Usually, symptoms are minimal, although corneal clouding is likely.

Diagnosis

Diagnosis is confirmed by an acid phosphatase level that is increased in plasma and tissues. The lipid blood level is normal. An increased level of *transcobalamin II*, a circulating vitamin B_{12}–binding protein in blood, also points to the diagnosis. An increased serum angiotensin-converting enzyme level and a decreased level of beta-glucosidase in leukocytes are seen. The platelet count is low.

Histopathology

Histologic analysis shows clusters of swollen, foamy histiocytes with an irregularly shaped, streaked cytoplasm resembling wrinkled tissue paper (**Gaucher's cells**) located on and within the retina. The periodic acid–Schiff test is positive.

Treatment

Treatment for Gaucher's disease consists of genetic counseling and enzyme replacement therapy. Splenectomy is an alternative intervention.

Suggested Reading

Arshinoff SA, Leung K. Gyrate Atrophy. In W Tasman, EA Jaeger, MM Parks (eds), Duane's Clinical Ophthalmology, vol 3. Philadelphia: Lippincott–Raven, 1996;25:1–16.

Baker RH, Trautmann JC, Young BR, et al. Late juvenile onset Krabbe's disease. Ophthalmology 1990;97:1176–1180.

Kaiser-Kupfer MI, Caruso RC, Valle D. Gyrate atrophy of the choroid and retina. Arch Ophthalmol 1991;109:1539–1543.

14

Toxic Retinopathy

Chloroquine Retinopathy

Chloroquine retinopathy is a degeneration of the macula and occurs in patients undergoing long-term therapy with chloroquine (Aralen), an aminoquinoline (total dose, 110–300 g or more). This agent is used as an antimalarial; in such collagen diseases as rheumatoid arthritis and systemic lupus erythematosus; in amebiasis; or in sarcoidosis. The disorder is caused by the direct effect of chloroquine or such of its derivatives as hydroxychloroquine (Plaquenil), which produces a macular retinal pigment epithelium (RPE) atrophy and damage to the retinal ganglion cell layer.

In the early stage, chloroquine retinopathy appears as a perifoveolar ring of pigment accompanied by loss of the foveal light reflex and by irregular and nonspecific mild granularity appearing as pigment mottling and stippling in the macula. As the lesion progresses, a fine granular pigment accumulates in the center of the macula and later becomes a hyperpigmented, dark-red, typically horizontal oval lesion, more pigmented inferiorly (Figure 14-1). In a later stage, patchy depigmented areas may surround the macula in a circular fashion. In time, another area of hyperpigmentation occurs in the perifoveolar region; it is similar to an advanced tapetoretinal degeneration and gives rise to a lesion resembling a target or a bull's-eye. This **bull's-eye macula** is irreversible and usually asymmetric and is characterized by more atrophy inferiorly located as a *half-moon pattern*. Arteries are attenuated and, in the end stage, become narrowed (threadlike) and may exhibit sheathing. There may be nonspecific pigmentation at the peripheral retina, and the disc may be waxy and pale.

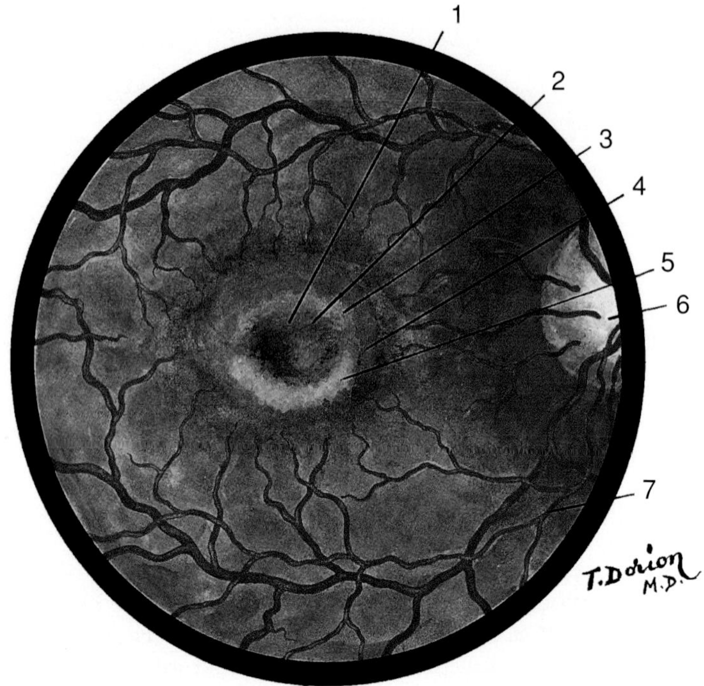

Figure 14-1. *Chloroquine retinopathy. (1) Loss of foveal light reflex. (2–5) Bull's-eye macula: (2) granular pigment accumulation in the center of the macula; (3) depigmented retinal pigment epithelium atrophy surrounding the macula; (4) perifoveolar hyperpigmentation; (5) half-moon retinal pigment epithelium atrophy, located inferiorly. (6) Pallor of the disc. (7) Attenuated, narrowed arteries.*

Symptoms

Symptoms include night blindness, decreased visual acuity, and loss of central vision, which is irreversible.

Diagnosis

An abnormal visual field examination with central, paracentral, and peripheral scotomas and peripheral field constriction confirm the diagnosis of chloroquine retinopathy. Static perimetry shows an elevation of the threshold. Electroretinography (ERG) is extinguished, and dark adaptation may be normal or may show minimally abnormal final thresholds. Color vision may reveal a red-green defect on the pseudoisochromatic Ishihara plates, on the polychromatic Stilling plates, on the Hardy-Rand-Ritter test, or on the Farnsworth-Munsell 100-hue test. Electro-oculography is supranormal, and photostress is abnormal. Fluorescein angiography may reveal a round area of hyperfluorescence around the macula, due to a window defect corresponding to RPE atrophy.

Differential Diagnosis

Considerations for the differential diagnosis include cone dystrophy, Spielmeyer-Vogt-Batten-Mayou syndrome, Stargardt's disease (or fundus flavimaculatus), or Laurence-Moon-Bardet-Biedl syndrome. Age-related macular degeneration may be a factor contributing to the disorder. Leber's congenital amaurosis and retinitis pigmentosa inversa are other considerations.

Histopathology

Histologic examination reveals an RPE atrophy on the macula, with pigment dispersion and disorganization. There are hyperpigmented areas beneath the foveola. Ganglion cells of the retina may have clusters of curvilinear structures and intracytoplasmic bodies. The rod and cone layer (photoreceptors) may be destroyed.

Treatment

No treatment is effective for chloroquine retinopathy. Discontinuation of the drug is strongly recommended.

Quinine Retinopathy

Quinine retinopathy is an acute, usually bilateral retinal edema that occurs after antimalarial therapy with quinine sulfate or after use of this agent as a relaxant for muscle cramps (sometimes after a single dose), after drug abusers' use in combination with heroin, in suicide attempts, or in attempted abortion. The disorder is due mostly to the direct toxic effect of quinine and (to a lesser degree) to pathologic damage by a primary retinal vasoconstriction.

Quinine retinopathy appears as a milky, creamy, opalescent cloudy area of intercellular ischemic retinal edema located at the posterior pole and occasionally involving the macula. A small **cherry-red spot** may appear in the macula with central artery emboli. It may resolve in several weeks after discontinuation of the drug, leaving marked retinal attenuation, extreme spastic narrowing of the arteries, a diffuse pigmented area, a pale disc, and (in a late stage) papilledema or optic atrophy.

Symptoms

Symptoms include blurred vision and severely decreased visual acuity (rarely to bilateral total blindness) with no light perception. Other symptoms are amblyopia, progressive tinnitus, and deafness. Onset may cause nausea, vomiting, diarrhea, and fever. Hypotension, cardiac irregularities, anuria, convulsions, and even coma can ensue.

Diagnosis

The visual field examination may reveal marked constricted field defects (to a central area of 5–10 degrees in diameter) that may remain permanently. Dark adaptation is impaired. Usually, fluorescein angiography is normal, except for a mild venous dilatation. Electro-oculography may be diminished, and ERG may reveal a reduction in the a-wave.

Differential Diagnosis

Considerations for differential diagnosis include central retinal artery occlusion and chloroquine retinopathy. Filix mas intoxication and ergot poisoning also can be considered.

Histopathology

Histologic appraisal reveals an alteration of the retinal ganglion layer, of the photoreceptors, and of the RPE. There is edema of the retina of varying degree. Optic atrophy may be present in the late stage.

Treatment

Treatment calls for discontinuation of the drug. Removal of the drug is effected by lavage or emesis. Renal excretion is promoted by fluids (2–4 liters daily). Anuria and shock should be treated appropriately. Vasodilators and adrenocorticotropic hormone therapy are medical options, as is stellate ganglion block.

Thioridazine Toxicity

Thioridazine toxicity is a retinopathy that occurs with antipsychotic and sedative effects after the use of a psychotropic drug or phenothiazine compound (**thioridazine** [**Mellaril**]) in a dose greater than 1,000 mg/day (total dose, 85–100 g in excess of 8 weeks) for treatment of schizophrenia or other psychotic disorders. The disorder is caused by the retinotoxic effect of this drug, especially on RPE.

Thioridazine toxicity may occur in either of two types: acute or chronic. **Acute** thioridazine toxicity affects patients receiving large doses (2,000 mg/day) and results in an acute decrease in the central vision. **Chronic** thioridazine toxicity appears in patients receiving lower doses for a long period and produces a peripheral visual field loss although maintaining good central vision.

The disorder may appear as a **salt-and-pepper** pigmentation or as pigment clumping in a plaquelike pattern. At a later stage, multiple aggregates and conglomerates of pigment (dispersed more frequently in the macula) may form an area of hyperpigmentation alternating with hypopigmentation (called *bull's-eye macula*). Also, coarse granulation of pigment or larger pigment plaques may manifest throughout the posterior pole. Sometimes, rounded areas of RPE hyperplasia and depigmentation may be seen posterior to the equator (called *nummular retinopathy*). In time, larger geographic areas of atrophy of the retina, the RPE, and the choriocapillaris may enlarge, coalesce, and become more confluent. Arteries may be diffusely narrowed. These pigmentary changes progress even after the thioridazine is discontinued.

Symptoms

Blurred vision results from this disorder. Other symptoms include nyctalopia and brownish vision.

Diagnosis

Fluorescein angiography may reveal a hyperfluorescence in a lobular confluent pattern. Visual field testing may show central or ring scotoma and generalized constriction. ERG may reveal diminished photopic and scotopic response or a depressed or extinguished ERG. Farnsworth-Munsell 100-hue test for color vision evaluation should confirm the diagnosis.

Differential Diagnosis

Considerations for the differential diagnosis are gyrate atrophy, retinitis pigmentosa, syphilis, and trauma.

Histopathology

Histologic evaluation shows a marked RPE atrophy with pigmentary disorganization.

Tamoxifen Retinopathy

Tamoxifen retinopathy may occur during the treatment of breast cancer with the nonsteroidal estrogen receptor antagonist tamoxifen (Nolvadex), even with regular doses of 20–30 mg/day PO. It may be associated with corneal deposits. The disorder is caused by the direct toxic effect of the drug, which produces deposition of an irreversible metabolite (probably of axonal origin) in the retina.

Tamoxifen retinopathy appears as bilateral, fine, white refractile crystals and yellow-white granules accumulated mostly in the perimacular area. There also may be scattered areas of retinal atrophy, irregular circular preretinal fibrosis, and cystoid macular edema. Rarely, small intraretinal hemorrhages may be seen.

Histopathology

Histologic analysis shows granular deposits at the level of the RPE in the macula or the posterior pole. Small, spherical intracellular inclusions (approximately 5–35 μm) are located in the retinal nerve fiber layer.

Nicotinic Acid Retinopathy

Nicotinic acid retinopathy, which is toxic, occurs after the use of nicotinic acid (niacin) in doses greater than 3 g/day as a peripheral vasodilator for headache, myalgia, neurologic disorders, or edema of the labyrinth or for treatment of hypercholesterolemia, in which it decreases the synthesis of low-density lipoproteins. The disorder appears as an atypical form of cystoid macular edema.

Symptoms

The predominant symptom is decreased visual acuity, which returns to normal after discontinuation of the drug.

Diagnosis

Fluorescein angiography reveals no capillary permeability alteration and no leakage of fluorescein.

Treatment

Treatment of nicotinic acid retinopathy mandates discontinuation of the nicotinic acid and of epinephrine-dipivefrin and niacin-containing medications. Possible drug interventions include such topical steroids as prednisolone 1%, 1 drop four times per day for 3 weeks, then tapered, and systemic steroids, such as prednisone, 40 mg/day PO for 5 days, then tapered.

Interferon Retinopathy

Interferon retinopathy is a retinopathy that occurs after therapy with human interferon, a glycoprotein with antineoplastic or antiviral action against RNA viruses and, to a lesser extent, against DNA viruses (inhibiting viral replication). This drug is used to prevent dissemination of early herpes zoster virus in immunocompromised patients, to delay reaction of herpes simplex, or to suppress viremia with hepatitis B virus. It also is used in the treatment of hairy-cell leukemia, Kaposi's sarcoma, the acquired immunodeficiency syndrome (AIDS), or condyloma acuminatum. It may be caused by an immune complex deposition of the drug in the retinal vessels.

Interferon retinopathy appears as multiple white-yellow, soft exudates with fluffy margins and variably sized cotton-wool spots scattered throughout the posterior pole. Several intraretinal, superficial, flame-shaped splinter hemorrhages (or occasionally) deeper dot-and-blot hemorrhages also may be present. The retinal vessels usually are normal, and the optic disc rarely is involved.

Interferon retinopathy may be asymptomatic. Decreased visual acuity may be evident, depending on the retinal area affected and the degree of macular involvement.

Histologic appraisal reveals a possible infarction in the retinal nerve fiber layer. Blood accumulation in the outer plexiform layer and nerve fiber layer also may be present.

Particulate Retinopathy

Also termed *talc retinopathy*, particulate retinopathy occurs after the parenteral, intravenous introduction by drug abusers of many thousands of crushed tablets of such easily available soluble substances as magnesium silicate (talc), methylphenidate (Ritalin), or cornstarch fillers. Usually, it is associated with a pneumopathy with occluded pulmonary capillaries.

The disorder is produced by the toxic effect of particulate matter that, after an intravenous injection, gains access to the systemic circulation, lodges in the capillaries of the lungs, and causes a granulomatous reaction and (subsequently) a shunt. This activity allows it to pass on to the eye, where it occludes retinal capillaries.

Particulate retinopathy appears as bilateral, tiny, glistening, crystalline white opacities that often adopt a vascular distribution and usually are located in small retinal vessels, the macula, the posterior pole, and (to a lesser extent) at the periphery. The macula may appear ischemic and edematous. Neovascularization may occur in the disc and, occasionally, vitreous hemorrhages are manifest. Tractional retinal detachment (more commonly rhegmatogenous) also may be present.

Symptoms

Particulate retinopathy usually is asymptomatic. However, loss of central vision may be evident.

Diagnosis

Diagnosis depends primarily on chest roentgenograms.

Differential Diagnosis

The differential diagnosis should consider sickle cell retinopathy, diabetes, sarcoidosis, Eales' disease, and radiation retinopathy.

Histopathology

Histologic examination may reveal the presence of emboli of refractile crystals in the inner retinal layers, the retinal vessels, the choriocapillaris, or the choroid.

Treatment

No treatment for the disorder is totally effective. Laser photocoagulation may be used for neovascularization and vitreous hemorrhages. Discontinuation of the drug is mandated.

Suggested Reading

Grant S. Toxic Retinopathy. In W Tasman, EA Jaeger, MM Parks, et al. Duane's Clinical Ophthalmology, vol 3. Philadelphia: Lippincott–Raven, 1996;33:1–14.
Grant WM. Drug Intoxications and Chemical Injuries. In A Sorsby (ed), Modern Ophthalmology, vol 2 (2nd ed). Philadelphia: Lippincott, 1972;661–684.
Guyer DR, Tideman J, Yannuzzi LA, et al. Interferon-associated retinopathy. Arch Ophthalmol 1993;111:350–356.

15

Systemic Retinopathy

Diabetic Retinopathy

Diabetic retinopathy is a bilateral vascular disorder of the retina and occurs often in long-standing diabetes mellitus; most of the changes involve the venous circulation. The disorder may be due to the loss of intramural pericytes of the capillaries, followed by outpouching of the capillary wall and then by an abnormal permeability of the capillaries, which may lead to retinal edema. Alternately, it may be due to a progressive capillary closure possibly elaborating a **vasoproliferative factor** that may stimulate the retinal neovascularization. Ultimately, the fibrovascular tissue may contract, producing vitreous hemorrhage and tractional retinal detachment.

Diabetic retinopathy can appear as one of two types: *nonproliferative* and *proliferative*. **Nonproliferative diabetic retinopathy** (NDR; Figure 15-1) can occur as a *minimal*, *mild*, *moderate*, or *severe* disorder. **Minimal NDR** (previously called *background diabetic retinopathy*) appears as microaneurysms only, scattered more commonly at the peripheral retina and the posterior pole. **Mild NDR** (also previously called *background diabetic retinopathy*) appears as microaneurysms, a few superficial and deep retinal hemorrhages, several cotton-wool spots, and hard exudates and drusen throughout the entire fundus.

Moderate NDR (previously called *transitional diabetic retinopathy*) appears as retinal hemorrhages and microaneurysms grouped together, several cotton-wool spots, venous beading, and intraretinal microvascular abnormalities.

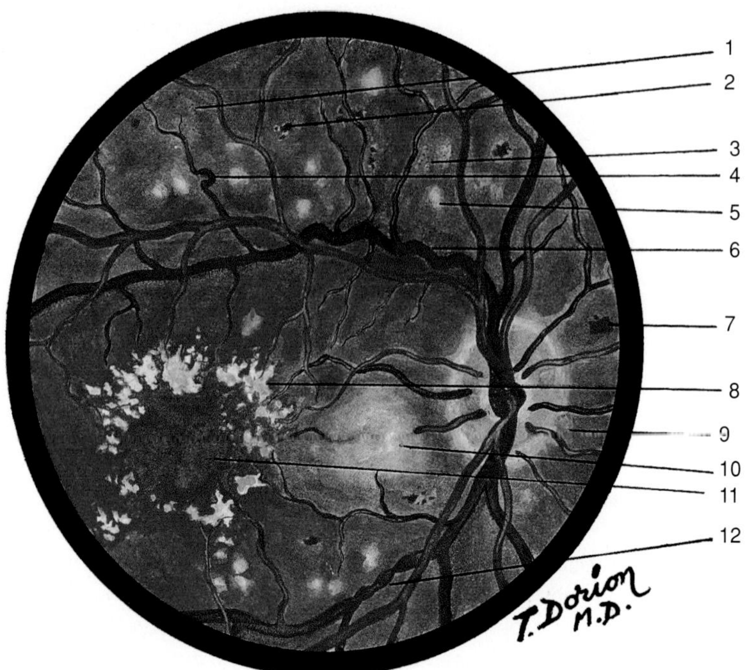

Figure 15-1. *Severe nonproliferative diabetic retinopathy. (1) Microaneurysms. (2) Deep retinal hemorrhage. (3) Intraretinal microvascular abnormalities. (4) Venous loop. (5) Cotton-wool spots. (6) Tortuous veins. (7) Superficial retinal hemorrhage. (8) Hard exudates, as circinate maculopathy. (9) Drusen. (10) Retinal edema. (11) Cystoid macular edema. (12) Venous beading.*

Severe NDR (previously called *preproliferative diabetic retinopathy*) appears as multiple hemorrhages and microaneurysms located in all four quadrants and intraretinal microvascular abnormalities located in two or more quadrants. At this stage, other changes may take place (e.g., cystoid macular edema, peripheral retinal edema near or temporal to the macula, dilated kinked and tortuous retinal vessels, venous loops, venous beading, and vascular shunts). Hard exudates as circinate maculopathy, drusen, and cotton-wool spots also are present.

Proliferative diabetic retinopathy (PDR; Figure 15-2) can occur as *early*, *high-risk*, or *advanced* disorder. **Early PDR** appears as a neovascularization of the disc (NVD), neovascularization of the retina elsewhere

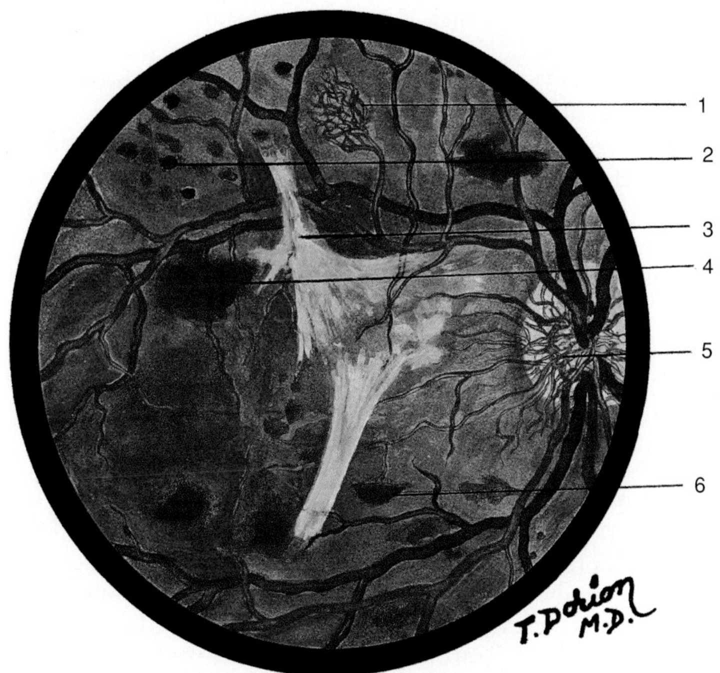

Figure 15-2. *Proliferative diabetic retinopathy. (1) Neovascularization elsewhere. (2) Intraretinal hemorrhages. (3) Fibrous retinitis proliferans. (4) Vitreous hemorrhage. (5) Neovascularization of the disc. (6) Preretinal hemorrhage.*

(NVE), preretinal hemorrhages, and vitreous hemorrhages. **High-risk PDR** appears as an NVD on or within 1 dd of the disc margin, equaling or exceeding one-fourth to one-third of the optic disc area; NVE larger than 0.5 dd; preretinal hemorrhages; and vitreous hemorrhages. **Advanced PDR** appears with all of the foregoing signs plus tractional macular detachment and intensive vitreous hemorrhages. If the blood remains in the subhyaloid space, it is called *swallow's-nest hemorrhage* and offers a good prognosis for resorption. If the blood breaks into the vitreous, it is called *intra-gel hemorrhage* and represents a guarded prognosis. At a later stage, the new vessels may become fibrous and may exhibit surrounding connective tissue proliferation, which may result in tractional retinal detachment and produce fibrous **retinitis proliferans**.

Diabetic retinopathy may be considered as either *juvenile* or *senile*. **Juvenile diabetic retinopathy** appears as a *triad* formed by (1) **wonder**

net or **rubeosis retinae**, which is a hypertrophy and a frondlike neovascularization especially of the retinal veins; (2) **saccular dilatation** of the veins; and (3) **microaneurysms**. Bright circumscribed areas of retinal ischemia also may be evident.

Senile diabetic retinopathy appears as a *triad* formed by (1) punctate and striate **retinal hemorrhages**; (2) **hard exudates** at the posterior pole, mostly between the nerve fiber bundles; and (3) **arteriosclerosis**, which appears as variations in the lumen diameter and the thickness of the vessel wall. The retina may appear *dry*, without edema. The disc may have sharp margins, good color, and occasional drusen. Asteroid hyalosis or lipemia retinalis sometimes may develop.

Diagnosis

Fluorescein angiography may show extensive microvascular changes with capillary nonperfusion, capillary closure, and diffuse capillary dilatation with massive vascular leakage. Hyperglycemia is evident. Diagnostic tools include a glucose tolerance test determining glycosuria and ketonuria and elevated serum lipid levels; indirect ophthalmoscopy; B-scan ultrasonography; visual evoked potentials for tractional macular detachment; and computed tomography (CT) scan of sinuses, orbit, and brain. Biopsy of any skin necrosis and a history of amphotericin B treatment for mucormycosis infection can confirm diagnosis.

Differential Diagnosis

Considerations for the differential diagnosis include central retinal vein occlusion, branch retinal vein occlusion, hypertension, sickle cell retinopathy, sarcoidosis, emboli, effects of radiation therapy, or orbital infection by mucormycosis.

Histopathology

Histologic analysis reveals a loss of pericytes of the retinal capillaries, outpouching of the capillary walls that form microaneurysms, and thickening of Bruch's membrane (Figures 15-3, 15-4). Capillary closure, intraretinal cysts, hypertrophy and atrophy of the endothelial

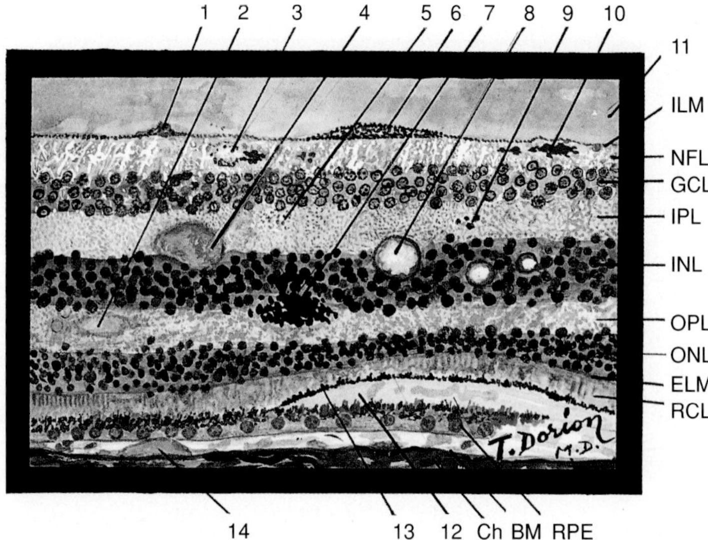

Figure 15-3. *Histopathologic findings in nonproliferative diabetic retinopathy. (1) Fixed folds on the internal limiting membrane. (2) Hard exudates (lipid) in the outer plexiform layer. (3) Microinfarcts in the nerve fiber layer (cotton-wool spots). (4) Drusen. (5) Intraretinal microvascular abnormalities. (6) Preretinal fibrovascular membranes. (7) Deep intraretinal hemorrhage. (8) Intraretinal cystic spaces. (9) Outpouchings of the capillary wall (microaneurysms). (10) Superficial retinal hemorrhages in the nerve fiber layer. (11) Vitreous. (12) Retinal detachment. (13) Loss of villi of retinal epithelial cells, with portions of pigment granules. (14) Drusen on Bruch's membrane. (ILM, internal limiting membrane; NFL, nerve fiber layer; GCL, ganglion cell layer; IPL, inner plexiform layer; INL, inner nuclear layer; OPL, outer plexiform layer; ONL, outer nuclear layer; ELM, external limiting membrane; RCL, rod and cone layer [photoreceptors]; RPE, retinal pigment epithelium; BM, Bruch's membrane; Ch, choroid.)*

cells, and intraretinal microvascular abnormalities (IRMAs) are visible. Lipid deposits are seen in the outer plexiform layer of the retina, often surrounded by fat-laden phagocytes. Also possible are neural tissue destruction, drusen deposition at or anterior to the Bruch's membrane, and thinning or hypopigmentation of the retinal pigment epithelium (RPE). Preretinal and intraretinal hemorrhages also may be present.

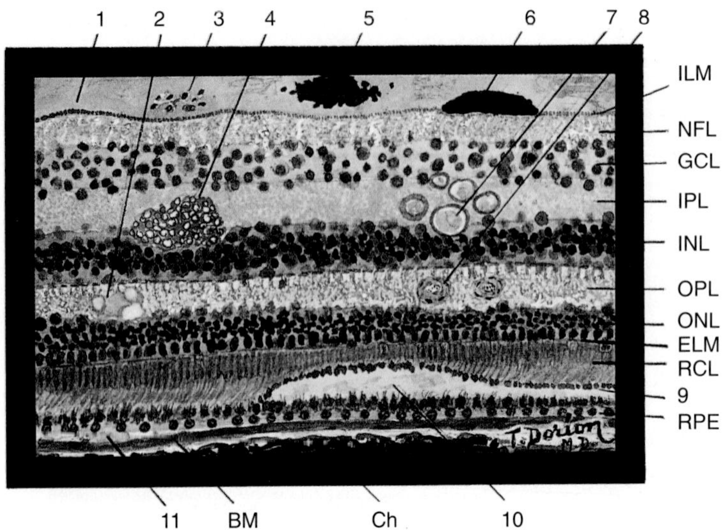

Figure 15-4. *Histopathologic findings in proliferative diabetic retinopathy. (1) Vitreous. (2) Lipid deposits in the outer plexiform layer, surrounded by macrophages. (3) Vascular cell migration. (4) Neovascularization elsewhere in the retina. (5) Vitreal hemorrhage. (6) Preretinal hemorrhage. (7) Intraretinal cysts. (8) Fibrosed vessels. (9) Apical villi and pigment from RPE. (10) Tractional retinal detachment. (11) Drusen on Bruch's membrane. (ILM, internal limiting membrane; NFL, nerve fiber layer; GCL, ganglion cell layer; IPL, inner plexiform layer; INL, inner nuclear layer; OPL, outer plexiform layer; ONL, outer nuclear layer; ELM, external limiting membrane; RCL, rod and cone layer [photoreceptors]; RPE, retinal pigment epithelium; Ch, choroid; BM, Bruch's membrane.)*

Treatment

Treatment for diabetic retinopathy includes laser photocoagulation and focal or panretinal photocoagulation (usually with argon laser) for high-risk PDR and for clinically significant macular edema, or microaneurysms. Possible surgical interventions are pars plana vitrectomy (for persistent nonclearing vitreous hemorrhage, tractional or rhegmatogenous retinal detachment involving the macula, fibrovascular proliferation, macular epiretinal membranes, and severe neovascularization) and scleral buckling for retinal detachment. Treatment should be managed by an internist. Strict blood glucose control in type I diabetes may prevent the onset of diabetic retinopathy and may reduce the progression of the nephropathy and neuropathy, as will a controlled diet. Hypoglycemic agents may be administered. Treatment of associated diseases is a consideration.

Sarcoidosis

Sarcoidosis is variously termed *Besnier-Boeck sarcoid*, *lupus pernio*, *Schaumann's disease*, and *Darier-Roussy syndrome*. A bilateral granulomatous chorioretinopathy is part of this generalized systemic chronic progressive reticulosis that occurs more often in young black women (20–40 years), especially in the southern United States and in Sweden. It involves multiple systems and organs, such as kidney, lungs, liver, muscle, bones, central nervous system, and eye. Its etiology is unknown.

Sarcoidosis appears as a chorioretinitis, periphlebitis retinae, choroidal or disc granuloma, optic neuritis, optic atrophy, papilledema, or vitritis (Figure 15-5). When sarcoid uveitis is associated with a facial nerve palsy, it is called *Heerfordt's syndrome*.

Sarcoid granuloma may occur as either a solitary or multiple, elevated, yellowish-white nodules; they are round or oval, slightly irregular, and scattered throughout the fundus. Usually, the disorder appears as any of three types: (1) **exophytic**, which grows outward of the retinal surface; (2) **sessile**, which is attached by a base and is not pedunculated; and (3) **endophytic**, which extends inward into the retina.

The disorder may appear as multiple patchy nodular choroidal infiltrates that resemble *Dalen-Fuchs nodules* in sympathetic ophthalmia. Their size may vary, starting at less than 1–2 dd. The retinal veins may appear surrounded by small, discrete, yellow exudates and fluffy opacities (called *candle wax drippings of Franceschetti* or *tache de bougies*) located at the inferior and equatorial retina, cuffing the vessels. Often, there are numerous spherical, grayish-white, fluffy, vitreous opacities (called *snowballs*) of different sizes (from small particles to one-third disc diameter scattered along the veins). Frequently, they are seen in chains, like a *string of pearls* in the lower vitreous and casting onto the retina. Also, peripheral neovascularization (as a **sea fan**) or an NVD appears and, occasionally, there may be preretinal nodules, called *Landers' sign*. The disorder also may produce intraretinal or subretinal hemorrhages or white-centered hemorrhages (called *Roth's spots*). Arteriovenous anastomoses, serous retinal detachment, or cystoid macular edema occasionally may be present.

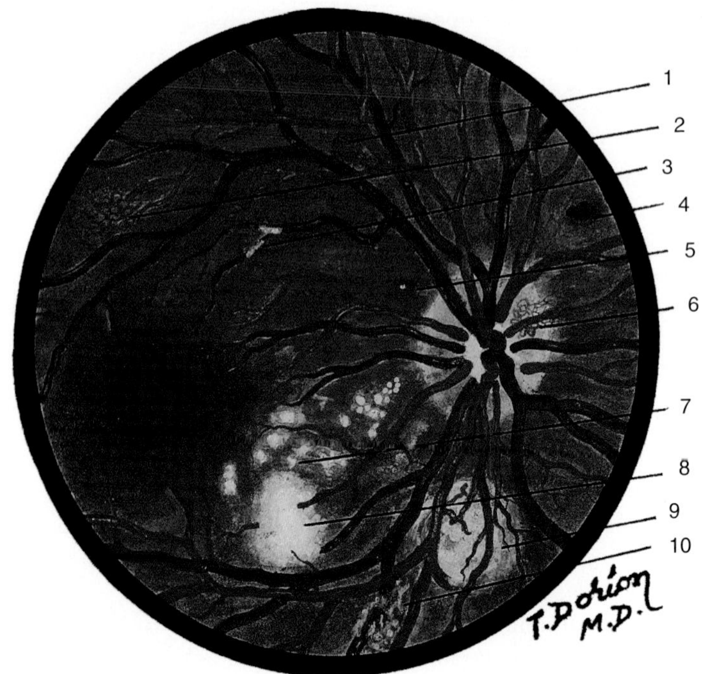

Figure 15-5. *Sarcoidosis. (1) Sea fan. (2) Neovascularization elsewhere. (3) Venous sheathing. (4) Intraretinal hemorrhage. (5) Roth's spot. (6) Neovascularization of the disc. (7) Nodular choroidal infiltrates. (8) Snowball. (9) Sarcoid nodule. (10) Candle wax drippings.*

Symptoms

Sarcoidosis may be asymptomatic. However, it may be accompanied by decreased vision, photophobia, and pain.

Diagnosis

In the acute stage, chest roentgenograms may show bilateral hilar adenopathy and, in the chronic stage, a diffuse pulmonary interstitial fibrosis. A gallium scan may show an increased uptake. Axial and coronal CT scans of the orbit may reveal infiltrating lesions. Biopsy from the conjunctiva, the salivary and lacrimal glands, the lymph nodes, and skin, liver, gastrocnemius muscle, or bronchi may show a *noncaseating granuloma.* Early-stage fluorescein angiography may reveal a diffuse staining and segmental irregular leakage around the veins; in a later stage, the test may reveal a hyperfluorescence of the new vessel walls (usually at the edge of a capillary closure); microangiopathy; excessive nonperfusion, telangiectasia, and ischemia; and staining of the optic disc and peripapillary spots. Visual field examination may show a large blind spot.

The tuberculin reaction is negative, but the Kveim skin test is inconclusive. The angiotensin-converting enzyme level is increased, and hypercalcemia may be evident. Serum and urine neuraminidase (lysozyme) levels may be high. The serum collagenase may be increased, the albumin-globulin ratio is abnormal (normal, 2:1), and serum protein electrophoresis shows hypergammaglobulinemia. The erythrocyte sedimentation rate is increased, and pulmonary functions may be abnormal, as are liver enzymes. Leukopenia and a slight eosinophilia may be present.

Differential Diagnosis

The differential diagnosis should consider tuberculosis, sickle-cell disease, pars planitis, and ocular lymphoma. Other diagnostic possibilities are retinitis pigmentosa, retinoblastoma, and amyloidosis.

Histopathology

The most common histologic finding in sarcoidosis is **retinal vasculitis with noncaseating tubercles**. This vasculitis is surrounded by a thin ring of lymphocytes and (rarely) displays a central necrosis *but not caseation.* The whole lesion is called *naked granuloma.* These nodules and tubercles frequently exhibit multinucleated giant cells, epithelioid cells, and spherical or basophilic laminated bodies (called *Schumann bodies*). Also, periphlebitis (or *candle wax drippings*) composed of chorioretinal granuloma, epithelioid cells, and lymphocytes appear as granulomatous material wrapped around the veins. RPE atrophy also may be present. Granulomatous inflammatory nodules may be present between the RPE and Bruch's membrane (similar to *Dalen-Fuchs nodules* from sympathetic ophthalmia).

Treatment

Treatment for sarcoidosis includes such agents as corticosteroids (topical prednisolone 1%, 1 drop OU four times per day; subconjunctival and periocular methylprednisolone, 20–40 mg, or triamcinolone via sub–Tenon's capsule, 40 mg for 4 weeks; and systemic prednisone, 60–100 mg/day PO for several weeks) and cycloplegics (atropine, homatropine, cyclopentolate 2%, and scopolamine 0.5% 1 drop OU twice per day). An antiulcerative agent such as the H_2-blocker ranitidine (Zantac), 150 mg PO twice per day, should be used during corticosteroid therapy. Immunosuppressive drugs such as the antibiotic cyclosporine A, 2.5–5.0 mg/kg/day with milk, is recommended. Antimetabolite drugs such as azathioprine, or alkylating drugs such as cyclophosphamide, are not helpful. Laser panretinal photocoagulation for retinal neovascularization is an alternate intervention.

Albinism

Albinism is known by many names: *oculocutaneous albinism*, *albinoidism*, *Nettleship-Falls syndrome*, *Forsius-Erikson syndrome*, *Bergsma-Kaiser-Kupfer syndrome*, *Apert's syndrome*, *Hermansky-Pudlak syndrome*, and *Bard-Waardenburg-like syndrome*. This disorder is a benign congenital anomaly consisting of bilateral hypopigmentation of the fundus (Figure 15-6) that also may involve the iris, skin, and hair. It is designated as either of two types: **true albinism** (both *ocular* and *oculocutaneous*) and **albinoidism.**

Albinism (except Nettleship-Falls syndrome, which is X-linked) is an autosomal recessive disease. Oculocutaneous albinism may be *tyrosinase-positive*, in which case the pigmentation of the skin and the fundus generally are normal, or *tyrosinase-negative*, in which case the skin and fundus completely lack pigmentation. Albinoidism is an autosomal dominant disease with incomplete penetrance.

The disorder may be caused variously by a defect in the **melanin** synthesis, with a reduction or absence of the pigment melanin; by an irregular distribution of normal *melanosomes* that are decreased in number; or by a disturbance in the melanosome structure.

Tyrosinase-negative albinism is due to a deficiency in tyrosinase, which cannot catalyze the conversion of tyrosine to dopa to form

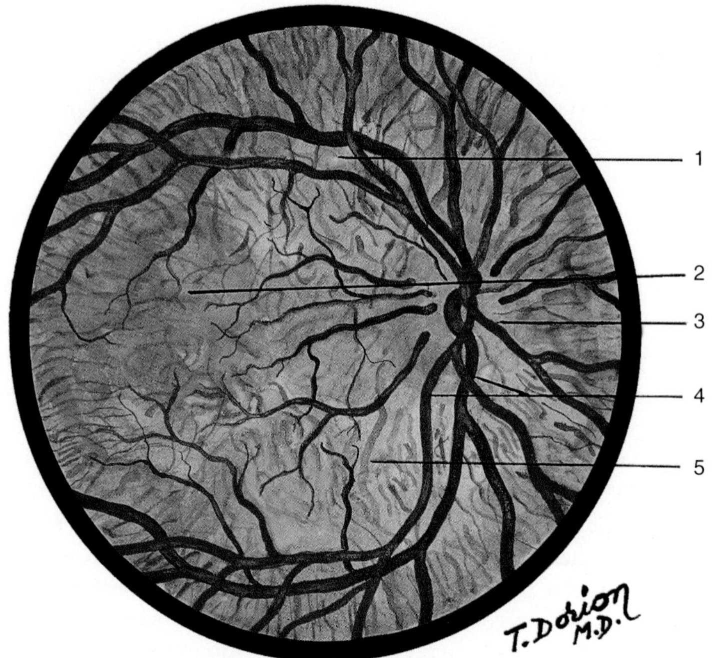

Figure 15-6. *Albinism. (1) Depigmented fundus. (2) Hypoplasia of the macula. (3) Hypoplasia of the disc. (4) Normal retinal vessels. (5) Prominent highly visible choroidal vessels.*

melanin. *Tyrosinase-positive albinism* is due to an abnormality in which tyrosinase cannot penetrate the melanocytes that contain melanin.

The disorder appears as a bilateral light, depigmented fundus (**blonde fundus**) of variable intensity and dispersed peripheral RPE mosaicism. Occasionally, areas of **salt-and-pepper** fundus may be present. The macula appears indistinct, hypoplastic, and not clearly identifiable, with a dull or absent foveal reflex, or it may be mottled, with stippling. Retinal vessels are normal, and the choroidal vessels are prominent and highly visible. Patches and streaks of hypopigmented RPE may appear in midperiphery, adjacent to a normal (or even pigment-clustered) fundus, and optic hypoplasia or (as in Apert's syndrome) optic atrophy may be present.

Symptoms

Symptoms include photophobia, searching nystagmus, reduced visual acuity (to approximately 20/200), strabismus, and myopia or hypermetropia.

Diagnosis

Diagnosis is confirmed by electroretinography (ERG) and supranormal amplitudes on electro-oculography.

Histopathology

Histologic analysis shows a macular hypoplasia or aplasia. The RPE may be absent or may exhibit decreased pigmentation. The number of normal melanosomes may be reduced, or the melanin pigment normally deposited in the melanosomes may be absent or reduced. Rarely, RPE cells may exhibit giant melanin granules called **macromelanosomes**. The retinal ganglion cell layer may be normal but is usually thick. The choroid may have abnormal granules in the monocytes and polymorphonuclear leukocytes, and choroid vessels are very prominent. The **Chédiak-Higashi syndrome** precipitates a granulomatous choroiditis, with optic neuritis and optic disc infiltration and cells resembling the immature lymphocytes. In **Bergsma-Kaiser-Kupfer syndrome** (**punctate oculocutaneous albinism**) there are window defects in the RPE.

Treatment

Dark sunglasses can ameliorate the symptoms, as can tinted contact lenses with an artificial pupil. Correction of refractive errors and strabismus is attempted. Low-vision aids and genetic counseling should be offered.

Waldenström's Macroglobulinemia

Waldenström's macroglobulinemia is a disorder of the reticuloendothelial system (or plasma cell dyscrasia or monoclonal gammopathy) that includes a bilateral retinopathy and that occurs in persons older

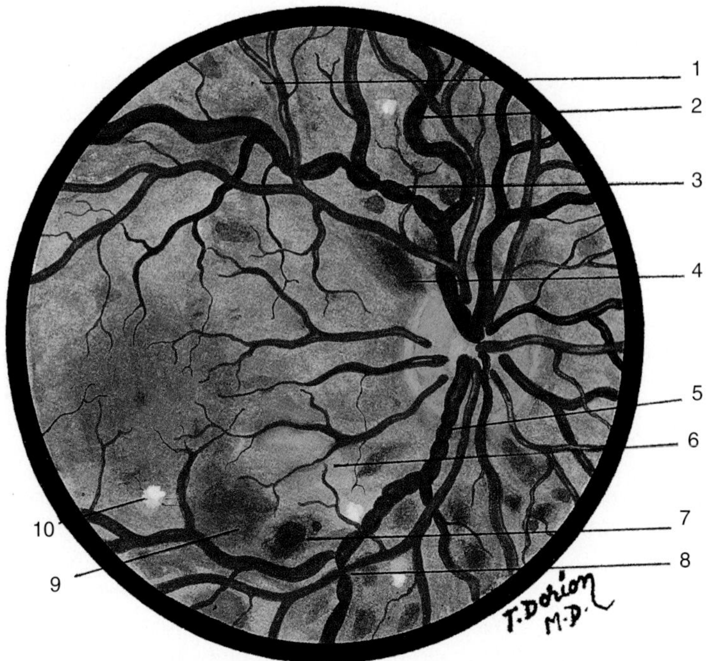

Figure 15-7. *Waldenström's macroglobulinemia. (1) Microaneurysms. (2) Dilated, tortuous veins. (3) Sausagelike vein constrictions. (4) Flame-shaped hemorrhages. (5) Venous beading. (6) Retinal edema. (7) Retinal hemorrhages. (8) Narrowed arteries and nicking. (9) Vitreous hemorrhage. (10) Cotton-wool spot.*

than 50 years. It is classified among the **hyperviscosity syndromes**, together with polycythemia vera and multiple myeloma.

The disorder is due to a vascular stasis and a secondary hypoxia, with sludging of the blood flow, and to an increase in the lateral pressure caused by the presence of an abnormal immunoglobulin (IgM; molecular weight, approximately 1 million, as compared with the normal hemoglobin of 150,000). This condition gives rise to *cryoglobulins* and to serum viscosity. As a result of an insufficient delivery of oxygen and metabolites to the tissues, the stasis leads to dilatation and occlusion of larger veins and to retinal hemorrhage.

Waldenström's macroglobulinemia appears as markedly dilated, tortuous veins, with *beading* and *sausagelike* constrictions (Figure 15-7).

Arteries are narrowed, and nicking is evident. Multiple, superficial flame-shaped or deep intraretinal hemorrhages extend to the periphery. Also, microaneurysms are evident at the peripheral retina, in addition to vitreal hemorrhage and occasional neovascularization, resembling a bilateral central vein occlusion. Sometimes, cotton-wool spots, retinal edema, and exudative retinal detachment may be present.

Symptoms

The predominant symptom of Waldenström's macroglobulinemia is decreased vision.

Diagnosis

Serum viscosity is increased to five times that of water (normal water-serum ratio is 1.2:1.6). Total serum globulin is increased as high as 7 g/dl (normal, 2.0–3.6 g/dl). Diagnosis is strengthened by an increased serum protein (normal, 6–8 g/dl). Protein electrophoresis reveals a sharp peak. Urinalysis may show *Bence Jones protein*, and the *Sia water (euglobulin) test* is positive, revealing an electrophoretic mobility in the gamma region.

Differential Diagnosis

A central retinal vein occlusion should be considered in the differential diagnosis. Multiple myeloma also is a possibility.

Histopathology

Histologic appraisal demonstrates venous dilatation, fibrinoid arterial degeneration, intraretinal hemorrhages, microinfarcts in the nerve fiber layer, exudates in the outer plexiform layer, and microaneurysms.

Treatment

Treatment is effective with chemotherapy: chlorambucil, 0.1–0.2 mg/kg/day once a month; melphalan, 0.25 mg/kg/day once a month; and prednisone, 60 mg/day PO. Plasmapheresis and cytotoxic drugs are additional medical interventions.

Rubella

Rubella (*German measles retinopathy*, *three-day measles*, or *Gregg's syndrome*) is a systemic disease involving a bilateral congenital retinopathy. Usually, it is stationary, although it may progress. It occurs after an infection with a ribonucleic (RNA) *togavirus* (*German measles virus*) in the first trimester of pregnancy (especially in the first month). It may be associated with such cardiovascular defects as patent ductus arteriosus, deafness, genitourinary disorders, cataract, searching strabismus, iritis, uveal coloboma, diabetes, osteomyelitis, hepatomegaly, congenital and infantile glaucoma, and microphthalmia. Pupillary anomalies and mental retardation also may ensue. **Expanded rubella** syndrome includes thrombocytopenic purpura, hemolytic anemia, and central nervous system diseases.

Rubella probably is due to the direct effect of the virus on the RPE, causing a *melanin* pigment disturbance. The disorder appears as a diffuse pigmentation (Figure 15-8) that can be exclusively *peripheral*, *macular*, or *sectorial*. The retina appears mottled with discrete, fine, granular alternating areas of pigmentation and depigmentation called *salt and pepper* (coarser in the macula and more granular elsewhere). Sometimes, a blotchy pigmentation, spicules, or speckles may be found at the posterior pole. The foveal reflex may be lost. Occasionally, choroidal neovascularization, retinal hemorrhages, and macular disciform scarring may occur. The retinal vessels are normal, although the disc may be pale.

Symptoms

Usually, rubella is asymptomatic.

Diagnosis

Fluorescein angiography may reveal a diffuse hyperfluorescence of the RPE. The antirubella antibody titer may be increased.

Differential Diagnosis

The differential diagnosis should consider congenital syphilis, blunt ocular trauma, and retinitis pigmentosa.

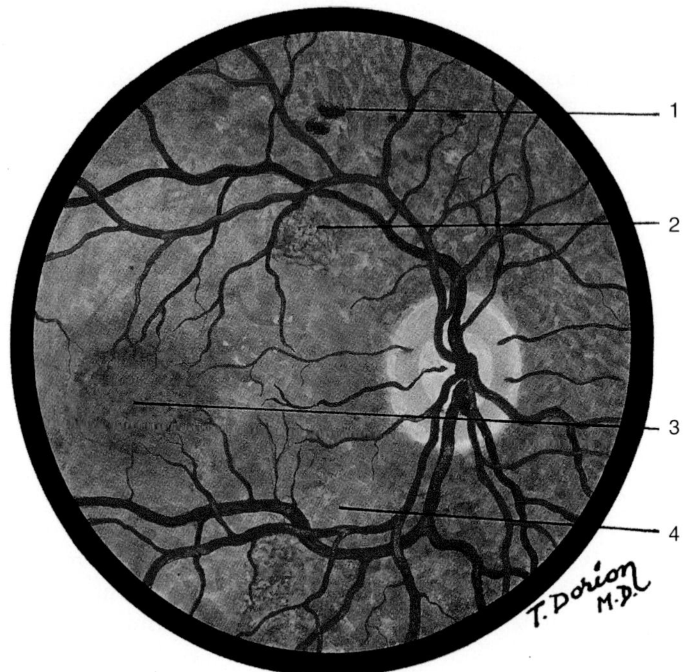

Figure 15-8. *Rubella. (1) Retinal hemorrhage. (2) Choroidal neovascularization. (3) Foveal reflex lost. (4) Salt-and-pepper pigmentation.*

Histopathology

Histologic examination reveals a possible moderate disruption of the RPE, occasionally with pigment clumping. Areas of atrophy alternate with hypertrophy of the RPE. Numerous foci of increased and decreased pigmentation usually are present.

Treatment

Treatment of glaucoma caused by this disorder is effected by administration of acetazolamide, 15 mg/kg/day. Beta-blockers also are effective. Goniotomy or trabeculotomy, filtration surgery with mitomycin D or fluorouracil, and cyclocryotherapy are surgical interventions.

Gardner's Syndrome

Gardner's syndrome is a hereditary, autosomal dominant, grouped-pattern pigmentation of the ocular fundus. It occurs in a systemic disease as a familial polyposis of the large bowel with supernumerary teeth, fibrous dysplasia of the skull, osteoma, fibroma, and epithelial cysts, and carries a very high risk for colon adenocarcinoma.

The disorder appears as multiple, bilateral, flat areas of hyperpigmentation (called *bear tracks*) similar to those in congenital hypertrophy of RPE and usually located peripherally but sometimes in the perimacular or peripapillary areas. The characteristic feature is a halo of RPE atrophy appearing as a depigmented surrounding area. Rarely, the bear tracks may be white and thus are called *polar bear tracks*.

Symptoms

Gardner's syndrome may be asymptomatic.

Histopathology

Histologic appraisal reveals hypertrophy of the RPE.

Treatment

No ocular treatment is needed for Gardner's syndrome.

Alport's Syndrome

Alport's syndrome comprises, among other abnormalities, a retinal detachment and a retinal dystrophy. It is an autosomal dominant trait with incomplete penetrance and varying expressivity of the mutant gene, and the disorder occurs more frequently in the male population. It appears as a progressive familial hematuric nephritis, with neuronal perceptive deafness, cataract, and thrombocytopenia. Rarely, it may be X-linked recessive, and usually it is fatal in 5 years. It may be due to a defect in Bruch's membrane formation.

Alport's syndrome appears as scattered, polymorphous, dystrophic, gray-white patches at the posterior pole and in the midperiphery, with areas of retinal detachment. The macula may exhibit a diminished foveal reflex, discrete pigmentation, macular holes, superficial perimacular white flecks, and crystalline deposits in the inner retina in a lacy configuration. The optic disc may contain drusen. The disorder may be accompanied by an **oil-droplet reflex** (an early sign of anterior lenticonus), and the vitreous may show neovascularization.

Symptoms

Symptoms of Alport's syndrome include decreased vision, increased myopia, irregular astigmatism, and anterior subcapsular cataract. Other possible symptoms are microspherophakia and rubeosis iridis.

Histopathology

Histologic analysis shows a disorganized and detached retina. Sometimes, the retina is neovascularized. Occasionally, the optic disc develops drusen, and pigment accumulation in the macular area may be present.

Subacute Sclerosing Panencephalitis

Also called *Dawson's inclusion body encephalitis*, subacute sclerosing panencephalitis manifests as a rare focal chorioretinitis with low-grade inflammation. It appears after measles or measles vaccination in a chronic, slowly progressive, lethal encephalitis in children 6–14 years old (more frequently boys). Probably it is caused by *measles virus*.

The disorder appears as a bilateral, not necessarily simultaneous, small, ground-glass whitening of the retina (Figure 15-9) in and around the macula. Sometimes, it results in areas of macular opalescent swelling or cystoid macular degeneration. Cotton-wool spots, papilledema, or optic atrophy may be present. Retinal vessels may appear narrowed and exhibit periphlebitis, and areas of necrotizing retinitis also may be seen. There may be hemorrhage in an early stage of the disease. A mild posterior uveitis with intraretinal infiltrates, hard exudates, preretinal membrane, and retinal folds may be present. The late-stage disorder may produce mottling of RPE and pigment proliferation, nonspecific chorioretinal scars, pigmentary atrophy, or gliosis.

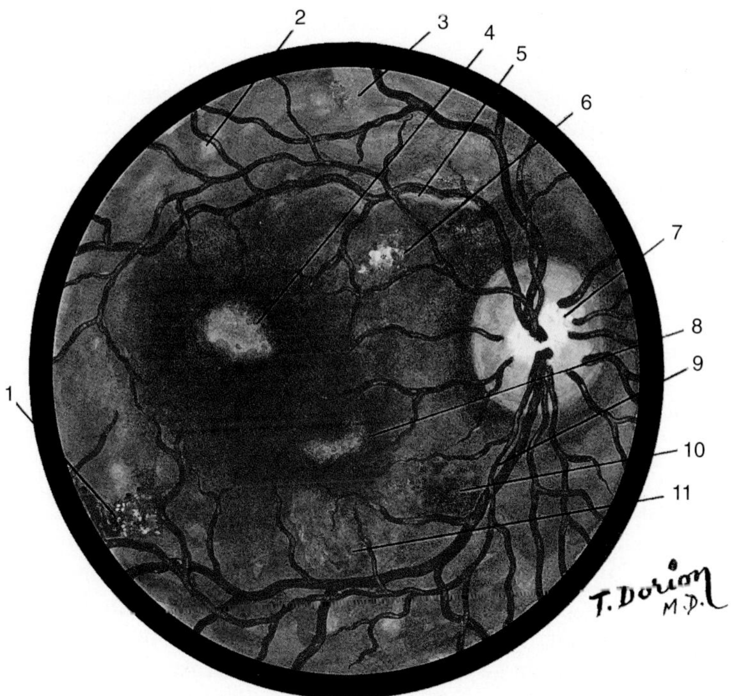

Figure 15-9. *Subacute sclerosing panencephalitis. (1) Necrotizing retinitis. (2) Cotton-wool spots. (3) Retinal infiltrates. (4) Small ground-glass retinal whitening, opalescent areas in the macula. (5) Periphlebitis. (6) Hard exudates. (7) Optic atrophy. (8) Nonspecific chorioretinal scars (9) Narrowed retinal vessels. (10) Mottling pigment proliferation. (11) Retinal folds.*

Symptoms

Subacute sclerosing panencephalitis may be asymptomatic for a long time. *Ocular symptoms may precede the neurologic signs.* Cortical blindness, nystagmus, myoclonic jerks, and mental retardation are additional indicators of this condition.

Diagnosis

An electroencephalogram is definitive. A lumbar puncture for cerebrospinal fluid (CSF) evaluation is performed to confirm the diagnosis.

Histopathology

Histologic examination shows a necrotizing retinitis, with atrophy of the inner retinal layers and cystoid degeneration of the outer plexiform layer. There is an intranuclear infiltration of the retina, with the nuclear chromatin clumped in the periphery. The cytoplasm contains agglomerations of multinucleated *inclusion bodies* and filamentous microtubules, probably **viral nucleocapsid.** Lymphocytic infiltration also is present.

Treatment

There is no treatment for subacute sclerosing panencephalitis.

Acquired Immunodeficiency Syndrome

Among the abnormalities that accompany the acquired immunodeficiency syndrome (AIDS) is a retinal vasculopathy attributable to the *human immunodeficiency virus (HIV-1).* The syndrome is caused by an RNA retrovirus in a systemic, devastating disease, usually is lethal in approximately 10 years, and occurs in such risk groups as homosexual or bisexual men, intravenous drug abusers, sexual partners of HIV-positive persons, prostitutes, infants from mothers afflicted with AIDS, hemophiliacs, and transfusion recipients. It may be associated with retinopathies such as occur in cytomegalovirus, *Pneumocystis carinii*, toxoplasmosis, herpes simplex, histoplasmosis, candidiasis, progressive outer retinal necrosis, and cryptococcosis. Currently, it is associated also with Kaposi's sarcoma, non-Hodgkin's lymphoma, and papovavirus-mediated demyelinating disease. (The specific pictures of the fundus are described elsewhere in this text for most of the foregoing diseases.)

Generally, the fundus lesions in AIDS-related diseases are microaneurysms, intraretinal hemorrhages, flame-shaped or dot-and-blot hemorrhages, Roth's spots, cotton-wool spots, retinal vasculitis, and periphlebitis. The disc may exhibit an optic neuritis, papilledema, or optic atrophy. The macula may show an ischemic maculopathy or a macular edema. The retina and the choroid may exhibit areas of opacification, necrosis, and edema.

Symptoms

AIDS may be asymptomatic. Poor vision, strabismus, follicular conjunctivitis, nongranulomatous iritis, and punctate or geographic ulcerative keratitis all may be seen in AIDS patients.

Diagnosis

Diagnostic evaluation includes a serologic test for HIV. There is an increased concentration of immune complex–dissociated HIV-1 p24 antigen and an elevated level of plasma virion RNA. The number of proviral cDNA in cells is increased. A polymerase chain reaction assay is performed to measure the viral load in the infected cells. A conjunctival biopsy can confirm Kaposi's sarcoma. Isolation of HIV is determined from tears and from the conjunctiva, cornea, aqueous humor, retina, and vitreous. Severe lymphopenia is demonstrated (frequently lower than 500/mm^3; normal, 1,200–3,900/mm^3). The ratio of helper to suppressor T lymphocytes is reversed to less than 0.5 (normal, 1.5 or greater), and the number of T lymphocytes is reduced to less than 30% (normal, 74–86%). Diagnostic tools include an enzyme-linked immunosorbent assay, a Western blot analysis, and a radioimmunoprecipitation procedure. Other definitive tests are immunofluorescent and immunochemical methods, using monoclonal or polyclonal antibodies, and a Southern blot hybridization procedure.

Differential Diagnosis

The differential diagnosis should consider diabetes, hypertension, collagen vascular diseases, and retinal vein occlusion.

Histopathology

Histologic evaluation reveals that the RPE may have HIV-positive cells, macrophages, and viral antigens. Bruch's membrane may be thickened, and lymphocytic and neutrophilic infiltration and swollen endothelial cells may be observed in the retina. Microinfarcts may occur in the nerve fiber layer from the high level of circulating immune complexes. The capillaries may be narrowed, the optic disc may be degenerated or atrophic, and macular edema may be present.

Treatment

Antiretroviral antimetabolite therapy for AIDS includes zidovudine (azidothymidine, Retrovir), 200 mg PO every 8 hours; didanosine (Videx), 125–200 mg PO twice per day; zalcitabine (Hivid), one 0.750-mg tablet PO every 8 hours; or stavudine (Zerit), one 40-mg tablet PO twice per day at a 12-hour interval between doses. Treatment of HIV-related diseases is mandated.

Polycythemia Vera

Also called *Osler-Vaquez disease*, polycythemia vera is classified as a *hyperviscosity syndrome* and occurs mostly in middle-aged persons. It features a chronic vascular retinopathy of unknown etiology. Usually, it is associated with kidney tumors or cysts, cerebellar hemangioblastoma, uterine myoma, and hepatoma. The disorder may occur as either of two types: *primary* and *secondary*.

Primary polycythemia is due to a hyperplasia of the *erythroblasts* in the bone marrow, which may cause a hyperviscosity of the blood and a resultant red cell count from 6–12 million/mm^2. **Secondary polycythemia** is due to a chronic ischemia or to an increased level of *erythropoietin* in such conditions as emphysema or congenital heart disease.

The disorder, a cyanotic fundus, appears as dark red to blue. The veins are engorged and markedly tortuous and exhibit dark-purple blood, venous stasis, and arteriovenous crossing defects. The arteries also may be dilated, and occlusions may occur in the central or branch retinal arteries and veins. Retinal hemorrhages and microaneurysms may be present, areas of retinal edema may be seen, and the choroid is thickened and red brown. The disc may be hyperemic and swollen, and optic atrophy may be seen.

Symptoms

Polycythemia vera causes mild blurring of vision and dusky redness of the conjunctiva, lips, and fingernails. Malaise, fatigue, weakness, a florid face, and headache are additional possible symptoms. Hearing loss and pain in the fingers and toes may ensue.

Diagnosis

A complete blood cell count (CBC) reveals red blood cells increased 6–12 million/mm^2, an increased hemoglobin level above 20 g/dl (normal, 14–18 g/dl in men, 12–16 g/dl in women), and an increase in the alkaline phosphatase level. The platelet count may be elevated above 1 million/µl (normal, 150,000–400,000/µl).

Histopathology

Histologic evaluation shows dilatation of veins (slightly overfilled). Sheets of blood representing hemorrhagic infarctions in the retinal inner layers are present. Pigmented deposits of **hemosiderin** in the retina commonly are present. The rod and cone layer (photoreceptors) usually is normal.

Treatment

An internist should handle any treatment. Additional interventions are radioactive phosphorus (^{32}P), 3–5 mCi IV, then increased by 25%, and venesection.

Pernicious Anemia

In pernicious anemia (or *megaloblastic anemia*), a hemorrhagic retinopathy is seen that usually occurs in adults older than 35 years. The disorder strikes those of Scandinavian, English, and Irish ancestry (but rarely Asians) in a hematologic disease accompanied by macrocytic anemia and thrombocytopenia. It may be associated with previous gastrectomy, regional ileitis, and fish tapeworm disease.

Pernicious anemia is due to a deficiency of absorption of vitamin B_{12}, a condition caused by a defect in production of the *intrinsic factor* in the walls of the stomach, with a consequent reduction of the platelet count to 40,000–100,000/µl (normal, 150,000–400,000/µl); a decrease in the red blood cells, which become hyperchromic and enlarged, to less than 2.5 million/µl (or as low as 500,000/µl; normal, 4–6 million/µl), and a diminishment of the hemoglobin to as low as 2–10 g/dl (normal, 14–18 g/dl).

Pernicious anemia appears as retinal hemorrhages (e.g., superficial flame-shaped or linear splinter hemorrhages) scattered throughout the fundus or the peripapillary region. Preretinal hemorrhage (boat-shaped and exhibiting a horizontal fluid level) may be present, or there may be spindle-shaped hemorrhages (usually horizontal) demonstrating a centered white area (called *Roth's spot*) resulting from the accumulation of degenerating leukocytes. Choroidal hemorrhages also are present. The fundus shows a generalized pale background, and blurring of the normal texture of the ocular fundus is possible, as is retinal edema appearing as an accentuation of the relative pallor of the choroidal reflex. Rarely, the disorder may cause a retinal detachment, owing to an intense transudation from the choroidal vessels. It usually reattaches spontaneously as the anemia recovers.

Bilateral optic neuropathy or optic atrophy are possible effects, in addition to small, variably sized and irregularly shaped, pale or yellow-white, soft exudates. These exudates with fluffy margins (*cotton-wool spots*) are caused by swollen nerve fibers resulting from a capillary ischemia, are located mainly at the posterior pole along the major arteries, and spare the macula. There may be chronic, wax-colored hard exudates (lipophilic deposits) with more delineated margins; they may coalesce, involving the macula, creating a series of radiating folds with edema residues, and giving rise to a **macular star**. Also, the retinal veins may be engorged.

Symptoms

Decreased visual acuity, nystagmus, and palpebral edema are symptoms of pernicious anemia. Rarely, ophthalmoplegia is considered. *Tobacco amblyopia* is seen in heavy smokers. Pallor, anorexia, dyspepsia, and symmetric numbness of feet are additional symptoms.

Diagnosis

Cataract and Horner's syndrome aid in making the diagnosis. A CBC is performed for pancytopenia, oval macrocytes, and hypersegmented neutrophils. A megaloblastic bone marrow test is confirmatory.

Histopathology

Histologic analysis reveals blood pockets in the retinal nerve fiber layer, in the arterioles, and in the capillary region. Also, blood may be accumulated in the subhyaloid area between the retina and the overlying posterior face of the vitreous. Hemorrhagic infarctions in the nerve fiber layer may be present. Lipophilic deposits in the outer plexiform layer also may be seen. The internal limiting membrane may exhibit discontinuities or may be lifted up at the macula into a series of radiating folds.

Treatment

Cyanocobalamin (vitamin B_{12}) is administered IM (100-μg doses) weekly for 2 months and then monthly for life.

Thrombocytic Thrombocytopenic Purpura

Thrombocytic thrombocytopenic purpura, a bilateral hemorrhagic retinopathy and a severe illness with a poor prognosis, represents an idiopathic form of **disseminated intravascular coagulopathy**. This disorder may be caused by a thrombotic occlusion of the choriocapillaris and adjacent choroidal arteries and veins in the macular and peripapillary areas. That condition consequently may produce a fibrinoid necrosis of the RPE, which becomes incompetent; the result is a breakdown of the blood-retina barrier, allowing large accumulations of subretinal serous fluid and altered viscous serum with an elevated fibrinogen level.

Thrombocytic thrombocytopenic purpura appears as boat-shaped preretinal hemorrhages (usually located superior to the disc) and as numerous paravenous retinal hemorrhages along both temporal vascular arcades. Sometimes, there are fine granular dots that suggest thrombi; also, there are scattered choroidal hemorrhages. Occasionally, areas of retinal discoloration and undulating folds of a diffuse secondary serous retinal detachment may be seen. Retinal edema, commonly near the optic disc, or even a papilledema also may be present.

Symptoms

Symptoms include decreased vision, fatigue, palpitations, and fainting. Hematemesis, jaundice, purpura, and fever also are manifest. Neurologic signs, such as disorientation, motility disturbances, even fatal cerebral hemorrhages, may be present.

Diagnosis

Fluorescein angiography may reveal focal leakage of the dye and a later staining of the discolored areas. Hemolytic anemia results, as do thrombocytopenia and azotemia. The Coombs' test is negative. Immunodeficiency may be revealed by low levels of IgM and absence of isohemagglutinin, but with normal levels of IgG and IgA.

Histopathology

Histologic examination shows areas of RPE necrosis exhibiting vacuolization. There are occlusions of the choriocapillaris and adjacent choroidal vessels by platelet thrombi, hyaline, and fibrillar material. Also revealed are areas of endothelial cell proliferation and areas of recanalization in the retina. Submacular choroidal and retinal hemorrhages may be present.

Treatment

Treatment should be managed by an internist. Fresh-frozen plasma is administered. Plasmapheresis is an additional intervention.

Pregnancy Retinopathy

Pregnancy retinopathy is a vascular retinopathy that may occur either in *normal pregnancy* or in such resultant complications as *pre-eclampsia* or *eclampsia.* **Retinopathy of normal pregnancy** occurs after the twenty-eighth week of a pregnancy in which the blood pressure is elevated (systolic above 160, diastolic above 100). This disorder usually appears as a narrowing of retinal arteries, especially of the nasal vessels.

Retinopathy of pre-eclampsia occurs in this complication of the pregnancy (either latent or manifest) in which marked hypertension is associated with edema or proteinuria. It appears initially as a segmental retinal narrowing on the nasal peripheral retina; it spreads toward the disc and is followed by a generalized arterial attenuation. Usually, the *artery-to-vein ratio* is increased (normal, 2:3, the vein being wider). Occasionally, multiple pigmentary spots (called *Elschnig's spots*) are seen along the vessels, or atrophic linear areas (called *Siegrist's streaks*) due to an anterior choroidal ischemia may occur. Rarely, a retinal detachment (usually located inferiorly) or retinal striae may be present. After delivery, all these changes may reverse to complete remission.

Retinopathy of eclampsia occurs in a more severe complication of the pregnancy and has the symptoms of pre-eclampsia plus convulsions, often uremia, and coma.

In an early stage, pregnancy retinopathy appears as a marked attenuation in the retina and in the nasal periphery and becomes generalized. The arteries are tortuous, resembling a corkscrew or a *beaded pearl necklace*. Occasionally, there is a localized, marked narrowing of the vessels, called *focal spasm*. In a late stage, an advanced arterial sclerosis may develop.

The disorder may be accompanied by a central serous choroidopathy due to a localized detachment of the retina and exhibiting a clear serous fluid at the macula. It may resolve completely after delivery or abortion. At the optic disc, there may be a complete absence of the retinal vessels over a distance of a few millimeters from the disc. Either an ischemic optic neuropathy or an optic atrophy may be present. Retinal ischemia, flame-shaped hemorrhages, cotton-wool spots, and macular star exudates also may occur. Sometimes, a bilateral subretinal edema may be observed; initially, it appears as a gray, patchy, cystic elevation located beneath the retinal vessels at varying intervals. The retina may appear gray, wet, or milky white and edematous and, along with the cotton-wool spots, gives rise to a pattern called *shot silk*. Some areas of retinal edema eventually may coalesce and, at the posterior pole, form a nonrhegmatogenous retinal detachment that also may involve the macula. They may increase in size, become globular, and gravitate inferiorly. Rarely, there may be a retinal arterial occlusion due to an amniotic fluid embolization.

Symptoms

Symptoms include blurred vision and difficulty in reading. Transient visual obscuration or complete vision loss are experienced. Cortical blindness may ensue.

Diagnosis

Diagnosis is confirmed by the presence of hypertension, proteinuria, seizures, and changes in refractive error. Visual field examination may reveal scotomas.

Treatment

Treatment of pregnancy retinopathy includes observation. Hypermetropic eyeglasses are prescribed as a temporary aid. Rarely, laser photocoagulation is performed. Termination of the pregnancy also is considered.

Vogt-Koyanagi-Harada Syndrome

Vogt-Koyanagi-Harada (VKH) syndrome (*uveo-meningoencephalitis syndrome*) is a rare bilateral uveitis of uncertain etiology (probably viral) that is part of a multisystemic disease involving the cerebrum, hair, skin, ears, and eyes. It occurs more frequently in Italy or in the Eastern Asia (especially in Japan) and in darkly pigmented persons such as Native Americans or Asian Indians of 20–50 years of age. The syndrome usually is associated with alopecia, vitiligo, poliosis, hearing defects, tinnitus, meningismus, ataxia, central nervous system abnormalities, seizures, extraocular muscle palsy, secondary glaucoma, anterior uveitis with mutton-fat keratic precipitates, acute or chronic iridocyclitis, peripheral anterior synechiae, and phthisis bulbi.

VKH syndrome may be due to a direct effect of a granulomatous or a nongranulomatous inflammatory process on the uvea. It occurs in three clinical stages: *prodromal*, *ophthalmic*, and *convalescent*. The **prodromal stage** is free of funduscopic findings.

In the **ophthalmic stage**, multiple, cloudy choroidal infiltrates are scattered unevenly throughout the fundus of both eyes (Figure 15-10). There may be several *Dalen-Fuchs nodules*, similar to those in sympathetic ophthalmia. Areas of RPE detachment of various sizes, mottling, and scarring at the posterior pole may be seen. Multiple zones of punctate pigment atrophy, also similar to those in sympathetic ophthalmia, may be present at the peripheral retina. Several areas of oval and circumscribed or large and acute exudative retinal detachment that gravitates inferiorly as a *teardrop* may be present. These detachments commonly resolve spontaneously with total retinal reattachment. Choroidal folds, exudates, and retinal hemorrhages or edema may also be seen. Sometimes, the fundus appears dark, earning the name *brunette fundus*. There may be macular edema or disciform macular degeneration. The optic disc may be congested, or papilledema may occur. The vitreous may be hazy and may exhibit cells.

The **convalescent stage** appears as a diffuse depigmentation of the retina owing to marked pigment loss; this is called *sunset glow* or *set-*

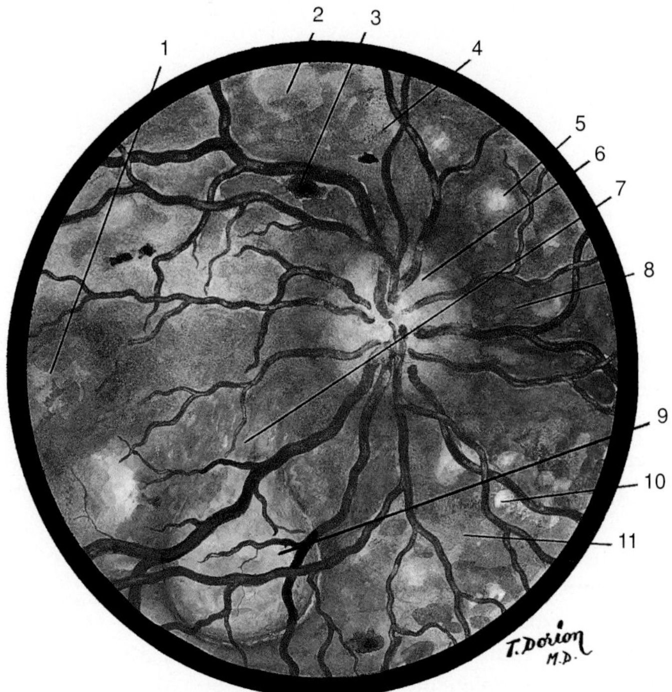

Figure 15-10. *Vogt-Koyanagi-Harada syndrome. (1) Macular edema. (2) Choroidal infiltrates. (3) Retinal hemorrhages. (4) Punctate retinal pigment epithelium atrophy. (5) Dalen-Fuchs nodules, similar to those in sympathetic ophthalmia. (6) Mild papilledema. (7) Choroidal folds. (8) Retinal pigment epithelium detachment. (9) Exudative retinal detachment, as a teardrop. (10) Mottling and scarring at the posterior pole. (11) Vitreous haze with cells.*

ting-sun fundus. Mottled white spots are interspersed with pigment deposits at the peripheral retina, mainly at the equator (*leopard spots*). Occasionally, areas of old chorioretinal scarring alternate with areas of active chorioretinitis. There may be a macular mottling depigmentation.

Symptoms

Prodromal fever, headache, stiff neck, nausea, malaise, dysacousia, tinnitus, and vertigo are all symptoms of VKH syndrome. Specific ocular symptoms include bilateral severe decreased visual acuity, photophobia, redness, and ocular pain.

Diagnosis

HLA testing may reveal HLA-BW22J and HLA-LDWa in Japanese patients and HLA-Dw-54 and HLA-DQw3 in Latin American and white patients. Antiretinal antibody titer will be increased in serum, and total T-cell counts (helper and suppressor) will be lower than normal. The circulating interferon gamma level is high in the setting of VKH syndrome. Skin tests, such as purified protein derivative of tuberculin (PPD) testing with anergy panel, may be undertaken to rule out diseases that present with similar symptoms.

Fluorescein angiography in the active phase may reveal areas of masking, which correspond to RPE lesions and multiple pinpoint areas of hyperfluorescence; in a later phase, leakage of fluorescein, window defects, disc staining, subretinal neovascularization, and occasional arteriovenous anastomoses are seen. Digital indocyanine green angiography may reveal multiple fluorescent spots and later hyperfluorescent foci, which may represent active leakage. ERG and electro-oculography are abnormal. Complete blood cell count (CBC), the rapid plasma reagin test (RPR), the fluorescent treponemal antibody absorption test (FTA-ABS), chest roentgenograms, angiotensin-converting enzyme levels, and PPD testing are useful clinically. CT scanning and magnetic resonance imaging might demonstrate important findings. A lumbar puncture may reveal CSF pleocytosis with increased levels of lymphocytes, mononuclear cells, and protein. Blood culture with Gram's and methenamine silver staining also may indicate the diagnosis.

Differential Diagnosis

In the differential diagnosis, syphilis, sympathetic ophthalmia, acute posterior multifocal placoid pigment epitheliopathy, sarcoidosis, and tuberculosis should be considered.

Histopathology

On histologic assessment, the choroid is seen to be diffusely thickened with granulomatous infiltration of nests of epithelioid cells surrounded by T lymphocytes, plasma cells, macrophages, and melanocytes. The choroid may be detached, blood may fill the suprachoroidal spaces, and scarring may be evident. The choriocapillaris may be obliterated, *not spared as in sympathetic ophthalmia.*

Usually, the retina is markedly gliotic, with striae and wrinkling of its internal limiting membrane. The RPE may occasionally be detached, or it may proliferate focally as granulomas that migrate into a disorganized retina. Occasionally, neovascular nodules that contain few inflammatory cells may extend into the vitreous. There may be a serous macular detachment or a total bullous retinal detachment. A thick preretinal or epiretinal membrane may also be present.

Treatment

Systemic corticosteroids are a therapeutic mainstay. Prednisone, 200 mg PO in the morning with breakfast for 7–10 days and then every other day for 2 weeks, followed by 100 mg/day PO for weeks or months, is the agent of choice. H_2-blockers (antiulcerative agents) include ranitidine, 150 mg PO twice a day. Prednisolone 0.125%, 1 drop hourly, is a first-choice topical steroid. Scopolamine 0.25%, 1 drop three times daily, is an effective cycloplegic. Immunosuppressive therapy might consist of cyclosporine A, 6-mercaptopurine, methotrexate, azathioprine, or chlorambucil.

Surgical interventions include lentectomy combined with vitrectomy. Laser photocoagulation is used to eliminate neovascular networks.

Whipple's Disease

A chronic retinochoroidopathy is seen in Whipple's disease, a rare, insidiously progressive intestinal lipodystrophy of unknown etiology that occurs mostly in middle-aged men. The disease mainly involves the gastrointestinal tract (with malabsorption) but also affects the musculoskeletal system (as arthritis), the central nervous system, and the eye. Whipple's disease appears as a bilateral retinitis displaying intraretinal hemorrhages, cotton-wool spots, retinal vasculitis, exudates over the pars plana, asteroid hyalosis, chronic vitritis with small white vitreous opacities, multifocal choroiditis with whitish choroidal lesions and choroidal folds, and papilledema. Any of these lesions may relapse.

Symptoms

Patients with Whipple's disease are likely to experience nystagmus, occasionally as unilateral pendular convergence nystagmus associated with a synchronous cocontraction of masticatory movements, called **oculomasticatory myorrhythmia.** Keratitis, chronic iridocyclitis, and ophthalmoparesis (predominantly vertical) are other ocular signs. Abdominal pain, diarrhea, arthritis that is recurrent and nondeformational, sacroiliitis, spondylitis, fever, malaise, and weight loss are other symptoms. Pneumonia or pleuritis may be seen. Other associated conditions include pericarditis, thyroiditis, progressive dementia, and skin hyperpigmentation.

Diagnosis

Jejunal mucosal biopsy and vitreous biopsy by pars plana vitrectomy can aid in establishing the diagnosis. CSF analysis also is useful in this regard.

Histopathology

In the inner retina and vitreous, and occasionally along the internal limiting membrane, is a *granuloma*, an accumulation of foamy macrophages having a pale blue cytoplasm, eccentric or paracentral small nuclei, and intracellular granules, which stain positively for periodic acid–Schiff. Sometimes, the granulomas exhibit serpiginous stacks of membranous structures. Tiny, rod-shaped, degenerated bacilli, which may be encased in phagocytic vacuoles, are found within and adjacent to the macrophages. These macrophages may be densely packed in the retinal nerve fiber layer, adjacent to the macula. A preretinal membrane may cause wrinkling of the internal limiting membrane. Outer and inner nuclear layers are relatively spared.

Treatment

Antibiotics are administered for at least 6 months and usually will succeed in inducing remission of this formerly lethal disease: Penicillin G (600,000 units PO twice per day), streptomycin (1 g IM twice per day), or tetracycline (250 mg PO four times per day) are the recommended agents. Another option is chloramphenicol, 50–100 mg/kg PO or IV in divided doses four times daily.

Behçet's Disease

Behçet's disease is a sometimes simultaneous, bilateral retinochoroidopathy that is part of a chronic inflammatory multisystemic disease of unknown etiology involving the eyes, skin, genitalia, and oropharyngeal membranes and occurs more frequently in men in Japan and the Middle East. It usually is associated with HLA-B51, which suggests that it may be an immune-mediated occlusive vasculitis associated with phlebitis, polyarthritis, cardiovascular lesions such as inferior vena cava thrombosis, and cerebral vasculitis. Behçet's disease may be due to an idiopathic obliterative vasculitic process that, in the past, was thought to be produced by a virus.

Behçet's disease appears in the acute phase as a marked retinal arterial attenuation with venous dilatation and tortuosity, intraretinal multifocal blotchy hemorrhages and infarctions, perivascular sheathing, and both periarteritis and periphlebitis at the posterior pole, more commonly involving the inferotemporal vessels. Dense perivascular exudates occasionally may obstruct the vessels completely, especially as a central retinal artery or branch retinal vein occlusion. After repeated attacks, the arteries may become narrowed as fine threads. There are areas of intense focal retinal ischemia and retinal necrosis.

Deep, focal, yellow-white, inflammatory intraretinal exudates may be scattered throughout the fundus. Neovascularization of the retina and retinal detachment may also be present. There is usually a severe vitritis with hazy vitreous, cells, and snowballs. Cystoid macular edema may be seen. The optic disc may be hyperemic, and sometimes papilledema develops.

In the chronic phase, a more diffuse posterior uveitis is seen. The macula appears pigmented and degenerated, with lipid deposits. Vascular sheathing worsens, optic disc hyperemia lessens, and papilledema, ischemic optic neuropathy, and optic atrophy may develop.

Symptoms

There is a *triad* of mucocutaneous uveal involvement: *uveitis*, with recurrent painful *oral aphthous ulcers* (canker sores), and *genital ulcer-*

ations. Visual acuity decreases to no light perception in approximately 5 years if the disease is not treated. Recurrent hypopyon are seen, but the eye typically is not red. Meningoencephalitis and cranial palsies; skin lesions such as erythema nodosum with a high fever, thrombophlebitis, and pyoderma; and gastrointestinal diseases such as colitis are known to occur in association with Behçet's disease.

Diagnosis

Fluorescein angiography in the acute phase reveals a marked capillary dilatation, diffuse leakage from small veins, and localized occlusions. In the later phase, leakage from larger vessels and the optic disc may be seen. The levels of circulating immune complexes are raised, whereas the complement level is reduced in the acute phase. Behçet's skin puncture test for pathergy and the HLA-B51 immunogenetic test might assist in making the diagnosis. The erythrocyte sedimentation rate may be elevated, as is the level of IgG during exacerbations of the disease. IgA is decreased in the acute disease phase but is elevated in the convalescent phase.

Histopathology

Chronic, nongranulomatous choroiditis is found in patients with Behçet's disease. Leukocytic, lymphocytic, and histiocytic perivascular infiltrates are seen on histologic evaluation. Endothelial cell proliferation and adventitial infiltration with thickening of the arterial walls also are present. The vascular lumina may undergo fibrinoid degeneration, with thrombosis and obliteration. Capillaries may demonstrate a proliferative endotheliitis. Hemorrhagic infarction usually is present. Areas of retinal detachment my be seen occasionally. In the vitreous, cells or microabscesses are usual findings.

Treatment

Immunosuppressive therapy consists of alkylating agents such as chlorambucil (Leukeran), 0.1–0.2 mg/kg/day PO, or cyclophosphamide, 1–2 mg/kg/day PO, for approximately 1 year. Antimetabolites such as azathioprine (Imuran), with an initial dose of 3–5 mg/kg/day, then reduced to 1–3 mg/kg/day in one or divided doses, are used. Prednisone tablets, 1 mg/kg/day PO, are the corticosteroid of choice. Antibiotics that might be used include cyclosporin A (Seromycin), 2.5–5.0 mg/kg/day PO with milk or juice, to a maximum of 10 mg/kg/day, and dapsone, 50 mg/day PO. Levamisole (Ergamisole), an immunostimulant drug, 50 mg PO four times a day for 3 days, may be beneficial. Consultation with an internist is recommended.

Systemic Lupus Erythematosus

Systemic lupus erythematosus (SLE) involves an arterial occlusive retinopathy that occurs mostly in black women of 20–40 years in conjunction with a chronic inflammatory disease of the connective tissue. SLE is associated with skin discoid butterfly lesions, Sjögren's syndrome, pericarditis, Raynaud's phenomenon, kidney diseases such as glomerulonephritis, nephrotic syndrome, and renal failure, arthritis, neurologic disorders, diplopia, nystagmus, hemolytic anemia, splenomegaly, thrombocytopenic purpura, HLA-DR2 and HLA-DR3, leukopenia, lymphopenia, and thyroiditis. The disease is due to a hyperactive immune system, which may synthesize anticell, anticytoplasmic, and antinuclear antibodies, thereby causing failure of the regulatory mechanism of the autoimmune system that prevents the body's attack of its own cells.

SLE appears as a retinal vasculitis in which the larger arteries are occluded and reduced in caliber to a fibrotic thread, the lumina are filled with white material, and the veins exhibit excessive sheathing and are congested, dilated, and beaded (Figure 15-11). Cotton-wool spots are scattered throughout the fundus. There are also deep and superficial flame-shaped hemorrhages, some of which have a white center (called **Roth's spots**). Occasionally, areas of bullous subretinal fluid, retinal edema, retinal exudative detachment, or venous stasis are present. The optic disc may be hazy and show blurred margins and a mild papilledema, which may obscure the details entirely, or there may even be a secondary optic atrophy.

Symptoms

Decreased visual acuity, blurred vision, amaurosis fugax, photophobia, and conjunctivitis all are symptoms of SLE.

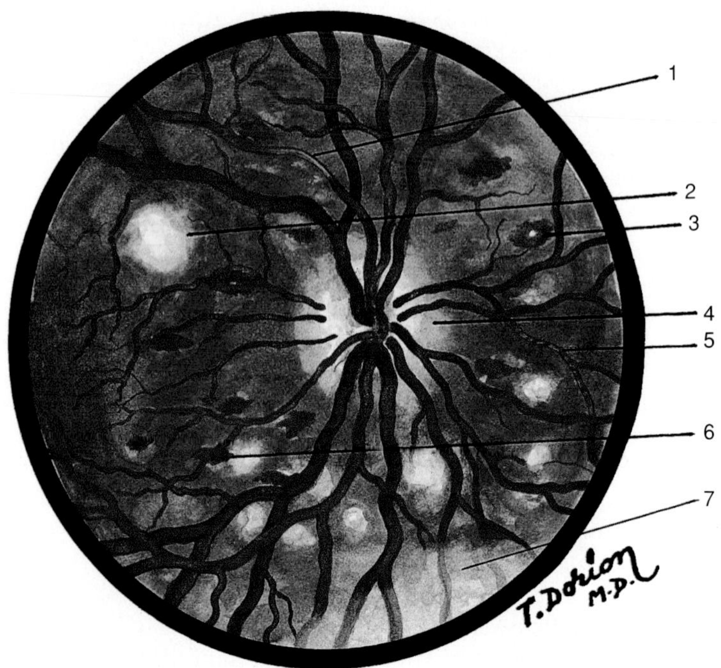

Figure 15-11. *Systemic lupus erythematosus. (1) Occluded large artery. (2) Cotton-wool spots. (3) Roth's spot. (4) Peripapillary edema. (5) Perivenous sheathing with beading veins. (6) Flame-shaped hemorrhage. (7) Retinal edema.*

Diagnosis

The antinuclear antibody (ANA) test is positive in SLE. A decreased hemoglobin and platelet count are seen. Leukopenia occurs owing to a decrease in the number of mononuclear cells. Testing for lupus erythematosus factor is positive. Hypergammaglobulinemia is present. The level of the third component of serum complement to native DNA (C3) is decreased (normal, 90–250 mg/dl), but often returns to normal in remission.

A Coombs' test will prove positive, as will a flocculation test. The erythrocyte sedimentation rate and fibrinogen level will be elevated. Tests for syphilis may be positive.

Fluorescein angiography may reveal neovascularization, serous elevation of the RPE and, in a late phase, staining of the retinal vessels, especially the arteries, and nonperfusion.

Differential Diagnosis

Among conditions to be considered in the differential diagnosis are rheumatoid arthritis, scleroderma, drug-induced lupus (procainamide and hydralazine), and chronic active hepatitis.

Histopathology

Histologic examination will reveal retinal arteries that might appear occluded by an amorphous material and little inflammatory reaction. The retina appears thickened, with areas of serous elevation of the RPE and sensory retina. There are retinal infarctions with cystoid bodies, as well as albuminous material with a hyaline center. Superficial and deep hemorrhages may be seen in the retinal nerve fiber and inner plexiform layers. Occasionally, there is granular degeneration in the rod and cone layer (photoreceptors), with accumulation of subretinal fluid. Choroidal arteries may be hypertrophic. There may be isolated foci of mild choroiditis, with infiltration by lymphocytes and round cells. The optic disc may exhibit infarcts, areas of demyelinization, or optic atrophy with loss of axons and foci of total nerve destruction.

Treatment

Corticosteroid therapy consists of prednisone, 40–60 mg/day PO. Immunosuppressive drugs include cyclophosphamide, azathioprine, and chlorambucil.

Tuberculosis

Tuberculosis (TB) is a systemic disease of which chorioretinopathy (usually bilateral) is a part. The disease may manifest itself ocularly as *tubercles*, *granulomas*, *choroiditis*, or *retinitis* and may involve the *optic disc* (Figure 15-12). It may be produced by an immune reaction to, or by hematogenous spread of, the bacillus *Mycobacterium tuberculosis homini of Koch*.

The **TB tubercle** may be solitary or conglomerated. A *solitary tubercle* appears as a pearly white or grayish creamy or hyalinized isolated choroidal mass, elevated from 1 to 2 D. It is of variable size, irregular,

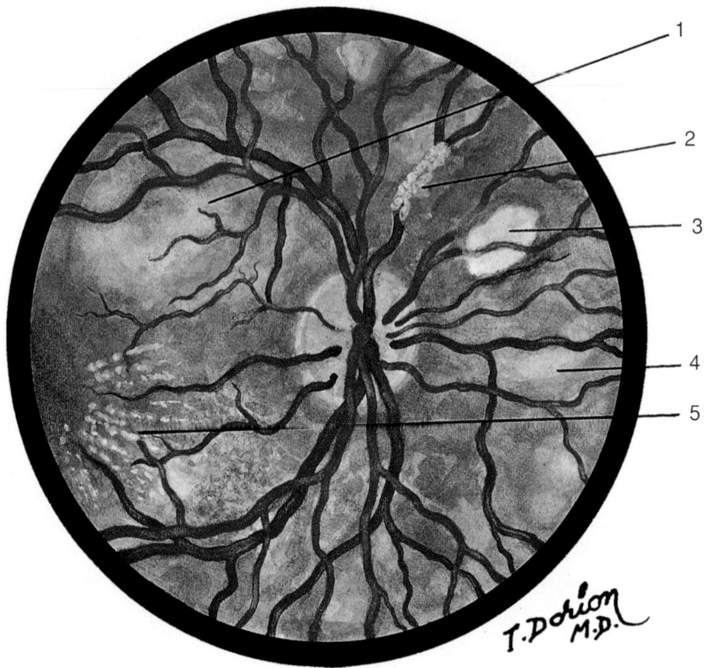

Figure 15-12. *Tuberculosis. (1) Granuloma. (2) Periphlebitis. (3) Choroidal atrophy. (4) Tubercle. (5) Macular star.*

and round or oval and displays a sharp delineated contour. Located at the posterior pole, it more commonly is seen in the perifoveolar region.

Conglomerated tubercles appear as large, white-gray choroidal masses, usually covered by exudates and hemorrhage, at the posterior pole. These may result from breakdown of a solitary tubercle, from fusion of miliary tubercles, or from extension of a spreading choroiditis.

TB granuloma may be *solitary* or *multiple*. Granulomas may appear as yellowish, round to oval nodules with ill-defined borders, approximately 0.5–2.0 mm in diameter, located anywhere in the fundus.

TB choroiditis may be circumscribed, miliary, or disseminated. *Circumscribed choroiditis* appears as a localized, gray-white lesion at the posterior pole, sometimes involving the macula as an ill-defined exudate. It does not spread, remains circumscribed, and heals with pigment heaping around the lesion.

Miliary choroiditis appears as several small, discrete, yellow-white or pink nodules or tubercles with little or no inflammation but sometimes with surrounding capillary congestion. There may be peripheral retinal and subretinal neovascularization. The choroiditis may remain localized and eventually heals, leaving superficial retinal exudate residues as a **macular star**.

Disseminated or *spreading choroiditis* appears as extensive gray-white lesions and heavy cloudiness of the vitreous, multiple areas of choroidal atrophy (occasionally with exposure of the choroidal vessels), and gliosis. Sometimes, necrosis and caseation progress rapidly, producing perforation of the globe.

TB retinitis may be exudative or may manifest as periphlebitis. *Exudative retinitis* appears as multiple, superficial, circumscribed, white-gray patches of variable size on the retina. In *periphlebitis*, there is white-yellow sheathing of exudates along the dilated retinal veins, often associated with recurrent hemorrhages that may extend into the vitreous, producing glial bands which, by contraction, may cause retinal detachment.

TB of the optic disc appears in the early stages as an optic neuritis and in the late stage as an optic atrophy.

Symptoms

Blurred vision, photophobia, and moderately injected eyes may be symptoms of ocular TB.

Diagnosis

Chest roentgenograms and a PPD skin test (5-TU [tuberculin unit]) will assist in the diagnostic workup. If TB is present, a Mantoux test will be positive. Fluorescein angiography may show hyperfluorescence of the choroidal lesions or perivascular staining of periphlebitis.

Differential Diagnosis

Sympathetic ophthalmia and sarcoidosis should be ruled out.

Histopathology

Histologic examination reveals a chorioretinopathy with zones of granulomatous reaction around areas of coagulative necrosis, called *caseation*

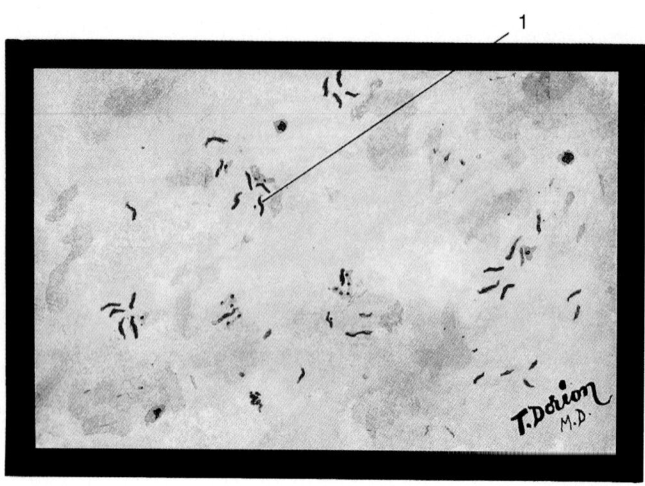

Figure 15-13. *Tuberculosis in sputum. (1) Small, red, acid-fast bacilli of* Mycobacterium tuberculosis *of Koch, the etiologic agent, shown in parallel alignment, or as serpentine cord.*

necrosis. The necrosis may be discrete in miliary TB or extensive in disseminated TB. In acute stages, there usually are numerous nests of deep epithelioid cells and tubercles. Retinal veins may be thrombosed, with varicosities, aneurysmal dilatations, and perivascular infiltration. The choroid usually is intensely infiltrated with lymphocytes and epithelioid cells. Small acidophilic bacilli of Koch may be seen by *Ziehl-Neelsen* coloration (Figure 15-13). In miliary choroiditis, these areas of infiltration are reduced and may or may not exhibit necrosis or caseation. In the late stage of TB, there is nonspecific retinal scarring. Tubercles often are present within the optic disc.

Treatment

An antituberculous combination of four drugs consists of *isoniazid (INH)*, *rifampin*, *pyrazinamide*, and either *ethambutol* or *streptomycin*. INH is administered in a dose of 300 mg/day PO, with added vitamin B_6 (pyridoxine), 10 mg/day PO, to prevent peripheral neuritis. Rifampin (Rifadin) is given 1–2 hours before or after meals; the dose is 300 mg PO twice per day. The dose of pyrazinamide is 0.75 g PO twice per day.

Ethambutol (Myambutol), 15 mg/kg/day PO, taken with food, may decrease visual acuity. Streptomycin is administered as 1 g IM two to three times weekly for months.

Other agents include *p*-aminosalicylic acid, 8–12 g/day PO, and capreomycin (Capastat), 1.5 mg/day IM. Prednisone, 40 mg/day PO, is the systemic steroid of choice. Cycloplegics may be added to TB therapy. Vitrectomy is an option.

Syphilis

A chorioretinopathy occurs in secondary and tertiary stages of both congenital and acquired syphilis (also known as *lues*), more frequently in nonwhite men. The disease is due to a systemic infection by the spirochete *Treponema pallidum*.

In **congenital syphilis**, bilateral, multiple, widespread, bright black and brown, round, star-shaped, or **bone-spicule** (retinitis pigmentosa–like) punctate dots are located at the posterior pole or in any isolated quadrants. Alternatively, focal pigmentation and atrophy, called *salt-and-pepper fundus*, might be seen in the peripheral retina (Figure 15-14). There are areas of hypopigmentation, chorioretinal atrophy, gliosis, retinal detachment, scattered retinal hemorrhages, and periphlebitis. Choroidal and retinal vessels may appear narrowed, with perivascular inflammation and sheathing. Clumps of cells and inflammatory changes may be present in the vitreous.

In **acquired syphilis**—usually in the secondary stage—unilateral or bilateral, diffuse, gray-yellow exudates appear more commonly along the retinal vessels and around the optic disc. There are also areas of necrotizing retinitis, with marked periarterial sheathing, thickening of vessel walls, segmentation of the blood column, constriction of the arterial lumen, vasculitis, or obliteration and sclerosis of both arteries and veins. As the inflammation subsides, blood empties from the vessels, resulting in *ghost vessels*. Scattered flame-shaped hemorrhages and areas of cloudy, edematous retina are seen. Occasionally, neovascularization of the retina and retinitis proliferans may develop. There also may be areas of active choroiditis, with multifocal infiltrates. Papilledema, ischemic optic neuropathy, and optic neovascularization may be seen. The vitreous may appear hazy, with cells and fine punctate exudates.

Other clinical forms of syphilis also exhibit ocular signs. These are *Förster's chorioretinitis*, *neuroretinitis papulosa*, *syphiloma* or *syphilis gummata*, and *tabetic optic atrophy*.

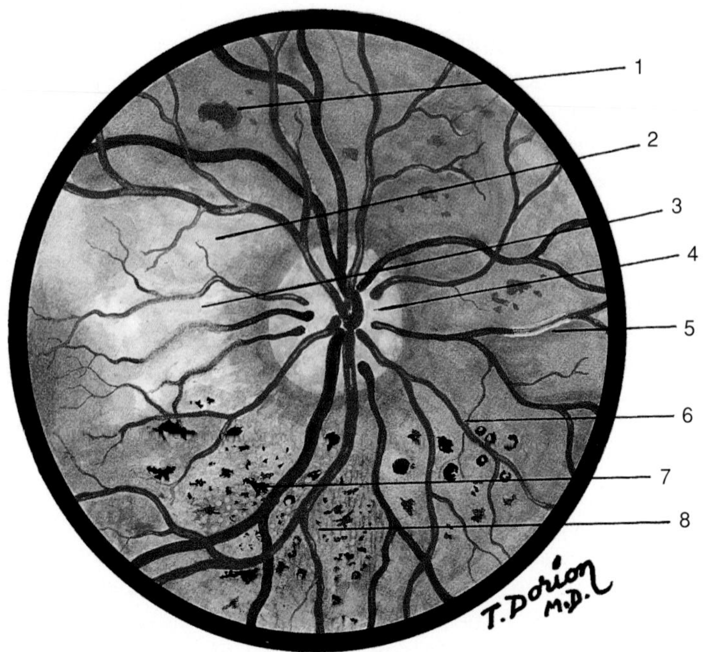

Figure 15-14. *Congenital syphilis. (1) Retinal hemorrhages. (2) Hypopigmented area. (3) Retinal edema. (4) Pale disc. (5) Periphlebitis. (6) Sclerosed vessels. (7) Bone-spicule pigmentation. (8) Salt-and-pepper fundus.*

Förster's chorioretinitis can occur in late secondary or tertiary syphilis. It is bilateral and appears as grayish areas at the posterior pole, which in time may become pigmented. Also, punched-out lesions of choroidal atrophy, gliosis, pigment clumping, or perivascular sheathing may develop. The optic disc appears inflamed and very hazy. The vitreous is cloudy and full of fine, dustlike opacities.

Neuroretinitis papulosa appears as a *triad* of *disseminated chorioretinitis*, *periphlebitis*, and *optic neuritis*. Occasionally, there may also be a peripapillary retinitis.

Syphiloma or **syphilis gummata** can occur in tertiary syphilis as a late benign lesion. It appears as a bluish or greenish mass with a rubbery center of variable size, with or without retinal detachment. It is thought to be due to the localization of *Treponema pallidum* into the choroid.

Tabetic optic atrophy occurs usually 15 or 20 years after the initial infection, in a slowly progressive parenchymatous syphilis called *tabes*. It may be primary or secondary. *Primary tabetic optic atrophy* involves those small nutrient vessels in the walls of larger arteries and veins called **vasa vasorum**. The optic disc is pale and yellowish white, with well-defined borders. *Secondary tabetic optic atrophy* occurs sometimes after hydrocephalus or basal meningitis. The disc is pale initially and then becomes grayer near the lamina cribrosa; it displays sharp margins.

Symptoms

Vision may be diminished.

Diagnosis

The diagnosis depends on positive tests for syphilis, including the VDRL test, RPR, microhemagglutination for *Treponema pallidum* (MHA-TP), treponemal passive hemagglutination assay (TPHA), FTA-ABS, and complement fixation test (Wassermann, Kolmer). Lumbar puncture is performed for CSF analysis, total protein, gamma globulin, and VDRL. Argyll-Robertson pupil is seen in neurosyphilis. Fluorescein angiography may show foci of epithelial degeneration.

Histopathology

Either a nongranulomatous or a granulomatous posterior choroiditis is evidenced on histologic examination. *Nongranulomatous posterior choroiditis* may be apparent in the outer retinal layers as disseminated, large atrophic scars. The RPE and choriocapillaris may be absent. Bruch's membrane may be folded and broken into a sclerosed choroid. Scattered lymphocytes and plasma cells may also be seen in the choroid.

Granulomatous posterior choroiditis may be marked by epithelioid cells, lymphocytes, and plasma cells around the vessels. RPE migration and pigment-laden macrophages may be found. The optic nerve may be atrophic. Coagulative necrosis, surrounded by epithelioid cells, lymphocytes, fibrotic cells and, occasionally, giant cells, may be present in the syphilitic gumma. Sometimes, *Treponema pallidum* is found within the choroid.

Treatment

Treatment is undertaken by an internist or dermatovenereologist. Systemic penicillin G benzathine, erythromycin, or tetracycline is administered, as are topical steroids and cycloplegics. Timolol (Timoptic), 0.5% 1 drop OU twice per day; levobunolol (Betagan), 0.5% 1 drop OU twice per day; or carteolol (Ocupress), 1% 1 drop OU twice per day, is used to control intraocular pressure.

Sturge-Weber Syndrome

Sturge-Weber syndrome (known also as *nevus flammeus*, *encephalo-oculoangiomatosis*, *encephalotrigeminal angiomatosis*, *encephalocavernous hemangiomatosis*, *port-wine stain*, and *claret stain*) is a unilateral, slowly progressive, choroidal hemangioma associated, as part of the syndrome, with an intracranial vascular malformation, a hemangioma of the ipsilateral leptomeninges and brain, with dural shunts. *It is the only phakomatosis that lacks a hereditary tendency.* The syndrome usually is fatal before age 30 years.

Sturge-Weber syndrome may increase the episcleral venous pressure (normal, 9–10 mm Hg) that is transmitted to the eye and may result in a *back pressure* that increases intraocular pressure (a secondary glaucoma). The ocular manifestations of the syndrome are a broad, red-orange, yellowish, relatively flat thickening of the choroid that measures up to several disc diameters; alternatively, the choroidal thickening might be diffuse and located at the posterior pole, temporal to the disc, may lack pigment, and might exhibit poorly delineated borders. Cystoid retinal degeneration may overlie the lesion, and this degeneration may cause secondary serous retinal detachment. Sometimes, the posterior pole appears more red than the background, a condition known as *tomato-ketchup fundus*. RPE alterations, which present a retinitis pigmentosa–like picture, are possible. Occasionally, the ocular sign of the Sturge-Weber syndrome is a juxtapapillary angioma.

Symptoms

Progressively decreased vision is symptomatic of the Sturge-Weber syndrome. A unilateral facial port-wine stain (called *nevus flammeus*) is seen over the distribution of the first and second branches of the fifth cranial (trigeminal) nerve. Facial hemihypertrophy and hematoma of the upper eyelid, episclera, ciliary body, and iris occur. Hemiparesis of the contralateral side may be seen. Unilateral, congenital, infantile, secondary open-angle glaucoma, due to an angle anomaly or elevation of the episcleral venous pressure, occurs on the affected side. Monocular buphthalmos, progressive hypermetropia, hemianopia, heterochromia iridis, megalocornea, and malformation of the anterior chamber are common. Jacksonian convulsive seizures, due to a corresponding angiomatous involvement of meninges and brain (leptomeningeal angiodysplasia), and subnormal intelligence or mental retardation all are associated with this syndrome.

Diagnosis

Visual field examination may reveal an arcuate field defect, gonioscopy may demonstrate blood in Schlemm's canal, and fluorescein angiography may reveal a rapidly developing hyperfluorescence. Thermography might be a useful diagnostic aid. B-scan ultrasonography may reveal a characteristic high internal acoustic reflectivity as a result of multiple changes in the tissue density, which is diagnostic. A pulsatile blood flow may be evident on Doppler scanning. Skull roentgenograms, CT scans (axial and coronal), and magnetic resonance imaging may reveal characteristic linear, serpiginous intracerebral calcifications of the meninges and, occasionally, a hemicortical atrophy. Karyotyping may reveal trisomy 22.

Differential Diagnosis

Choroidal melanoma, posterior scleritis, and choroidal metastasis should be ruled out.

Histopathology

On histologic evaluation, a choroidal hemangioma—a hamartoma composed of tissue that normally is found in the choroid—is seen. Also visible are engorged spaces and endothelium-lined, walled vessels that lack a capsule and are filled with red blood cells.

Treatment

Initially, the hypermetropic amblyopia should be treated. Cyclodiathermy is used for glaucoma. External-beam or plaque radiotherapy may prove beneficial. Argon laser photocoagulation is used to reduce the size of the hemangioma or to repair secondary retinal detachment. Anticonvulsant therapy is administered to control seizures: Among the effective agents are barbiturates (phenobarbital, 30–120 mg/day PO in two or three divided doses), benzodiazepines (clorazepate [Tranxene], 30 mg/day PO in divided doses), or hydantoin derivatives (phenytoin [Dilantin], 100 mg PO three times per day).

Tularemia

Tularemia is a systemic infectious disease caused by a gram-negative coccobacillus, *Francisella (Pasteurella) tularensis*, and transmitted from animals to humans by contact with wild rodents (e.g., rabbits, ground squirrels, chipmunks, rats, mice), fox, beavers, birds, sheep, and calves, via the bite of blood-sucking insects (e.g., wood ticks, deer flies, mosquitoes, lice), by consumption of infected, undercooked meat, or by drinking of contaminated water. The ocular manifestation is a hemorrhagic retinopathy, which appears as deep intraretinal hemorrhages, Roth's spots, and superficial perivascular infiltrates throughout the fundus. At the macula, there may be a submacular inflammatory focus with radiating striae. Optic neuritis also may develop.

Symptoms

Tularemia may be asymptomatic. More commonly, a host of symptoms occurs, including severe headache, nausea, fever, a local lesion (an ulcerative papule at the site of inoculation), conjunctivitis, limbal nodules with pannus, corneal ulcers with perforation, and dacryocystitis. Atypical pneumonia, lung abscess, enteritis, stupor, delirium, and splenomegaly all are possible. In **Parinaud's oculoglandular tularemia**, granulomatous conjunctivitis is accompanied by lymphadenopathy involving the preauricular, parotid, submaxillary, and cervical lymph nodes.

Diagnosis

The diagnosis is made on the basis of demonstration of the organism on blood culture, lymph node aspirate, or culture from the ulcerated lesion. The agglutination test is positive at a raised titer of 1 to 80 in the second week of infection. The skin test is considered positive if more than a 5-mm induration is seen.

Differential Diagnosis

Rickettsial infections, meningococcal infections, cat-scratch disease, pneumonia, and fungal diseases all are considered in the differential diagnosis.

Histopathology

The histologic picture is of a granulomatous inflammatory reaction involving the retinal vessels, retina, macula, and optic disc.

Treatment

Medical therapy consists of streptomycin (0.5 g IM every 8 hours for 7 days), chloramphenicol (0.5 g PO every 8 hours), or tetracycline (0.5 g PO every 8 hours). Drainage of suppurated lymph nodes is indicated.

Aicardi's Syndrome

Aicardi's syndrome is a systemic, congenital, X-linked dominant condition that, in girls, manifests as mental retardation, infantile spasms, and seizures but that, in boys, is lethal. A lacunar chorioretinopathy is part of this syndrome complex.

The syndrome is due to an intrauterine insult, probably not infectious, that occurs in the fourth to fifth week after conception and that is characterized by agenesis of the corpus callosum, with ectopic projections of abnormal brain tissue into the ventricles and chorioretinopathy. The ocular anomaly appears as multiple, circumscribed, well-delineated, round or oval areas of pigmented and depigmented, whitish lacunae, which usually involve the choroid and the RPE and are scattered mainly at the posterior pole. At the lacunar edges, RPE may proliferate. Sometimes, these areas appear as *punched-out lesions* of the choroid. Occasionally, there is total retinal detachment. A large juxtapapillary choroidal coloboma may extend to the optic disc. A dark gray optic nerve atrophy may also be present.

Symptoms

Visual impairment, mental retardation, seizures, and spasms are symptoms seen in Aicardi's syndrome.

Diagnosis

Electroencephalography usually shows high-amplitude, hypsarrhythmic waves.

Differential Diagnosis

Toxoplasmosis or choroidal coloboma should be considered in the differential diagnosis.

Histopathology

On histologic assessment, a disorganized retinal dysplasia is seen, and the retina is usually entirely detached. Extensive areas of gliosis and scattered rosette lesions may be present. A coloboma may be visible in the choroid. There may also be a coloboma of the optic disc, with proliferation of RPE at its edges and extensive tubular and papillary projections that may extend along the meninges of the optic nerve, surrounding the disc. The optic disc may be pale and atrophic. Papillae, lined by a markedly thinned and attenuated RPE, might be located along lacunae in the choroid. Retinal vessels likely will appear dilated. The choriocapillaris usually is intact.

Laurence-Moon-Bardet-Biedl Syndrome

Laurence-Moon-Bardet-Biedl syndrome is a hereditary, autosomal recessive, systemic disease (with a high rate of consanguinity) that comprises mental retardation, spastic paraplegia or hemiparesis, midbrain hypophyseal disturbances, adiposogenital syndrome with a fat-moon shape, short stature, truncal obesity and hypogonadism, polydactyly, retinitis pigmentosa, and deaf-mutism. A generalized atypical pigmentary retinopathy is a part of the syndrome complex.

The retinopathy appears as a pigmentary degeneration of the peripheral retina, similar to that in retinitis pigmentosa, or macular disturbances similar to those of juvenile amaurotic idiocy (Spielmeyer-Vogt-Batten-Mayou syndrome). There is thinning and sheathing of the arteries. Extensive chorioretinal atrophy, similar to that in choroideremia, is seen. In addition, optic atrophy may be present.

Stickler's Syndrome

Stickler's syndrome, otherwise known as *arthro-ophthalmopathy*, is a hereditary, progressive, autosomal dominant, degenerative disease consisting of ocular, orofacial, and skeletal abnormalities with *marfanoid* habitus. The ocular sign is a perivascular pigment deposit along the major retinal arteries and veins at the posterior fundus. There may be areas of circumferential and radial lattice degeneration. At the optic disc, vessels usually are dragged. Several small retinal breaks, areas of rhegmatogenous retinal detachment, and retinoschisis may be seen. There also may be multiple posterior vitreoretinal adhesions and, occasionally, proliferative vitreoretinopathy, vitreous cortical condensation, empty optic vitreous, vitreous veils usually located around large dehiscences, or lacunae of the vitreous gel. A thin layer of vitreous cortex sometimes is present behind the lens. Bands of collagen traversing the vitreous and adhering to the retina may be seen as well.

Symptoms

Stickler's syndrome may be signaled by micrognathia, epiphyseal dysplasia, cleft palate, midfacial flattening with large philtrum of the upper eyelid, glossoptosis, and decreased hearing. Loose or enlarged joints, hyperflexibility, and ataxia are common. Patients are likely to suffer from arthritis and to have long fingers with grooved nails. Cataract, ectopia lentis, glaucoma, high myopia, and strabismus are ocular signs and symptoms.

Diagnosis

ERG response is depressed.

Histopathology

At the RPE, pigment disorganization and clumping occur. Histologic workup may reveal areas of RPE atrophy. The vitreous cortex is condensed, and retinal detachment and retinal breaks may be seen.

Bassen-Kornzweig Syndrome

The Bassen-Kornzweig syndrome (also called *abetalipoproteinemia* and *acanthocytosis*) is a rare, hereditary, autosomal recessive, RPE dystrophy accompanied by abetalipoproteinemia and avitaminosis A in the retina and liver. The condition occurs usually in the first decade of life but might not be manifest until one's teenage years. It is commonly associated with celiac syndrome with acanthocytosis. The syndrome may be lethal.

The Bassen-Kornzweig syndrome appears as a pigment accumulation initially in the macula and slowly progressing toward the periphery. Alternatively, it sometimes merely resembles retinitis pigmentosa, with bone-spicule pigment. Retinal vessels are attenuated. There may be scattered angioid streaks, subretinal neovascularization, and generalized retinal atrophy. There also may be a pericentral pigmentary retinopathy or a retinitis punctata albescens. The optic disc may be pale and waxy, and cataract may occur.

The syndrome may be caused by a defect in the microsomal *triglyceride transfer protein*, with inability to synthesize very-low-density lipoproteins, chylomicrons, or *apolipoprotein B*, which in turn may produce a malabsorption of fat-soluble vitamins A, D, E, and K.

Symptoms

Vision loss progresses to blindness. Night blindness (nyctalopia) occurs early. There is dissociated nystagmus on lateral gaze, progressive palsy of the medial rectus muscles (with exotropia), and ophthalmoplegia. Abdominal distension, steatorrhea, and fat intolerance may signal the Bassen-Kornzweig syndrome. Patients suffer muscle weakness, retarded growth, skeletal deformities, peripheral progressive neuropathy, cerebral ataxia, and spinocerebellar degeneration.

Diagnosis

Serum abetalipoproteinemia levels should be ascertained to aid in making the diagnosis. A cholesterol count below 80 mg/dl signals this syndrome (normal, 150–250 mg/dl). Phospholipid and triglyceride levels also will be low. Low-density lipoproteins, very-low-density lipoproteins, and chylomicrons are absent. In the cerebrospinal fluid, the protein level will be increased. Findings of intestinal malabsorption, diarrhea, hypovitaminosis A and D, and cardiac conduction defects are indicative of the Bassen-Kornzweig syndrome. ERG is abnormal, up to extinction of the wave in late-stage disease. Fluorescein angiography may reveal a tapetochoroidal dystrophy. Abnormal, crenated erythrocytes (*acanthocytosis*) are seen.

Histopathology

On histologic evaluation, photoreceptor loss is seen. The RPE is attenuated or lost, although usually the macula is spared. There may be an accumulation of *lipofuscin* in the macular RPE.

Treatment

Treatment of the Bassen-Kornzweig syndrome consists of a fat-restricted diet, with medium-chain triglycerides included in the diet. Vitamin A (25,000 USP units PO twice per day for 2 months) and vitamin E (1,000 USP units PO daily) supplementation is indicated.

Suggested Reading

Bacal DA. Vogt-Koyanagi-Harada syndrome. Ophthalmol Times 1994;11:31.

Bylsma SS, Achim CL, Willey CA, et al. The predictive value of cytomegalic encephalitis in acquired immunodeficiency syndrome. Arch Ophthalmol 1995;113:89–95.

Chew EY, Klein ML, Ferris FL III, et al. Association of elevated serum lipid with retinal hard exudate in diabetic retinopathy. Arch Ophthalmol 1996;114: 1079–1084.

Condon PJ. Pregnancy and Its Complications. In A Sorsby (ed), Modern Ophthalmology, vol 2 (2nd ed). Philadelphia: Lippincott, 1972;607–616.

Deschenes J, Seamone C, Cha SB. Tuberculosis and Atypical Mycobacteria. In W Tasman, EA Jaeger, MM Parks, et al., Duane's Clinical Ophthalmology, vol 4. Philadelphia: Lippincott–Raven, 1996;58:5–7.

Gass JDM, Braunstein RA, Chenoweth RG. Acute syphilitic posterior placoid chorioretinitis. Ophthalmology 1990;97:1288–1297.

Ginsburg HL, Aiello LM. Diabetic retinopathy: classification, progression and management. Focal Points 1993;7:2–13.

Kahn M, Pepose JS, Green WR, Foos RY. Immunologic findings in a case of Vogt-Koyanagi-Harada syndrome. Ophthalmology 1993;100:1191–1198.

Lilley ER, Bruggers CS, Pollock SC. Papilledema in a patient with aplastic anemia. Arch Ophthalmol 1990;108:1674–1676.

Nesburn AB, Wood TR. Rubella and Viral Infections. In A Sorsby (ed), Modern Ophthalmology, vol 2 (2nd ed). Philadelphia: Lippincott, 1972;33–41.

O'Donnell FE Jr, Green WR. The Eye in Albinism. In W Tasman, EA Jaeger, MM Parks, et al., Duane's Clinical Ophthalmology, vol 4. Philadelphia: Lippincott–Raven, 1996;38:1–16.

O'Neill D, Bell J. Ocular Manifestations of Gastrointestinal Disorders. In W Tasman, EA Jaeger, MM Parks, et al., Duane's Clinical Ophthalmology, vol 5. Philadelphia: Lippincott–Raven, 1996;30:5–10.

Simpson GV. Sarcoidosis. In A Sorsby (ed), Modern Ophthalmology, vol 2 (2nd ed). Philadelphia: Lippincott, 1972;151–162.

Stenson SM, Friedberg DN. AIDS and the Eye. New Orleans: Contact Lens Association of Ophthalmologists, 1995;18–113.

Wang FM. Perinatal Ophthalmology. In W Tasman, EA Jaeger, MM Parks, et al., Duane's Clinical Ophthalmology, vol 5. Philadelphia: Lippincott–Raven, 1996;39:9–12.

Westlake WH, Heath JD. Sarcoidosis involving the optic nerve and the thalamus. Arch Ophthalmol 1995;113:669–670.

Wilhelmus KR. Common venereal diseases and the eye. Focal Points 1987;3:2–14.

Woods AC, Sorsby A. Ocular Tuberculosis. In A Sorsby (ed), Modern Ophthalmology, vol 2 (2nd ed). Philadelphia: Lippincott, 1972;105–143.

Glossary

ablatio retinae — See *commotio retinae.*

acanthocyte — a distorted erythrocyte with irregular protoplasmic projections, having a thorny appearance

acanthocytosis — presence of acanthocytes in the blood, with abetalipoproteinemia

accommodation — adjustment of the lens power for various distances; at near work (e.g., reading), the refractive power of the lens, its thickness, and its curvature are increased through contraction of the ciliary muscle (cranial nerve III [oculomotorius])

acidophil — a cell or tissue staining readily (in red) with acid dyes

adventitia — the outermost coating of a vessel

AIDS — acquired immunodeficiency syndrome, produced by the human immunodeficiency virus (HIV)

AION — anterior ischemic optic neuropathy

alkylating agents — highly reactive compounds that substitute alkyl groups for the hydrogen atoms of cer-

	tain organic substances; cytotoxic; used as antineoplastic agents
allele	an alternative form of a gene that can occupy a specific chromosomal locus
amaurosis fugax	temporary episode of unilateral loss of vision, occurring without apparent lesion of the eye, lasting usually approximately 10 minutes and rarely up to 2 hours
amaurotic cat's eye	unilateral blindness, with bright reflection of the pupil; often indicative of retinoblastoma
amblyopia	decreased central vision without any detectable organic lesion of the eye; commonly called *lazy eye*
amotio retinae	See *commotio retinae.*
Amsler's grid	a target test for detecting defects of the central visual field, consisting of evenly spaced horizontal and vertical lines and a central dot for fixation
ANA test	antinuclear antibody test, which is positive in systemic lupus erythematosus
angioblast	a vessel-forming cell
angiosclerosis	hardening of the walls of blood vessels
angiospasm	a sudden but transitory constriction of the blood vessels
angiotensin-converting enzyme (ACE)	peptidyl-dipeptidase A, an enzyme of a family of vasopressor hormones formed by the catalytic action of renin on renin substrate
anterior chamber	a space in the eye between cornea anteriorly and iris and pupil posteriorly, filled with aqueous humor
antimetabolite drug	a substance that structurally closely resembles a substance required for normal physi-

ologic functioning and that exerts its effect by interfering with utilization of the essential metabolite

antioxidant a synthetic or natural substance added to a product to prevent or delay its degradation by action of oxygen in the air

aphakia absence of the lens of the eye

apoptosis fragmentation of a cell into particles that then are eliminated by phagocytosis

Argyll-Robertson pupil a pupil that responds to accommodation by becoming miotic but that does not respond to light; usually present in neurosyphilis

ARMD age-related macular degeneration; previously called *senile macular degeneration*

A-scan a visual display on a cathode ray tube of ultrasonographic echoes, in which one axis represents the time required for return to the echo and the other represents the strength of the echo; determines the distance from the front of the cornea to the back of the retina (the axial length) and, possibly, the depth of intraocular structures; used in calculating the power of the intraocular lenses in cataract surgery

assay determination of amount of a constituent of a mixture or of the biological or pharmaceutical potency of a drug

astigmatism error of refraction in which there is an unequal curvature of the surface of the eye, so that the refracting power of the eye is not the same in all meridians; hence, a point of light cannot be brought to a point focus on the retina but is spread over a diffuse area

astrocyte a neuroglial cell with fibrous, protoplasmic, or plasmatofibrous processes

atrophy a diminution in the size of a cell, tissue, organ, or part; a wasting away

autologous related to self; originating within an organism itself

autosomal dominant inheritance in which the gene is located on any chromosome that is not a sex chromosome and is phenotypically expressed when present either in homozygous or heterozygous form

autosomal dominant with high penetrance maximum frequency of expression of a genotype (equal to 100%)

autosomal recessive inheritance in which the gene is located on any chromosome that is not a sex chromosome and is phenotypically expressed only in homozygous or hemizygous form

A/V ratio ratio between the artery and vein; normal, 2 to 3, the vein being wider

a-wave in ERG, a small negative deflection that occurs after stimulus presentation, related to activity of photoreceptor processes

backward retinopathy retinopathy that occurs after trauma, demonstrating venous alterations

bag of worms plexiform fibroma of the eyelid, as part of neurofibromatosis

banking abnormal dilatation and swelling of a vein, peripheral to the arteriovenous crossings, which appears as an hourglass constriction on both sides of the crossing and is produced by impeded circulation

basophil cells and tissues staining readily with basic dyes, appearing blue-black

beacon of lights in fluorescein angiography, focal transmission defects in sub-RPE area, occurring usually in central serous chorioretinopathy

beaded vessels having the appearance of strings of beads

bear's track	nonfamilial pigmented degeneration of retina, with no clinical significance
beaten bronze	macular atrophy with patchy pigmented areas and brownish spots, usually appearing in Stargardt's disease
Bence Jones protein	abnormal plasma or urinary protein, with unusual solubility properties, precipitating on heating at 50°C, redissolving at 100°C, and again precipitating and redissolving on cooling
Bergmeister's papilla	small remnant glial mass that surrounds the hyaloid artery at the optic disc
Berlin's edema	See *commotio retinae.*
beta-blockers	drugs that induce blockage of beta-adrenergic receptors, reducing the inflow and increasing the outflow in the eye, thereby decreasing the intraocular pressure; effects may slow the heart, precipitate cardiac failure, and cause asthma, hallucinations, and sleeplessness
blastopore	opening of the archenteron to the exterior of the embryo at the gastrula stage
Blessig-Ivanoff cysts	peripheral retinal cysts close to the ora serrata, without significant effect on the vision
blind spot of Mariotte	area of blindness in the visual field that represents the site at which the retina joins the optic nerve; not sensitive to light, as it lacks photoreceptors
blood-aqueous barrier	anatomic mechanism that prevents exchange of material between the eye and blood, allowing aqueous humor to pass into the bloodstream but preventing cells or fluid from blood from passing into the eye
B lymphocytes	cells primarily responsible for humoral immunity; precursor of plasma cells (antibody-producing cells)

brachytherapy radiation therapy in which the source is placed on the surface or a short distance from the eye; also called *contact therapy*

bradyzoite small, slow-growing, comma-shaped form of *Toxoplasma gondii*, found in tissues, muscles, and brain in chronic toxoplasmosis

BRAO branch retinal artery occlusion

Bruch's membrane inner layer of choroid that is in contact with RPE

brushfire retinitis slowly progressive necrotizing retinitis, in cytomegalovirus retinopathy, in immunocompromised patients with AIDS

BRVO branch retinal vein occlusion

B-scan a display on a cathode ray tube of ultrasonographic echoes, in which the position of the bright dot corresponds to the time elapsed and the brightness of the dot corresponds to the strength of the echo; used to determine the shape and depth of various intraocular structures, such as tumor or retinal detachment

buphthalmos enlarged and distended eye, usually due to an increased intraocular pressure in congenital glaucoma

b-wave in ERG, a high-amplitude, positive deflection that occurs immediately after the *a-wave*, related to the bipolar cell activity

calcospherite small globular particle formed during calcification by chemical union of calcium and albuminous organic matter of intercellular substance

candle wax drippings (of Franceschetti) granulomatous exudates around retinal vessels, generally occurring in sarcoidosis

CAPED central areolar pigment epithelial dystrophy

capsid shell formed of protein that protects the nucleic acid of a virus

caseation necrosis necrosis in which the tissue is transformed into a dry, amorphous mass resembling cheese

catecholamines biogenic amines with sympathomimetic action, such as epinephrine, dopa, dopamine

C/D ratio cup-to-disc ratio; ratio between the diameter of the cup and the diameter of the optic disc; normal, 1 to 3 (0.3), but can be as large as 1 to 9 (0.9)

CEA carcinoembryonic antigen

cellophane retinopathy wrinkled sheen over the macula, due probably to defects in the internal limiting membrane; also called *silk-screen retinopathy*

central vision vision elicited from stimuli that reach the macula directly

centrocecal scotoma area of blindness on the visual field that affects the central point (fixation point) and the blind spot (cecum)

cerclage surgical procedure consisting of encircling polyethylene bands or tubes; used in retinal detachment

cGy centigray, a unit of absorbed radiation dose equal to 1/100 of a gray, or 1 rad

choked disc See *papilledema.*

cholesterosis bulbi synchysis scintillans

choristoma a mass of tissue not normally belonging to the area in which it is located

chromatopsia color vision defect in which colored objects appear unnaturally colored and colorless objects appear colored

chromosome in the nucleus of a cell, a structure that contains DNA, which transmits genetic information

circle of Zinn annular ligament attached to the edge of the optic canal and superior orbital fissure; the common origin of ocular recti muscles

claret stain Sturge-Weber syndrome

clinically significant macular edema (CSME) retinal thickening or hard exudates at or within 500 μm of the center of the macula; or retinal thickening within 500 μm of the center of the macula associated with adjacent retinal thickening that may be outside the 500-μm limit; or retinal thickening of 1 dd or larger, any part of which is within 1 dd of the center of the macula

clivus slope as an oval ring at the concave floor of the macula

Cloquet's canal a fibrous structure, a passage running from the optic disc to the lens, which in the fetus transmits the hyaloid artery

CME cystoid macular edema

CMV cytomegalovirus

coagulative necrosis necrosis with formation of fibrous infarcts, in which a part of the tissue has been deprived of the blood supply by a coagulum plugging of its vessels

coloboma partial congenital absence of ocular tissue

commotio retinae macular edema and retinal hemorrhage primarily in the macula, after a recent orbital or ocular trauma; also called *Berlin's edema*

complement heat-labile factors in serum that produce immune cytolysis and other biological functions

complement fixation consumption of complement on reaction with immune complexes, used for detection of antigens and antibodies

conduction velocity speed, in meters per second, at which an impulse moves along a nerve fiber

contrecoup mechanism mechanism by which an injury is produced from a blow on the opposite side of the site of injury

Coombs' test antiglobulin test, in which an anitibody is directed against gamma globulin

cotton-wool spots small, fluffy, white retinal patches due to a microinfarct and edema in the retinal nerve fiber layer; also called *cytoid bodies*

CRAO central retinal artery occlusion

C-reactive protein globulin that forms a precipitate with the somatic C-polysaccharide of the pneumococcus in vitro

CRVO central retinal vein occlusion

cryopexy surgical procedure that attempts to fix a tissue by application of extreme cold with a freezing probe; used usually in retinal detachment

cryotherapy treatment that uses cold

CSME clinically significant macular edema

CT scan computed tomography scan; records the internal organ or body image according to a predetermined plan

cycloplegic drug that produces paralysis of the ciliary muscle and therefore paralysis of accommodation, resulting in pupil dilatation and failure of near vision

cystoid macular edema (CME) thickening of the retina in the macula after an extracellular accumulation of fluid in cystoid spaces

cytoid bodies See *cotton-wool spots.*

Dalen-Fuchs nodules inflammatory choroidal white exudates that usually occur in sympathetic ophthalmia and sarcoidosis

dark adaptation adjustment of vision in decreased illumination by increasing the sensitivity of the retina to dim light and the level of visual purple (rhodopsin) in the rods

daughter lesion lesion arising from or near another older lesion

degeneration deteriorating change to a lower or less functionally active tissue

deoxyribonucleic acid (DNA) nucleic acid having deoxyribose as a sugar, constituting the primary genetic material in the nucleus of all cells and the DNA viruses

dialysis a large break; see also *retinal dialysis*

diathermy therapy that uses application of currents of low tension and high amperage to warm the deeper parts of the body

disc sign of sickling tiny red spots of blocked vessels on the surface of the optic disc, as a result of sickle-shaped deformity of erythrocytes on deoxygenation, in sickle-cell disease

doll's-head maneuver on moving the head in one direction, the eyes turn in the opposite site direction

dopa an amino acid, dihydroxyphenylalanine, produced by oxidation of tyrosine, which is a precursor of dopamine and an intermediate product of epinephrine, norepinephrine, and melanin

Doppler ultrasonography visualization of deep structures of the body by recording the reflections of pulses of ultrasonic waves directed into the tissues; shift in frequency between emitted waves and their echoes is used to measure velocity of moving structures

drusen congenital or acquired hyaline amorphous deposits of the retina, the RPE, or the optic disc

dysplasia alteration in size, shape, and organization of adult cells or tissues

EBR external-beam radiation therapy

eclampsia state of convulsion, hypertension, edema, and proteinuria in a pregnant or puerperal woman

ectopia lentis displacement or malposition of the crystalline lens in the eye

ectropion eversion (turning outward) of the edge of the lower eyelid, resulting in a separation of the eyelid from the eyeball and exposing the palpebral conjunctiva

ectropion uveae twisting inside-out of the pupillary margin of the iris; also called *iridectropium*

edema abnormal accumulation of excessive fluid intercellularly

effusion escape of fluid into a part or tissue

EIA enzyme immunoassay

elastica elastic tissue in the tunica media of blood vessels

elastosis degeneration of elastic tissue

electroencephalography (EEG) recording of the electric currents developed in the brain

electro-oculography (EOG) method of measuring the electric potential changes by moving the eyes a constant distance between two points of fixation

electrophoresis separation of ionic solutes as a result of the difference in their rates of migration in an electric field

electroretinography (ERG) method of recording changes in the electric potential that follows stimulation of retina by light

electrostatic potential work per unit charge necessary to move a charged body in an electrostatic field from a point at infinity to another point, measured in volts

ELISA enzyme-linked immunosorbent assay

endophytic growing inward

endozoite tachyzoite

enophthalmos recession of the eyeball into the orbit

entropion inversion (turning inward) of the edge of the eyelid

entropion uveae inversion of the edge of the pupillary margin of the iris; inflammatory or congenital

EOG electro-oculography

equator imaginary line encircling the eyeball equidistant from the anterior and posterior poles

ERG electroretinography

erythroblast nucleated erythrocyte, an immature cell from which a red blood cell develops

erythropoietin glycoprotein hormone secreted by the kidney in the adult and by the liver in the fetus, which stimulates erythropoiesis (production of red blood cells) in the bone marrow

esotropia strabismus in which inward deviation of the nonfixating eye is manifest and occurs with both eyes open; also called *cross-eyes*

ESR erythrocyte sedimentation rate (Westergren method)

euglobulin globulin insoluble in water but soluble in saline solution

exophytic growing outward

exotropia strabismus with permanent outward deviation of the nonfixating eye; also called *wall-eyes*

expanded rubella rubella with thrombocytopenic purpura, hemolytic anemia, and central nervous system diseases

exudate fluid with a high protein or cell content that has escaped from blood vessels and has been deposited on the tissue surface or within tissue, usually as a result of an inflammatory process

Farnsworth-Munsell 100-hue test color vision test that contains 100 colored dots arranged in an increasing hue order

FAZ foveolar avascular zone

FBS fasting blood sugar test

fibrosis repair or replacement of parenchymatous structures by formation of fibrous tissue

flare excessive protein in the anterior chamber which is seen via the slit-lamp beam

fleurettes cells found in flowerlike clusters, exhibiting protrusion of processes of inner and outer segments of photoreceptors; usually present in retinoblastoma and retinocytoma

Flexner-Wintersteiner rosettes small round or polygonal cuboid cells, closely packed around a clear central core; present in retinoblastoma

floaters deposits in the vitreous seen by a patient as moving spots before the eye; may represent vitreous protein occurring as benign degenerative changes, shifting location when the gaze position is changed

fluorescein angiography radiographic visualization of vascular abnormalities of retinal and choroidal circulation, by intravenous injection of a contrast dye (fluorescein)

forward retinopathy retinopathy that may occur after trauma, marked by arterial alterations

Foster-Kennedy syndrome ipsilateral optic atrophy and contralateral papilledema occurring in tumors of the frontal lobe of the brain

fovea oval depression in the center of the macula

foveola small depression in the fovea, which is devoid of rods, has cones exclusively, and is vascular-free

FTA-ABS fluorescent treponemal antibody absorption test for syphilis

Fuchs' spot black, round macular lesion as a proliferation of RPE and choroidal degeneration, caused by a recurrent choroidal hemorrhage, with hemosiderin deposits, which occurs in high myopia

gene the biological unit of heredity, self-reproducing, and transmitted from parents to offspring

genome the full set of genes in an individual

genotype the entire genetic constitution of an individual

ghost vessel vessel containing no blood

glare visual discomfort or loss of central vision performance when bright light enters the visual field, especially when the eyes are adapted to dark

Goldmann perimetry technique of visual field examination that determines the borders of the field by presenting a test target (point of light) to the patient whose eyes are fixated on the middle of a white concave screen and who reports when the target becomes visible

goniotomy surgical procedure in which a narrow anterior chamber angle in glaucoma is opened via opening Schlemm's canal under direct vision using a contact lens

Gunn's sign deviation of vein at the arteriovenous crossing in hypertension

gyrate atrophy congenital metabolic chorioretinopathy due to a deficiency of the enzyme ornithine ketotransferase and a consequent increased level of the amino acid ornithine in blood, urine, cerebrospinal fluid, and aqueous humor

Haab's macula oval or transverse, asymmetric macular lesions with minimal pigment, in ARMD

half-moon pattern	circular atrophy of the macula, more marked inferiorly, present in bull's-eye maculopathy of chloroquine retinopathy
hamartoma	a benign mass composed of overgrowth of mature cells that normally belong to the area in which the mass is located
haplotype	genetic constitution of an individual at a set of alleles of closely linked genes, such as HLA complex
hemeralopia	decreased vision in bright light; day blindness
heterochromia	different color of the iris of one eye in relation to the other eye
heterophil antibody	antibody directed against a cross-reacting antigen that occurs in several species (heterophil antigen)
heterozygote	an individual possessing different alleles at a given focus
high water marks	deposits of proteinaceous material around the optic disc after resolution of papilledema
histospots	small, peripheral, chorioretinal atrophic lesions in histoplasmosis
HIV	human immunodeficiency virus; the pathogenic agent of acquired immunodeficiency syndrome (AIDS)
Homer-Wright rosette	cells found in clusters, in a circular grouping around a central area of neurofibrils, but lacking a clear center; usually occurs in retinoblastoma
homozygote	an individual possessing a pair of identical alleles to a given locus
humping	abrupt elevation of the vein over the artery, at the arteriovenous crossing, due to a thickening of the arterial wall
hyaline	a translucent, glassy substance

hyalinization	conversion into a hyaline substance resembling glass
hyaloid	membrane at the posterior face of the vitreous
hyaluronic acid	a glycosaminoglycan found in vitreous humor, blood vessels, cartilage, and some viscoelastic substances
hypercortisolism	complex of symptoms or signs due to excessive production or administration of hydrocortisone or its semisynthetic analogues; hyperadrenocorticism
hypermetropia	error of refraction in which the light beams entering the eye parallel to the optic axis are brought to a focal point behind the retina, the eye being too short; also called *farsightedness*
hyperviscosity syndromes	syndromes associated with increased viscosity of the blood, usually with spontaneous bleeding and neurologic and ocular disorders, such as polycythemia vera, Waldenström's macroglobulinemia, leukemia, hyperglobulinemia, and cryoglobulinemia
hyphae	filaments of threads that compose the mycelium of a fungus
immunoglobulins	glycoproteins that function as antibodies; divided into five classes on the basis of structure and biological activity: IgM, IgG, IgA, IgD, and IgE
interferon	glycoprotein that exerts virus-nonspecific but host-specific antiviral activity by inducing transcription of cellular genes coding for antiviral protein that selectively inhibits the synthesis of viral RNA and protein

intima — inner coat of blood vessels made up of endothelial cells surrounded by elastic fibers and connective tissue

intra-gel hemorrhage — hemorrhage of the subhyaloid space that breaks into the vitreous in advanced proliferative diabetic retinopathy

IOL — intraocular lens

IOP — intraocular pressure

iridescent spots — yellow, fine, glistening deposits of hemosiderin in the peripheral retina or the macula after hemorrhages resolve; seen in sickle cell retinopathy

Ishihara's pseudoisochromatic plates — device to test red-green color defects by recognizing numbers and trace lines made up of multicolored, variously sized round dots

Kaposi's sarcoma — malignant, bluish red nodules on skin, eyelids, and conjunctiva; associated with AIDS

karyotype analysis — photomicrograph of chromosomes arranged according to a standard classification

keratoconus — noninflammatory, bilateral, conical protrusion of the cornea

keratoglobus — enlarged globular protrusion of the cornea; megalocornea

keratomileusis — surgical procedure in which a slice of the patient's cornea is removed with a keratome, reshaped to a desired curvature after freezing, and then replaced on the cornea to correct optical error

Kolmer test — complement fixation test

lacquer cracks — breaks in Bruch's membrane through which connective tissue, hemorrhage, and choroidal neovascularization may pass beneath the RPE; seen in high myopia and Marfan's, Ehlers-Danlos, or Stickler's syndrome

lacuna a small pit or hollow cavity

lamina fusca avascular layer of elastic, collagenous lamellar fibers that connects sclera to choroid; also called *suprachoroid*

laminar dot sign deepening of the optic cup that causes the lamina cribrosa to bow posteriorly and its gray fenestrations to become visible; seen in glaucoma

Landers' sign preretinal nodules; seen in sarcoidosis

lattice framework of intersecting fine strips, usually regularly spaced

LDH lactate dehydrogenase

lenticonus abnormal, unilateral conical prominence of the lens surface, more frequently the posterior surface

leukokoria whitish reflex in the pupil caused by a mass; also called *cat's-eye reflex*

lipofuscin yellow to brown lipid pigment

Litten's sign See *Roth's spot.*

locus position of a gene on a chromosome

loop sharp curve or turn in a vessel or cordlike structure

lupus pernio sarcoidosis

lysosomal enzyme enzyme released into the cell after an injury of lysosome, which may damage the cell

lysosome minute body in a cell, containing hydrolytic enzymes and normally involved in the process of localized digestion

macula oval area at the posterior pole, just below and temporal to the optic disc, in which the rods and cones are densely packed; the site of fine central vision

macular star accumulation of intraretinal hard exudates in the macula, in a starlike pattern; seen in diabetes, hypertension, angiomatosis retinae, and resolving papilledema

Marcus-Gunn pupil pupil with impaired response to bright light, consisting of bilateral pupillary constriction when light is directed to the normal eye and of bilateral pupillary dilation when light is transferred rapidly to the affected eye

marfanoid habitus displaying the characteristic symptoms of Marfan's syndrome

Martegiani's area tunnel-shaped space at the optic disc surface that extends toward the vitreous and may become continuous with Cloquet's canal

media (1) middle coat of the blood vessels made up of elastic and muscle fibers; (2) transparent layers of the eye: cornea, aqueous humor, lens, and vitreous

melanin dark pigment of choroid produced by polymerization of oxidation products of tyrosine and dihydroxyphenyl compounds

melanosomes granules within melanocytes that contain tyrosinase and synthesize melanin

metamorphopsia distortion of objects seen

MHA-TP microhemagglutination for *Treponema pallidum*; test for syphilis

microaneurysm finer outpouchings of capillary walls in diabetes, Coats' disease, hyperviscosity syndromes, and periphlebitis

micropsia visualization of objects as smaller than they are

miotics drugs that constrict the pupil

Mittendorf's dot small circular opacity of the posterior capsule of the lens, which represents a remnant of the hyaloid artery and occurs only at the capsule's anterior lens insertion

mixed retinopathy a retinopathy that occurs after a distant trauma, marked by both arterial and venous alterations

morning-glory anomaly congenital, nonhereditary deformity of the optic disc, with spokelike, radiating vessels at the periphery that resemble a flower; associated with astigmatism, basal encephalocele, absence of corpus callosum, and hare lip and cleft palate

de Morsier's syndrome septo-optic dysplasia

mosaicism presence in an individual of two or more cell lines that are karyotypically or genotypically distinct and are derived from a single zygote

MRI magnetic resonance imaging

mucopolysaccharides polysaccharide that contains hexosamine, including glycosaminoglycan

mutation permanent transmissible change in the genetic material, which usually occurs in a single gene

mydriatics drugs that dilate the pupil

myoid basophilic region of inner segment of rod and cone processes, containing agranular endoplasmic reticulum and free ribosomes

myopia refractive error in which the light beams entering parallel to the optic axis are brought to a focal point in front of the retina, the eye being too long, or the refractive power of cornea and lens are too strong; also called *nearsightedness*

naked granuloma	granuloma formed by retinal vasculitis in which tubercles are surrounded by lymphocytes, rarely associated with central necrosis but not caseation
napkin ring	annular constriction around the optic disc by a subretinal membrane; seen in proliferative vitreoretinopathy, grade C, type C3 of the Retina Society classification
necrobiosis	swelling, basophilia, and distortion of collagen, sometimes with obliteration of normal tissue structure but short of actual necrosis; seen in diabetes
necrosis	morphologic changes that indicate cell death, caused by progressive degradative action of enzymes
neovascular glaucoma	secondary glaucoma caused by neovascularization of the anterior chamber angle
neuroepithelium	See *sensory retina.*
neuroretina	See *sensory retina.*
neuroretinal rim	portion of the optic disc between the margin of the cup and the margin of the disc
nicking	a localized constriction of blood vessels at the arteriovenous crossings, with a tapering concealment of the vein, which is narrow but in which the lumen is normal
Nissl granules	large basophilic bodies in the cytoplasm of neurons, composed of rough endoplasmic reticulum and free ribosomes, in retinal ganglion cells
nm	nanometer, a unit of linear measurement equal to one billionth of a meter (10^{-9} meter)

nonrhegmatogenous retinal detachment without a tear, break, or hole

notching pitlike enlargement of the optic cup or an erosion of the disc, usually in the upper temporal area; seen in glaucoma

nucleocapsid a nucleic acid protected by a shell of protein (capsid), which represents a structural unit of a virus

NVD neovascularization of the optic disc

NVE neovascularization of the retina elsewhere but not in the optic disc

nyctalopia decreased vision at night; also called *night blindness*

oncosphere larva of the tapeworm

operculum lid or covering structure

ophthalmoplegia paralysis of the ocular muscles: *ophthalmoplegia externa*, paralysis of extraocular muscles; *ophthalmoplegia interna*, paralysis of the muscles of iris and ciliary body; *total ophthalmoplegia*, paralysis of both intrinsic and extrinsic muscles

oral pertaining to the ora serrata

ora serrata anterior margin of the sensory retina, located at the junction of the choroid and ciliary body; the most peripheral area of the retina

orbital pseudotumor chronic inflammatory reaction of the orbit, with exophthalmos and swelling of eyelids, resembling a neoplasm

ornithine amino acid produced by urea's splitting off from arginine and converting into citrulline; level elevated in gyrate atrophy

panretinal photocoagulation laser technique to produce chorioretinal scars on the entire retina through condensation of protein material, by the absorption

	of a controlled intense beam of light and its conversion to heat by the RPE
papilledema	edema of the optic disc
papilloma	benign epithelial neoplasm with fingerlike projections
papovavirus	a family of DNA viruses
paracentesis	surgical puncture of a cavity for diagnosis and therapy; in *ocular paracentesis*, puncture of the anterior chamber
parallactic displacement	apparent displacement of an object's position owing to change in the position of the observer
paraneoplastic	symptoms or changes arising in a cancer-bearing patient and produced remote from a tumor or its metastases, which cannot be explained by local or distant spread of the malignancy
pars plana	outermost ring of the ciliary body; the site of incision used often for vitrectomy
pars planitis	inflammation of the retina and vitreous at the site of the pars plana; also called *intermediate uveitis*
Paul-Bunnell test	test for determination of highest dilution of patient's serum capable of agglutination of sheep erythrocytes; used in infectious mononucleosis
PCR	polymerase chain reaction
pendular nystagmus	involuntary, rapid, rhythmic tremors of the eyes, which occur independently of normal ocular movements and in which the oscillations of both eyes have an equal rate, amplitude, direction, and type of movement
penetrance	frequency of expression of a genotype
pericyte	contractile, elongated cell wrapped about precapillary arterioles

pericyte-to–endothelial cell ratio	normal, 1 to 1
perimetry	evaluation the extent of visual field
periodic acid–Schiff (PAS)	test for glycogen, mucin, neutral polysaccharides, and glycoproteins
peripheral vision	vision of objects outside the central region without turning the eyes toward them
peroxisome	intracellular microbodies rich in the enzymes peroxidase, catalase, D-amino acid oxidase, and urate oxidase, which participate in some metabolic oxidations
phakomatosis	congenital and hereditary anomalies having in common tissues of ectodermal origin and development of glial hamartomas (phakomas); seen in neurofibromatosis, tuberous sclerosis, Sturge-Weber syndrome, von Hippel–Lindau disease, and ataxia-telangiectasia
photic	pertaining to light
photocoagulation	laser technique of producing chorioretinal scars through condensation of protein material, by the absorption of a controlled intense beam of light and its conversion to heat by the RPE
photodisruption	morphologic defect of a tissue due to rapid molecular ionization caused by laser
photodynamic therapy	treatment with a photosensitive drug such as BPD-MA (benzoporphyrin derivate-monoacid) (Verteporfin), a liposomal benzoporphyrin derivative monoacid ring A; seen in ARMD
photophobia	abnormal intolerance of light, characterized by visual discomfort or ocular pain on exposure to bright light
photopia	vision in daytime in which the cones are perceiving the light and the rods are suppressed
photopsia	vision of flashing lights or sparks due to a disorder of the retina, optic nerve, or brain

photoreceptors rod and cone retinal layer

phototoxicity chemically induced type of photosensitivity that is nonimmunologic and is produced by the release of free radicals and lysosomal enzymes, which damage the retinal photoreceptors

phthisis bulbi shrinkage and wasting of the eye

pipecolic acid an amino acid that occurs as an intermediate of lysine degradation

plasmogen vital part of cytoplasm; also called *bioplasm*

pleocytosis excessive number of cells in the cerebrospinal fluid

plombage surgical procedure consisting of scleral buckling with silicone sponge in retinal detachment

plus disease form of retinopathy of prematurity characterized by progressive dilatation and tortuosity of retinal vessels

polymerase enzyme that catalyzes polymerization, especially of nucleotides to polynucleotides

PORN progressive outer retinal necrosis

posterior chamber a space in the eye between the iris anteriorly and the lens and suspensory ligament posteriorly, filled with aqueous humor

posterior pole area of the retina extending from the optic disc to the equator

PPD purified protein derivative of tuberculin, used in skin testing for tuberculosis

precapillary artery vessel lacking complete coats, intermediate between an arteriole and a true capillary; also called a *metarteriole*

pre-eclampsia state of hypertension, edema, or proteinuria (or all three) in a complicated pregnancy

prepapillary vascular loops congenital anomaly of retinal vessels consisting of loops in front of the surface of the optic disc

prethreshold disease early form of retinopathy of prematurity

primary vitreous vitreous associated embryologically with lens capsule formation and the hyaloid vascular system

proptosis abnormal protrusion of the eyeball from the orbit; also called *exophthalmos*

prostaglandin substances derived from unsaturated 20-carbon fatty acids, primarily arachidonic acid, that are extremely potent mediators of diverse physiologic processes

protanopia inability to distinguish red and green hues but retaining the sensory mechanism for blue and yellow

protein S plasma protein, which is vitamin K–dependent, inhibits blood clotting, and is a cofactor for activated protein C

pseudocoloboma a line or scar giving the appearance of an absence or defect of tissue of the eye (coloboma)

pseudo–Foster-Kennedy syndrome ischemic papillitis in one eye and optic atrophy in the other; seen in giant-cell arteritis (temporal arteritis)

pseudopapilledema congenital anomalous elevation of the optic disc that is not pathologic but simulates papilledema; seen in hypermetropia, astigmatism, and disc drusen

pseudophakia a post–cataract surgery state in which an intraocular lens was implanted

pseudoretinitis retinal disorganization, with pigmentary migration, in acute retinal pigment epitheliitis

pseudorosettes clustered cells in the perivascular region or surrounding tumor cells, or incomplete rosettes, found in retinoblastoma

pseudotumor cerebri — cerebral edema with increased intracranial pressure, papilledema, headache, nausea, and vomiting but without neurologic signs except occasional sixth cranial nerve (abducens) palsy

ptosis — drooping of the upper eyelid

purpura — hemorrhagic disease with decreased platelet counts

pyknosis — degeneration of a cell marked by shrunken nucleolus and a mass of condensed chromatin

Q-switched laser — laser that concentrates energy into short pulses, with filters that prevent the light from exiting until a specific energy threshold is attained

rad — unit of radiation-absorbed dose

radial keratotomy — refractive surgical procedure to flatten the cornea by radial incisions; used in myopia

relative afferent pupillary defect (RAPD) — relative afferent pupillary defect; decreased miosis to light in the affected eye in comparison with the normal eye, when using a swinging flashlight

retinal dialysis — congenital or traumatic separation of sensory retina from nonpigmented retinal epithelium at ora serrata

retinoschisis — congenital or acquired splitting of the retina

rhegmatogenous — retinal detachment with a tear, break, or hole

ribbon — dense lamella surrounded by a halo of vesicles found in the inner plexiform layer of the retina, at the synapses between the bipolar cells and ganglion cells

ribonucleic acid (RNA) — nucleic acid in which ribose is a sugar and that is the genetic material in RNA viruses, playing a role in genetic information

ribosome large molecular structure that is the site of protein synthesis

rip-off syndrome sudden loss of vision with simultaneous hemorrhage produced by tearing of the RPE detachment, which may flap back under itself

ROP retinopathy of prematurity

rosette focus of François large, yellow-green, irregular macular scar surrounded by black pigmentation; seen in congenital toxoplasmosis

rosettes small tumor cells in clusters around a central area, which can be a clear empty lumen, such as in *Flexner-Wintersteiner rosettes*, or an area with neurofibrillary material but no lumen, such as in *Homer-Wright rosettes*; seen in retinoblastoma

Roth's spot white-centered hemorrhage exhibiting a microabscess, plug of fibrin, leukemic cells, or fungi

RPE retinal pigment epithelium

RPR rapid plasma reagin test for syphilis

rubeosis iridis formation of new vessels and connective tissue on the surface of the iris; seen in diabetes and CRAO or CRVO

rubeosis retinae neovascularization in front of the optic disc, in retinitis proliferans, which usually leads to retinal detachment

rush disease fulminant progressive form of retinopathy of prematurity that may produce rhegmatogenous retinal detachment

Sabouraud's dextrose agar medium medium used for cultivation and identification of fungi

salmon patches preretinal and intraretinal hemorrhages that usually spare the visual axis; seen in sickle cell retinopathy

salt-and-pepper fundus slowly progressive, hyperpigmented and hypopigmented, punctate lesions or exudates of the posterior pole, which may heal spontaneously and do not recur; seen in rubella, congenital syphilis, cytomegalovirus retinopathy, and some other diseases

Salus' sign deviation of a vein at the arteriovenous crossing; seen in hypertension

satellite lesion new chorioretinal lesion that occurs next to an old scar; seen in acquired toxoplasmosis and cytomegalovirus retinopathy

scan visualization of the image of ultrasonic echoes from an organ under examination for size, structure, or defects

Schaumann's bodies basophilic, laminated, shell-like bodies; seen in sarcoidosis

scleral buckling surgical procedure for retinal detachment in which an elastic band is used to indent the retina to facilitate reattaching RPE to the sensory retina

scotoma area of blindness within the visual field due to a total or partial loss of retinal sensitivity

scotopia night or dim vision in which rods are sensitized with rhodopsin in the process of dark adaptation

sea-blue histiocyte granulated histiocyte that is morphologically distinct and sea blue in color

sea fan retinal arterial neovascularization in the shape of a small sector of a circle (fan); seen in sickle cell retinopathy

secondary vitreous develops after primary vitreous, is composed of densely packed fine fibrils, deriving probably from Müller cells

senile macular degeneration age-related macular degeneration (ARMD)

sensory retina comprises nine inner layers of the retina (all but the RPE); also called *neuroretina* or *neuroepithelium*

sessile not pedunculated but attached by a base

SGPT serum glutamate pyruvate transaminase, increased in liver diseases and infectious mononucleosis

shot-silk area of gray, wet retina and cotton-wool spots; seen in eclampsia

shunt passage, bypass, or anastomosis between two vessels

sickle-cell disease hereditary hemolytic anemia with sickle-shaped erythrocytes, markedly susceptible to changes in oxygenation; occurs almost exclusively in black patients

Siegrist's streaks clusters of fine pigment or yellow streaks as chains, representing pigmentary disturbances or chorioretinal atrophy; seen in malignant hypertension

silk-screen retinopathy cellophane retinopathy

silver-wire reflex increased light reflex of an arteriosclerotic artery, which appears as a whitish tube

situs inversus irregular vascular pattern of the origin of retinal vessels, which makes the vessels of the right eye resemble those of the left eye, and vice versa, in tilted disc

smoldering retinitis localized moving inflammatory process of the sensory retina; seen in cytomegalovirus retinopathy

Snellen's chart chart on which appear printed block letters in gradually decreasing sizes, constructed to subtend an angle of 5 minutes and in which each portion of a letter subtends an angle of

	1 minute at a given distance; used to test visual acuity against a reference value of 20/20 at a 20-ft (6-m) distance
snowballs	microabscesses in the vitreous; seen in sarcoidosis, pars planitis, and candidiasis; also called *snowbank*
staphyloma	ectasia and protrusion of the sclera lined with choroid
star folds	regular retinal folds that radiate centripetally toward a focal area of proliferative vitreoretinopathy, grade C, type C1 of the Retina Society classification
stratum opticum	retinal nerve fiber layer
sunset glow	bilateral depigmentation of the ocular fundus that occurs in the convalescent stage of Vogt-Koyanagi-Harada syndrome
swallow's-nest hemorrhage	hemorrhage in the subhyaloid space in advanced proliferative diabetic retinopathy
synchysis	softening or liquefaction of vitreous
synchysis scintillans	cholesterol crystals in the vitreous, after trauma, surgery, or vitreous hemorrhage; also called *cholesterosis bulbi*
syncytium	mass of protoplasm having multiple nuclei produced by merging of the cells
syneresis	collapse of the vitreous due to a metabolic or pathologic dissolution of the collagen network
tabes	neurosyphilis
tache de bougie	candle wax drippings; seen in sarcoidosis
tachyzoite	crescent-shaped, quickly multiplying form of *Toxoplasma gondii*, found in all tissues except nonnucleated erythrocytes, in acute toxoplasmosis; also called *endozoite*
tapetoretinopathy	hereditary degeneration of the RPE and the sensory retina

TB	tuberculosis
telangiectasia	permanent dilatation of capillaries, arteries, and veins
teletherapy	radiation therapy in which the source is distant from the eye or body
tertiary vitreous	zonule of Zinn, deriving from primary vitreous and nonpigmented epithelium of the ciliary body
thermography	technique that determines photographically the temperature of the body surface, based on self-emanating infrared radiation
T lymphocyte	thymus-dependent lymphocyte, responsible for cell-mediated immunity
tobacco amblyopia	nutritional or toxic impairment of visual acuity without any detectable organic lesion
togavirus	RNA virus that may cause rubella
TPHA	treponemal passive hemagglutination assay for syphilis
transudate	liquid with high fluidity and low protein or cell content that passes through the blood vessels as a result of hemodynamic forces and that is noninflammatory
threshold disease	form of retinopathy of prematurity, a neovascularization of the retina with progressive dilatation and tortuosity of the vessels and a ridge of fibrovascular proliferation into the vitreous
trilateral retinoblastoma	bilateral genetic retinoblastoma associated with a primary nonretinoblastoma malignancy, such as a pinealoblastoma
umbo	small central depression of the foveola, in the macula
Valsalva's maneuver	forcible exhalation effort against a closed glottis after heavy lifting, vomiting, coughing,

	or straining at stool, which rapidly increases the intrathoracic and intra-abdominal pressure, with a subsequent marked rise of retinal venous pressure, resulting in a hemorrhagic retinopathy called *Valsalva retinopathy*
vasa vasorum	small nutrient vessels, arteries, and veins located in the walls of larger vessels
venous beading	segmental, irregular dilatation of veins resembling a string of beads, due to increased venous pressure or to a markedly decreased intraocular pressure; seen in diabetes, hypertension, papilledema, occlusive carotid artery disease, and Alport's syndrome
virion	extracellular particle of a virus capable of infecting a living cell
visual evoked response (VER)	brain activity produced by a visual stimulus, measurable by electroencephalography
visual field	area of vision of objects or light stimuli when the eyes are in a straight-ahead position at a central fixation point
vitrectomy	surgical procedure to remove the vitreous humor
vitreoretinal symphysis	vitreous base
vitreous base	annular band of adhesion of vitreous that extends from the ora serrata to the pars plana anteriorly and to the retina posteriorly; also called *vitreoretinal symphysis*
wavelength	distance between the top of an electromagnetic wave and the identical top of a succeeding wave
Weigert's ligament	annular zone of adhesion between the anterior hyaloid and the posterior capsule of the lens
Weiss-Otto reflex	white reflex on the nasal side of the retina; seen in myopia

white with pressure change in color of the fundus to grayish white during a scleral depression; seen in elderly myopes, retinoschisis, posterior vitreous detachment, choroidal detachment, and retinal tears

white without pressure benign bilateral whitening of peripheral retina, with or without pressure, which has no clinical significance; seen in elderly patients, sickle-cell disease, lattice degeneration, and posterior vitreous detachment

wipe-out syndrome subacute neuroretinitis, which occurs in healthy young persons; also called *diffuse unilateral subacute neuroretinitis (DUSN)*

wonder net frondlike neovascularization of the retina, especially of the retinal veins, in juvenile diabetic retinopathy

X-linked inheritance inheritance in which a gene is carried on either an X or a Y (sex) chromosome

zygote cell resulting from union of a male and a female gamete (sperm and ovum)

Index